Endoscopic Surgery in Children

Springer
*Berlin
Heidelberg
New York
Barcelona
Hong Kong
London
Milan
Paris
Singapore
Tokyo*

N.M.A. Bax · K.E. Georgeson · A.S. Najmaldin · J-S. Valla
(Eds.)

Endoscopic Surgery in Children

With 182 figures and 13 tables

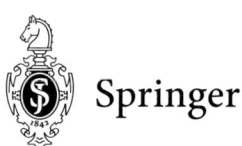 Springer

N.M.A. Bax, MD, PhD
Professor of Pediatric Surgery
Department of Pediatric Surgery
University Children's Hospital
Utrecht
The Netherlands

Azad S. Najmaldin, MS, FRCS
Senior Consultant
Department of Pediatric Surgery
St. James's University Hospital
Leeds
United Kingdom

Keith E. Georgeson, MD
Professor of Pediatric Surgery and
Director of the Division of
Pediatric Surgery
The Children's Hospital of Alabama
Birmingham
Alabama
USA

Jean-Stéphane Valla, MD
Professor of Pediatric Surgery and
Head of the Department of
Pediatric Surgery
Fondation Lenval
Hôpital pour Enfants
Nice
France

ISBN 3-540-64073-8 Springer-Verlag Berlin Heidelberg New York

Library of Congress Cataloging-in-Publication Data
Endoscopic surgery in children / N.M.A. Bax ... [et al.].
p. cm. Includes bibliographical references and index.
ISBN 3-540-64073-8 (alk. paper)
1. Endoscopic surgery. 2. Children--Surgery. I. Bax, N. M. A., 1944- .
[DNLM: 1. Surgical Procedures, Endoscopic--in infancy & childhood.
WO 505 E56 1999]
RJ51.E53E53 1999 617.9´8--dc21 DNLM/DLC
for Library of Congress 99-10448 CIP
ISBN 3-540-64073-8

This work is subject to copyright. All rights are reserved, whether the whole part of the material is concerned, specifically the rights of translation, reprinting, reuse of illustrations, recitation, broadcasting, reproduction on microfilm or in any other way, and storage in data banks. Duplication of this publication or parts thereof is permitted only under the provisions of the German Copyright Law of September 9, 1965, in its current version, and permission for use must always be obtained from Springer-Verlag. Violations are liable for prosectuion under the German Copyright Law.

© Springer-Verlag Berlin Heidelberg 1999
Printed in Germany

The use of general descriptive names, registered names, trademarks, etc. in this publication does not imply, even in the absence of a specific statement, that such names are exempt from the relevant protective laws and regulations and therefore free for general use.

Coverdesign: estudio Calamar, frido steinen-broo
Illustrator: Ingrid Janssen, University of Utrecht, Utrecht
Production: ProduServ GmbH, Verlagsservice, Berlin
Typesetting: MEDIO GmbH, Berlin

SPIN: 10554603   24/3020 - 5 4 3 2 1 0 – Printed on acid-free paper.

*To all sick children
of the world*

Preface

Pediatric surgeons have been involved in thoracoscopy and laparoscopy since at least the end of the 1960's (Gans and Berci 1971, 1973; Klimkovich et al. 1971; Kushch and Timchenko 1969; Rosenberg and Gognat 1971; Zeidler and Vogt-Moykopf 1972). Most of the procedures at that time were diagnostic. In 1973 a laparoscopic therapeutic procedure, the removal of a broken off ventriculo-peritoneal shunt, was published by Gans and Berci (1973) and in 1979 Morgan reported laparoscopic-assisted placement and repair of ventriculo-peritoneal shunts (Morgan 1979). The state of the art regarding pediatric endoscopy at the beginning of the 1980's is well described in *Pediatric Endoscopy*, edited by Gans (1983). Most of the chapters in Gans' book describe diagnostic endoscopy. During the rest of 1980's it remained quite in the area of pediatric thoracoscopy and laparoscopy.

In 1990 the first publications regarding laparoscopic clipping of the testicular vessels as the first step of a Fowler-Stephens orchidopexy for intra-abdominal testis appeared (Andze et al. 1990). In 1991 a large multicenter series regarding laparoscopic appendectomy in children was published (Valla et al. 1991). Also in 1991 the first reports of more extended multichannel laparoscopic operations in children (such as cholecystectomy) appeared in the literature (Holcomb et al. 1991; Newman et al. 1991). In contrast, the first reports concerning multichannel laparoscopic cholecystectomy in adults had been published 2 years earlier (Dubois et al. 1989; Reddick and Olsen 1989; Périssat et al. 1989). While pediatric surgeons traditionally have been more involved in diagnostic thoracoscopy and laparoscopy than their colleagues treating adults, pediatric surgeons have lagged behind in the development of thoracoscopic and laparoscopic therapeutic procedures for use in children.

This book presents the current state of the art in endoscopic surgery in children. As this type of surgery in children has been developed by many colleagues from all over the world, many of these experts have been invited to contribute to this book. They have been asked not to write about what can be done, but about what *has* been done, and whether one should continue along these lines. The book focuses primarily on the surgical endoscopic technique. Some differences in technique may emerge as the various authors present their personal techniques. They may also have different views regarding indications. These differences reflect the reality in medicine.

Part I deals with general aspects. It begins with a general discussion on the rationale of endoscopic surgery in children. General equipment and basic techniques are then described. One chapter is reserved for ergonomics and another for the training in and teaching of endoscopic techniques in children. Also, a chapter on anesthesia is included. Part II discusses thoracoscopic procedures, and Part III laparoscopic procedures. Each is subdivided into a section on diagnosis and a section on therapy. Unfortunately, complications associated with endoscopic surgery do occur, and a chapter dealing with this is included in Part III. Part IV focuses on the endoscopic approach of the urogenital tract, and Part V on the endoscopic approach of the vertebral column and of the brain. Part VI discusses the place of endoscopic surgical techniques in pediatric oncology. The book concludes with a view to the future.

The editors hope that this book fulfills a need and will help pediatric surgeons to become involved in and to advance with endoscopic surgery. It is the duty of all pediatric surgeons to think about less invasive surgical methods in treating children. The current state of endoscopic surgery is not as advanced as it should be, but at least the first steps have been taken, and they will spur on further progress.

This book could not have appeared without the support of many persons and institutions, principal of whom are those at Springer-Verlag. We are also very grateful to our artist, Ingrid Janssen, from the Audiovisual Department, University of Utrecht, The Netherlands, for her excellent restyling of the drawings. We are indebted to Karl Storz for the financial support in producing the figures.

N.M.A. Bax
K.E. Georgeson
A.S. Najmaldin
J-S. Valla

References

Andze GO et al (1990) La place de la laparoscopie thérapeutique dans le traitment des testicules intra-abdominaux chez l'enfant Chir Pediatr 31: 299–302

Dubois F, Berthelot G, Levard H (1989) Cholecystectomie par coelioscopie. Presse Med 18:980–982

Gans L, Berci G (1971) Advances in endoscopy of infants and children. J Pediatr Surg 6:199–233

Gans L, Berci G (1973) Peritoneoscopy in infants and children. J Pediatr Surg 8:399–405

Gans SL (1983) Pediatric endoscopy. Grune and Stratton, New York

Holcomb III GW, Olsen DO, Sharp KW (1991) Laparoscopic cholecystectomy in the pediatric patient. J Pediatr Surg 26: 1186–1190

Klimkovitch IG et al (1991) Torakoskopiia u detei. Khirurgiia Mosk 47: 19–24

Kushch NL, Timchenko AD (1969) Laparoskopiia u detei. Vestn Khir 102:92–94

Morgan WW (1979) The use of peritoneoscopy in the diagnosis and treatment of complications of ventriculoperitoneal shunts in children. J Pediatr Surg 14:18-181

Newman KD et al (1991) Laparoscopic cholecystectomy in pediatric patients. J Pediatr Surg 26: 1184-1185

Perissat J, Collet DR, Belliard R (1989) Gallstones: laparoscopic treatment, intracorporeal lithotripsy by cholecystostomy or cholecystectomy – a personal technique. Endoscopy 21 Suppl 1 : 373-374

Reddick EJ, Olsen DO (1989) Laparoscopic laser cholecystectomy. A comparison with minilap cholecystectomy. Surg Endosc 3: 131-133

Rosenberg D, Gognat M (1971) La coelioscopie dans l'enfance et l'adolescence. Gynecol Pract 22: 531-539

Valla JS et al. (1991) Appendicectomies chez l'enfant sous coelioscopie opératoire. 465 cas. J Chir Paris 128: 306-312

Zeidler D. Vogt-Moykopf I (1972) Die Endoscopie im Thoraxbereich beim Kind. Med Klin 67: 660-664

Contents

Part I Basics

Why Endoscopic Surgery in Children?
N.M.A. Bax 3
Instrumentation
K.E. Georgeson 8
Basic Technique
A.S. Najmaldin, D. Grousseau 14
Ergonomics of Task Performance in Endoscopic Surgery
G.B. Hanna, C. Kimber, A. Cuschieri 35
Training in Paediatric Endoscopic Surgery
A.S. Najmaldin 49
Basic Physiology and Anesthesia
M. Sfez 53

Part II Chest

Thoracoscopy in Infants and Children: Basic Technique
S.S. Rothenberg 73
Diagnostic Thoracoscopy in Children
B.M. Rodgers 84
Thoracoscopy in the Treatment of Empyema in Children
B.M. Rodgers 92
Therapeutic Thoracoscopic Procedures in Children:
Indications and Surgical Applications in Lung and Mediastinum
J-L. Michel, Y. Revillon 98
Thoracoscopic Repair of Hiatal Hernia in Children
S.S. Rothenberg 109
Closure of Patent Ductus Arteriosus
F. Laborde, T. Folliguet 114
Vascular Access
N.M.A. Bax, D.C. van der Zee 121
Endoscopic Transthoracic Sympathectomy in the Treatment
of Primary Palmar Hyperhidrosis in Children
G. Lotan, I. Vinograd 125
Video-Asssisted Repair of Esophageal Atresia
M. Robert, H. Lardy 130

Part III Abdomen
Diagnostic Laparoscopy

Diagnostic Laparoscopy
 J. Waldschmidt, N.M.A. Bax 137

Gastrointestinal Tract

Laparoscopic Treatment of Achalasia
 G. Mattioli, A. Cagnazzo, P. Buffa, V. Jasonni 157
Laparoscopic Nissen Fundoplication in Children
 A.S. Najmaldin, G.M.E. Humphrey............................. 163
Laparoscopic Toupet Fundoplication
 P. Montupet, G. Cargill, J.-S. Valla 174
Laparoscopic Thal Fundoplication in Infants and Children
 D.C. van der Zee, N.M.A. Bax................................. 184
Laparoscopic Gastrostomy
 K.E. Georgeson 191
Laparoscopic Antroplasty
 K.E. Georgeson 195
Laparoscopic Extramucosal Pyloromyotomy
 J.L. Alain, D. Grousseau 198
Laparoscopic Jejunostomy
 K.E. Georgeson 203
Laparoscopic Treatment of Anomalies of Intestinal Rotation in Children
 N.M.A. Bax, D.C. van der Zee 207
Laparoscopic Approach to Intestinal Obstruction in Children
 D.C. van der Zee, N.M.A. Bax 215
Laparoscopic Diagnosis and Treatment of Meckel's Diverticulum
 in Children
 J-S. Valla, H. Steyaert 221
Intussusception
 A.S. Najmaldin 229
Laparoscopic Appendicectomy in Children
 J-S. Valla, H. Steyaert 234
Laparoscopic Total Colectomy
 D.A. Beals, K.E. Georgeson.................................... 254
Laparoscopic Endorectal Pull-Through
 K.E. Georgeson 261
Laparoscopic Removal of the Aganglionic Bowel According
 to Duhamel-Martin
 N.M.A. Bax, D.C. van der Zee 272
Treatment of Hirschsprung's Disease by Laparoscopic Dissection
 of Bowel, Transanal Eversion and Perineal Resection
 F. Schier, J. Waldschmidt 281

Liver and Biliary Tree

Endoscopic Surgery for Liver Hydatid Cysts
F.J. Berchi 291
Laparoscopic Cholecystectomy
G.W. Holcomb III 297

Spleen

Laparoscopic Splenectomy
W.R. Thompson, E. Parra-Davila 311

Diaphragm

Laparoscopic Repair of Diaphragmatic Conditions in Infants and Children
D.C. van der Zee, N.M.A. Bax, J-S. Valla 323

Inguinal Hernia

Contralateral Groin Exploration During Inguinal Hernia Repair
K.E. Georgeson 331

Shunts and Catheters

Laparoscopic Approach to Ventriculoperitoneal Shunts
N.M.A. Bax, D.C. van der Zee, W.P. Vandertop 337
Laparoscopic Insertion of Peritoneal Dialysis Catheters in Children
C.K. Yeung, K. F. Yip 344

Complications

Complications in Laparoscopic Surgery in Children
N.M.A. Bax, D.C. van der Zee 357

Part IV Urogenital Tract

Transperitoneal Laparoscopic Nephrectomy
A.S. Najmaldin 371
Videosurgery of the Retroperitoneal Space in Children
J-S. Valla 379
The Nonpalpable Testis
F. Ferro 393
Laparoscopic Varicocele
G.A. MacKinlay 408
Adnexal Pathology
H. Steyaert, Y. Heloury, V. Plattner, J-S. Valla 415
Laparoscopy and Intersex
Y. Heloury, V. Plattner 427

Part V Orthopedics and Neurosurgery

Thoracoscopic Anterior Spinal Diskectomy and Fusion
  G.W. Holcomb III 433
Indications, Techniques and Results of Pediatric Neuroendoscopy
  J.A. Grotenhuis, W.P. Vandertop 443

Part VI Oncology

Endoscopic Surgery in Paediatric Oncology
  H.A. Steinbrecher, A.S. Najmaldin 465

Part VII Conclusion

The Future of Endoscopic Surgery in Children
  K.E. Georgeson 477

Subject Index 481

Contributors

Jean Luc Alain, MD
   Professor of Pediatric Surgery and Head of the Department of Pediatric Surgery, University of Limoges School of Medicine, University Dupytren Hospital, Limoges, France

Klaas(N) M.A. Bax, MD, PhD
   Professor of Pediatric Surgery, Department of Pediatric Surgery, University Children's Hospital, Utrecht, The Netherlands

Daniel A. Beals, MD
   Division of Pediatric Surgery, The University of Alabama at Birmingham, The Children's Hospital of Alabama, Birmingham, USA

Francisco J. Berchi, MD
   Professor of Pediatric Surgery and Head of the Department of Pediatric Surgery, Hospital Materno Infantil 12 de Octubre, University of Compultense, Madrid, Spain

Piero Buffa, MD
   Department of Pediatric Surgery, Giannina Gaslini Institute, University of Genoa, Genoa, Italy

Aldo Cagnazzo, MD
   Department of Pediatric Surgery, Giannina Gaslini Institute, University of Genoa, Genoa, Italy

Guillaume Cargill, MD
   Department of Pediatric Surgery, Hôpital Necker-Enfants Malades, Paris, France

Alfred Cuschieri, MD, ChM, FRCSEd, FRCSEng, FRCSGlas (Hon), FIBiol
   Professor of Surgery, Ninewells Hospital and Medical School, Dundee, Scotland

Fabio Ferro, MD
   Department of Pediatric Surgery and Urology, Bambino Gesù Children's Hospital, Rome, Italy

Thierry Folliguet
   L'Institut Mutualiste Montsouris, Paris, France

Keith E. Georgeson, MD
   Professor and Director, Department of Surgery, Division of Pediatric Surgery, The University of Alabama at Birmingham, The Children's Hospital of Alabama, Birmingham, USA

J. André Grotenhuis, MD
  Senior Consultant, Department of Neurosurgery, Academic Hospital Nijmegen, Nijmegen, The Netherlands
Dominique Grousseau, MD
  Senior Consultant, Department of Pediatric Surgery, University Dupytren Hospital, Limoges, France
George B. Hanna, MD
  Consultant, Department of Surgery, Ninewells Hospital and Medical School, Dundee, Scotland
Yves Heloury, MD
  Professor of Pediatric Surgery, Department of Pediatric Surgery, Centre Hospitalier Universitaire de Nantes, Hôpital Mère et Enfant, Nantes, France
George W. Holcomb, III, MD
  Associate Professor of Surgery, Department of Pediatric Surgery, Vanderbilt University Medical Center, Nashville, Tennessee, USA
Gill M.E. Humphrey, MB, ChB, MD
  Senior Registrar in Pediatric Surgery, Leeds United Teaching Hospitals, St. James's University Hospital, Leeds, United Kingdom
Ingrid Janssen, illustrator,
  Audiovisual Department, University of Utrecht, The Netherlands
Vincenzo Jasonni, MD
  Professor of Pediatric Surgery, Department of Pediatric Surgery, Giannina Gaslini Institute, University of Genoa, Genoa, Italy
Chris Kimber
  Research Fellow, Surgical Skills Unit, Ninewells Hospital and Medical School, Dundee, Scotland
François Laborde, MD
  L'Institut Mutualiste Montsouris, Paris, France
Hubert Lardy, MD
  Consultant, Department of Pediatric Surgery, Centre Hospitalier Universitaire, Clocheville, Tours, France
Gad Lotan, MD
  Department of Pediatric Surgery, "Assaf Harofeh" Medical Center, Zerifin, Israel
Gordon A. Mackinlay, MB, BS, LRCP, FRCS(Ed), FRCS
  Senior Lecturer in Clinical Surgery, University of Edinburgh; Consultant Paediatric Surgeon, The Royal Hospital for Sick Children, Edinburgh, Scotland
Girolamo Mattioli, MD
  Department of Pediatric Surgery, Giannina Gaslini Institute, University of Genoa, Genoa, Italy
Jean-Luc Michel, MD
  Department of Pediatric Surgery, Hôpital Necker-Enfants Malades, Paris, France
Philippe Montupet, MD
  Department of Pediatric Surgery, Hôpital Necker-Enfants Malades, Paris, France

Azad S. Najmaldin, MS, FRCS
  Senior Consultant, Department of Paediatric Surgery, St. James's University Hospital, Leeds, United Kingdom
Eduardo Parra-Davila, MD
  Chief Resident, Department of General Surgery, University of Miami, Jackson Memorial Hospital, Miami, Florida, USA
Véronique Plattner, MD
  Senior Consultant, Department of Pediatric Surgery, Centre Hospitalier Universitaire de Nantes, Hôpital Mère et Enfant, Nantes, France
Yann Revillon, MD
  Professor of Pediatric Surgery, Department of Pediatric Surgery, Hôpital Necker-Enfants Malades, Paris, France
Michel Robert, MD
  Professor of Pediatric Surgery and Head of the Department of Pediatric Surgery, Centre Hospitalier Universitaire, Clocheville, Tours, France
Bradley M. Rodgers, MD
  University of Virginia Health System, Department of Pediatric Surgery, Division of Pediatric Surgery, Charlottesville, Virginia, USA
Steven S. Rothenberg, MD
  Assistant Clinical Professor of Surgery, University of Colorado, Director of Pediatric Surgery, Columbia Presbyterian/St Luke's Medical Center, Denver, Colorado, USA
Felix Schier, MD
  Professor of Pediatric Surgery and Head of the Department of Pediatric Surgery, Friedrich-Schiller University Hospital, Jena, Germany
Michel Sfez, MD
  Senior Consultant Anesthetist, Paris, France
Henrik A. Steinbrecher, MS, FRCS
  Consultant, Department of Pediatric Surgery, Wessex Regional Centre for Paediatric Surgery, Southampton General Hospital, Southampton, United Kingdom
Henri Steylaert, MD
  Senior Consultant, Department of Pediatric Surgery, Fondation Lenval, Hôpital pour Enfants, Nice, France
W. Raleigh Thompson, MD
  Associate Professor of Surgery, Chief Division of Pediatric Surgery, University of Miami School of Medicine, Miami, Florida, USA
Jean-Stéphane Valla, MD
  Professor of Pediatric Surgery and Head of the Department of Pediatric Surgery, Fondation Lenval, Hôpital pour Enfants, Nice, France
David C. van der Zee, MD, PhD
  Senior Consultant, Department of Pediatric Surgery, University Children's Hospital, Utrecht, The Netherlands
W. Peter Vandertop, MD, PhD
  Senior Consultant, Department of Neurosurgery, University Hospital and University Children's Hospital, Utrecht, The Netherlands

Itzhak Vinograd, MD
   Department of Pediatric Surgery, "Assaf Harofeh" Medical Center, Zerifin, Israel

Jürgen Waldschmidt, MD
   Professor of Pediatric Surgery and Head of the Department of Pediatric Surgery, University Hospital Benjamin Franklin, Berlin, Germany

Chung Kwong Yeung, MD, FRCS, FRACS, DCH
   Professor of Pediatric Surgery and Head of the Department of Pediatric Surgery, The Chinese University of Hong Kong, Prince of Wales Hospital, Hong Kong, Republic of China

Kam-Fai Yip, MD
   Senior Consultant, Department of Pediatric Surgery, The Chinese University of Hong Kong, Prince of Wales Hospital, Hong Kong, Republic of China

Part I
Basics

CHAPTER 1

Why Endoscopic Surgery in Children?

N.M.A. Bax

The traditional hippocratic ethos provides the background of the idea that the less invasive procedure, the better. It is morally preferable, if possible, to avoid invading into the body of a patient (van Willigenburg 1995). This is in contrast with classic open surgery. Thanks to the invention of anesthesia in 1846, it became possible to open body cavities, and surgery, which had been limited to the treatment of external diseases became "internal" medicine (Haeger 1988). One of the principles of classic surgery, however, has been and still is adequate exposure, which often requires large incisions especially when a body cavity is to be opened. Classic surgery opens the body and externalizes the problem.

In conditions in which the body wall itself is not affected, it is a pity that the body wall must be opened, as body wall related complications do occur, for example, infection, dehiscence, and incisional hernia. Even in the absence of complications, opening of the body wall results in morbidity. The ensuing stress and pain should be regarded as morbidity. The larger the wound the more fascia, muscles and nerves are transected and the more morbidity can be expected. Pain related to the access wound may not only be limited to the early postoperative period but may become chronic. Long-term morbidity after a classical posterolateral thoracotomy is well known. Hypertrophic scars are not only important from the cosmetic point of view but also in terms of morbidity. These scars may be painful or may give the patient a feeling of traction and therefor limit movement. Other scars represent abnormal tissue as well and may cause discomfort. Some paresthesia is virtually always present around a scar.

Wide opening of the body wall results in loss of water and heat, which especially threatens small children. Drying out of the tissues and handling of the tissues causes trauma to them and impaired healing. Hypothermia and drying out of the tissues, however, can also happen during endoscopy surgery when a high flow is used. High flows should be avoided (Bessell et al. 1995; Mansvelt et al. 1995).

Due to the magnification and good illumination endoscopic surgery gives a much better view of the operative field than open surgery. On the other hand bleeding during endoscopic surgery should be avoided as much as possible as this is more difficult to control during endoscopic surgery than during open surgery. Moreover bleeding blurs the detailed endoscopic anatomy of the field and diminishes the available light by absorption. The endoscopic surgeon must therefore be meticulous and usually operates in a much less traumatic way than during open surgery.

One of the major problems of open surgery is the formation of adhesions between the intraabdominal contents and the laparotomy scar (Becker et al. 1996; Brill et al. 1995). While adhesions do not cause cosmetic impairment, they may give long-term morbidity. There is little doubt that the laparoscopic approach elicits fewer adhesions between the intraabdominal contents and the abdominal wall than after open surgery (Jorgenson et al. 1995a).

In endoscopic surgery the chance of direct contact between the body fluids of the patient and the surgeon is less than in open surgery, which makes endoscopic surgery more safe for the surgeon.

Many surgeons minimize the cosmetic impact of a scar. Parents regard each scar in their children as a scar on their soul. Even when a primary tooth breaks as a result of a fall, and the parents are told that this tooth will be replaced in time by a healthy permanent one, parents feel sad. Moreover, parents often start complaining about the scar as soon as the life-threatening event for which surgery was carried out fades from memory. It should not be forgotten that scars in children grow with the patient. During puberty body integrity becomes very important to the child and even the slightest abnormality as a touch of acnea is taken seriously by that child. Modern advertising takes advantage of this.

It seems obvious that the lesser the trauma, the quicker the recovery. However, how to prove this scientifically? Most clinical studies relate to cholecystectomy. Mealy found no significant difference in urinary urea excretion in the first 24 h between patients with open and laparoscopic cholecystectomy (Mealy et al. 1992). Moreover there appears no difference in serum cortisol concentrations and urinary cortisol excretion for the ensuing 48 h (Joris et al. 1992; Mealy et al. 1992). Similarly, the plasma catecholamine response does not appear to differ between the two types of surgery (Joris et al. 1992). Several studies found a higher C-reactive protein concentration after 24 h in patients undergoing open cholecystectomy (Joris et al. 1992; Mealy et al. 1992; O'Riordain et al. 1994), and both Joris et al. (1992) and Maruszinsky and Pojda (1995) found a higher interleukin-6 response. Other authors found a more heterogeneous interleukin-6 response in the laparoscopic group (O'Riordain et al. 1994; Roumen et al. 1992). From these studies the general conclusion that the laparoscopic approach is superior cannot be drawn. Two randomized trials, however, found that patients operated laparoscopically had less pain, had a quicker recovery and returned earlier to work (Barkun et al. 1992; McMahon et al. 1994). Majeed et al. (1996), in another controlled study, did not find such a difference. How can these different result be explained? The unique design of Majeed's study has been applauded (Horton 1996; Terpstra 1996). In this study laparoscopic cholecystectomy is compared with cholecystectomy through a minilaparotomy. This means that the classic open approach demanding a large exposure and therefor a large incision has been abandoned. Baguley et al. (1995) even studied in a randomized fashion the difference between a muscle cutting and a muscle splitting incision for open cholecystectomy. Fleshman et al. (1996) compared prospectively outcomes after minilaparotomy and laparoscopy for colorectal diseases and found no differences in early outcome. By minimizing the length of the incision in open surgery, the advantages of the minimal access in laparoscopic surgery regarding pain and cosmesis become less important. The question now arises: how long should an incision in classic surgery be to allow for good exposure and a safe operation?

Endoscopic approaches at present are still quite invasive. The use of CO_2 as a gas for insufflation causes profound local and general acid-base and hemodynamic changes (Chiu et al. 1995; Volz et al. 1996). Insufflation pressure on its own causes hemodynamic changes and prolonged insufflation of the abdomen causes a compartment syndrome (Hunter 1995). High flow causes drying of the tissues and hypothermia (Bessell et al. 1995; Mansvelt et al. 1995). No wonder that the neuroendocrine, the cytokine and the C-reactive protein systems are activated during endoscopic surgery.

Endoscopic surgery has only started. It is certainly not minimally invasive at the present, and many changes will be introduced in the future. The imaging system and instruments will further improve, and systems will be invented to increase the working space. At the time being studies are conducted regarding the use of other gasses for insufflation as helium (Declan Fleming et al. 1997; Rademaker et al. 1995a), while devices have been invented to lift the anterior abdominal wall so that endoscopic surgery is possible without insufflation (Chiu et al. 1995; Rademaker et al. 1995b). Together with these improvements, endoscopic surgery will find its proper place in medicine. At the time being one should be careful to implicate endoscopic surgery in the treatment of malignancies as many reports about implantation and growth of malignant cells at the port sites have been described, even after diagnostic procedures (Andersen and Steven 1995; Ash et al. 1995; Berends et al. 1994; Cirocco et al. 1994; Childers et al. 1994; Fry et al. 1995; Jorgesen et al. 1995; Walsh and Nesbitt 1995). Animal experiments have yielded conflicting results. Allendorf et al. (1995) found in a murine model that a laparotomy increased tumor establishment and growth when compared with laparoscopy, while Jacobi et al. (1997) in a rat model found that CO_2 insufflation increased tumor growth in vitro. Again in a murine model Allendorf et al. (1997) showed that postoperative cell mediated function varies inversely with the degree of surgical trauma, favoring the laparoscopic approach.

It leaves no doubt that the less invasive a procedure is, the better for the patient. The recent introduction of endoscopic surgery on a larger more therapeutic scale has changed the classic surgical idea that good exposure always requires large incisions. Thanks to modern anesthesia and technical innovations, sufficient exposure nowadays can be reached with smaller incisions.

This new surgical thinking should also be applied to children. It is our duty as surgeons involved with the medical care of children to make surgical procedures for children as minimally invasive as possible yet as safe as possible.

References

Allendorf JD et al (1995) Increased tumor establishment and growth after laparotomy versus laparoscopy in a murine model. Arch Surg 130:649–653

Allendorf JDF et al (1997) Postoperative immune function varies inversely with the degree of surgical trauma in a murine model. Surg Endosc 11:427–430

Andersen JR, Steven K (1995) Implantation metastasis after laparoscopic biopsy of bladder cancer. J Urol 153:1047–1048

Ash AK et al (1995) Laparoscopy and spread of ovarian cancer (letter). Lancet 346:709–710

Baguley PE, de Gara CJ, Gagic N (1995) Open cholecystectomy: muscle splitting versus muscle dividing incision: a randomized study. J R Coll Surg Edinb 40:230–232

Barkun SB et al (1992) Randomised controlled trial of laparoscopic versus minilaparotomy cholecystectomy. Lancet 340:116–119

Becker JM et al (1996) Prevention of postoperative abdominal adhesions by a sodium hyaluronate-based bioresorbable membrane: a prospective, randomized, double-blind multicenter study. J Am Coll Surg 183:297–306

Berends FJ et al (1994) Subcutaneous metastases after laparoscopic colectomy (letter). Lancet 344:58

Bessell JR et al (1995) Hypothermia induced by laparoscopic insufflation. A randomized study in a pig model. Surg Endosc 9:791–796

Brill AI et al (1995) The incidence of adhesions after prior laparotomy: a laparoscopic appraisal (comments). Obstet Gynecol 85:269–272

Childers JM et al (1994) Abdominal wall tumor implantation after laparoscopy for malignant conditions. Obstet Gynecol 84:765–769

Chiu AW et al (1995) The impact of pneumoperitoneum, pneumoretroperitoneum, and gasless laparoscopy on the systemic and renal hemodynamics. J Am Coll Surg 181:397–406

Cirocco WC, Schwartzman A, Golub RW (1994) Abdominal wall recurrence after laparoscopic colectomy for colon cancer. Surgery 116:842–846

Declan Fleming RY, Dougherty TB, Feig BW (1997) The safety of helium for abdominal insufflation. Surg Endosc 11:230–234

Fleshman JW et al (1996) Laparoscopic-assisted and minilaparotomy approaches to colorectal diseases are similar in early outcome. Dis Colon Rectum 39:15–22

Fry WA et al (1995) Thoracoscopic implantation of cancer with fatal outcome. Ann Thorac Surg 59:42–45

Haeger K (1988) The illustrated history of surgery. Nordbok, Göthenborg

Horton R (1996) Surgical research or comic opera: questions but few answers. Lancet 347:984–985

Hunter JG (1995) Editorial: Laparoscopic pneumoperitoneum: the abdominal compartment syndrome revisited. J Am Coll Surg 181:469–470

Jacob CA et al (1997) Inhibition of peritoneal tumor cell growth and implantation in laparoscopic surgery in a rat model. Am J Surg 174:359–363

Jorgenson JO, Lalak NJ, Hunt DR (1995a) Is laparoscopy associated with a lower rate of postoperative adhesions than laparotomy? A comparative study in the rabbit. Aust N Z J Surg 65:342–344

Jorgesen JO, McCall JL, Morris DL (1995b) Port site seeding after laparoscopic ultrasonographic staging of pancreatic carcinoma. Surgery 117:118–119

Joris J et al (1992) Metabolic and respiratory changes after cholecystectomy performed via laparotomy or laparoscopy. Br J Anaesth 69:341–517

Majeed AW et al (1996) Randomised prospective, single blind comparison of laparoscopic versus small incision cholecystectomy. Lancet 347:989–994

Mansvelt B et al (1995) Utilization of gas heater humidifier in the course of coelioscopies. Acta Chir Belg 95:100–102

Maruszynski M, Pojda Z (1995) Interleukin-6 (IL-6) levels in the monitoring of surgical trauma. A comparison of serum IL-6 concentrations in patients treated by cholecystectomy via laprotomy or laparoscopy. Surg Endosc 9:882–885

McMahon AJ et al (1994) Laparoscopic versus minilaparotomy cholecystectomy: a randomised trial. Lancet 434:135–138

Mealy K et al (1992) Physiological and metabolic responses to open and laparoscopic cholecystectomy. Br J Surg 79:1061–1064

O'Riordain M, Ross JA, Fearon KCH (1994) The inflammatory and metabolic response to open surgery and minimally invasive surgery. In: Patterson-Brown S, Garden J (eds) Principles and practice of surgical laparoscopy. Saunders, London, pp 7–21

Rademaker BM et al (1995a) Effects of pneumoperotoneum with helium on hemodynamics and oxygen transport: a comparison with carbon dioxide. J Laparoendosc Surg 5:15–20

Rademaker BM et al (1995b) Laparoscopy without pneumoperitoneum. Surg Endosc 9:797–801

Roumen RMH et al (1992) Serum interleukin-6 and C-reactive protein responses in patients after laparoscopic or conventional cholecystectomy. Eur J Surg 158:541–544

Terpstra OT (1996) Laparoscopic cholecystectomy: the other side of the coin. Br Med J 312:1375

van Willigenburg T (1995) Laparoscopic surgery: systematic appraisal of moral pro's and con's. Book of abstracts, international symposium: laparoscopic surgery in children: sense and non-sense, Utrecht, 7–8 April, p 14

Volz J et al (1996) Pathophysiologic features of a pneumoperitoneum at laparoscopy: a swine model. Am J Obstet Gynecol 174:132–140

Walsh GL, Nesbitt JC (1995) Tumor implants after thoracoscopic resection of a metastatic sarcoma. Ann Thorac Surg 59:215–216

CHAPTER 2

Instrumentation

K.E. Georgeson

Introduction

Instrumentation for pediatric endoscopic surgery has improved steadily over the past 5 years. Early endoscopic surgical procedures in children required the use of instruments and trocars designed for adults. These instruments were not only oversized in diameter but also too long for convenient use in small patients. Instruments are now available which facilitate application of endoscopic surgical procedures to infants and children.

Trocars

Trocars are the most frequently used instruments in endoscopic surgery. Both reusable and disposable trocars are in common use by pediatric surgeons. The reusable trocars are less expensive but lack safety shields and require more forceful insertion. Both types of trocars require fixation devices to avoid the frustration of unintentional in and out movement of the trocar during the surgical procedure.

Reusable trocars are frequently top heavy, which makes their use as working ports awkward. Light plastic ports or metal ports with light heads are much easier to use than top heavy ports.

Trocar valves should be carefully evaluated. Trocars with a manual trumpet valve or a very stiff valve decreases the working dexterity of endoscopic surgeons and diminishes task performance.

Trocars are inserted with an insertion spike. The spike can have either a cutting or conical tip. The cutting tip allows easier insertion but leaves a larger defect in the abdominal wall. The conical spike stretches the tissue leaving a smaller hole when the trocars are removed. The conical spike also induces a tighter fit between the trocar and the abdominal wall tissues allowing for less leakage of the pneumoperitoneum, an important factor in thin walled children.

A trocar can be fixed to the infant or child's abdominal wall using a 1- to 2-cm sleeve of Red Robinson catheter (see Fig. 1). The cut sleeve of the catheter is passed over the trocar. A 2-0 silk suture is passed through the substance of the catheter and through the skin securing the catheter and trocar to the abdominal

Fig. 1. 3.5- and 5-mm trocars used in pediatric laparoscopy. Note the catheter sleeves on the reusable trocars

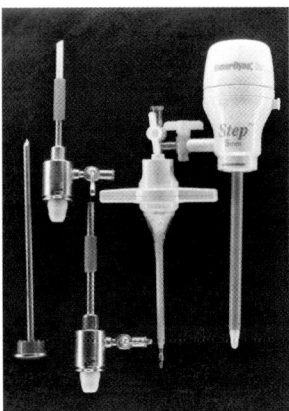

wall. This method of fixation also allows adjustment of the trocar's position during the operative procedure by sliding the trocar within the sleeve.

Disposable trocars are popular because of the ease of introduction into the peritoneal cavity. They usually have a safety shield which helps to prevent injury to underlying viscera during introduction of the trocar. Disposable trocars also need fixation devices to keep them from sliding during the operative procedure. Sutures, trocar screws, and catheter sleeves are all helpful techniques for fixing disposable trocars to the abdominal wall.

Expandable sleeve trocars are also useful in children (InnerDyne, Sunnyvale, Calif.). A stab wound is made in the abdominal wall and the expandable sleeve, which slips over a Veress needle, is passed into the peritoneal cavity. The Veress needle is then removed, and the trocar is passed through the expandable sleeve into the abdominal cavity. Expandable sleeve trocars produce a tight fit between the trocar and the abdominal wall, holding the trocar in place and diminishing the potential for gas leakage. Insertion safety is also increased with this technique as the initial placement of the sleeve can be carefully directed. The primary problems of expandable sleeve trocars are cost and the lack of availability of small sized trocars. A partially reusable expandable trocar is now available. The sleeve is disposable but the inside cannula is reusable.

Scopes

Scopes of 1–10 mm are useful for surgeons performing pediatric endoscopic surgery. Small scopes with excellent optics are available. However, the smaller the scope, the poorer the light gathering capability, producing a dim, less colorful picture on the video monitor. Every year a new generation of cameras allows the use of smaller scopes with an acceptable image. In the future, digital cameras with high definition capability will allow the use of 1- and 2-mm scopes for most pediatric surgical procedures.

Scopes come in various lengths and angles. Short scopes allow a more compact operating field. However, the bulk of the camera head is brought closer to the body wall, which sometimes interferes with operative manipulation of the endoscopic surgical instruments. Common scope angles include 0°, 30°, 45°, and 70°. Scopes of 33° and 45° allow the tip of operating scope to be above the operating field within the chest or abdomen. This position of the scope helps to prevent sword fighting of the scope with other instruments and frequently allows a better working view than can be achieved with a straight scope. Scopes of 0° and 30° are mandatory for pediatric endoscopic surgery. Scopes of 45° and 70° are also useful in specialized situations.

Cameras

Cameras currently come in one- or three-color computer chips. Three-chip cameras have much better color definition and are more useful in pediatric endoscopic surgical procedures. Three-dimensional cameras are also available and have been popular attractions at endoscopic surgical meetings. However, they do not yet appear to be refined enough to be useful in clinical applications for children. Obviously, evolution in 3-D technology should produce a useful camera in the future. Another promising technical improvement is the emergence of high-definition digital cameras. These digital cameras allow much greater picture resolution with smaller scopes and allow enhancement of the picture digitally.

Insufflators

Insufflators useful in adult endoscopic surgery are also satisfactory for most pediatric endoscopic procedures. Ideally, insufflators that allow gas flow both to and from the patient are best to maintain a constant intracavitary pressure. Unidirectional insufflation can overshoot the regulated pressure in the child's small volume peritoneal cavity causing prolonged exposure to high intracavitary pressures. The use of gases other than the carbon dioxide such as helium remains experimental. Gasless laparoscopy using corkscrew, wire, or metal struts as body wall lifters are evolving for use in pediatric endoscopic surgery. These lifting devices have theoretical advantages including simplification of trocars (no gas valve is necessary), no collapse of the field with suctioning and decreased cost. Further development is necessary before they achieve widespread application.

Instruments

Most instruments available for pediatric endoscopic surgery were originally designed for adults. They are frequently too long and too large in diameter. The

2 Instrumentation

ideal position of an instrument during endoscopic surgical procedures is to have two-thirds of the instrument inside the body cavity and the other one-third outside the body. This position allows economy of external motion and precision of internal motion. Adult length instruments frequently leave 75%–80% of the instrument outside the child and only 20% inside. This arrangement makes operative manipulation awkward and less precise. Because trocars are grouped closely together for pediatric endoscopic surgery, both short and long instruments sometimes clash with each other outside the abdomen.

Laparoscopic Instruments that function like open surgical instruments are usually best. Locking devices which require the use of two hands to lock or manipulate are much more difficult to use.

Figs. 2–5 show instruments useful for pediatric laparoscopy and are available commercially. Other instruments, with special functions, are also available. In general, reusable instruments are preferable to disposable instruments. Reusable instruments are made of much higher quality materials than disposable instruments and are also less expensive in the long run.

Graspers come with single and double action jaws. Double action jaws open wider and are easier to manipulate during dissection but have a groove that can

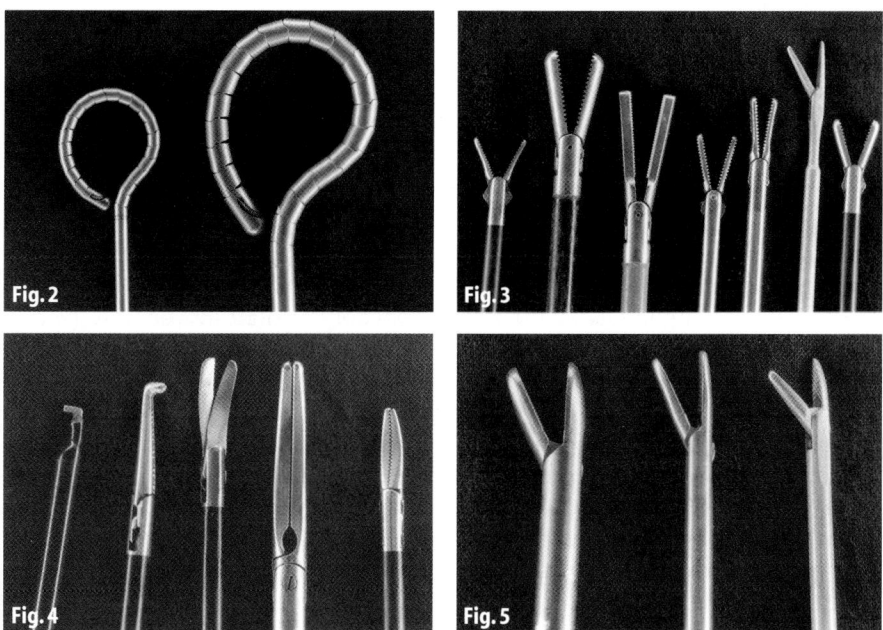

Fig. 2. 3- and 5-mm retractors
Fig. 3. 3- and 5-mm graspers
Fig. 4. 3- and 5-mm instruments useful for fine dissection and cauterization
Fig. 5. 3- and 5-mm coaxial needle drivers

trap sutures during knot tying. Single action jaws are less likely to have this suture-trapping groove and are useful for internal knotting.

Curved Metzenbaum scissors make an excellent dissecting tool. The points should be rounded for safer dissection. Many scissors have monopolar or bipolar electrocautery capability. With monopolar cautery it is usually best to close the scissors and use the tip as a cautery wand than to activate the blade while cutting. Activating the cautery during cutting dulls the cutting surfaces of the scissors and is also associated with less efficient cauterization.

Needle drivers have both straight and angled jaws. Angled jaws are superior for internal knotting. Endoscopic needle drivers function best if they are coaxial and have a locking mechanism. The Castro-Viejo locking mechanism preferred by many instrument companies makes internal knot tying awkward. Internal knot tying is better than external knot tying with a knot pusher when operating through the small trocars used in pediatric endoscopic surgery. The author favors a standard lock coaxial needle driver with a curved or angled tip, which is excellent for both internal suturing and knotting. A straight or curved instrument is also useful in the left hand for facilitating internal knot tying. Knot pushers for external knot tying come in a variety of configurations. Rapid application and reliability are important factors when selecting knot pushers.

Needles come in three basic configurations: curved, straight, and ski shaped. Straight needles are the easiest of the three to manipulate and pass through small diameter trocars. They do not utilize standard surgical wrist rotation and are usually considered inadequate for complex suturing tasks by experienced endoscopic surgeons. Curved needles do not pass through the small trocars used in pediatric endoscopic surgery. They are also harder to grasp, and align inside the body cavity. Curved needles can be passed through the body cavity wall, grasped internally and pulled inside. They are passed outside in reverse fashion.

Ski needles are popular among endoscopic surgeons because they can be easily grasped and aligned using the straight part of the shaft just behind the curvature of the needle. These allow rotational suturing using the curved portion of the needle. A working port large enough to allow passage of the ski needle is usually utilized to avoid making the suturing process tedious. Needles are often passed through the trocar by grasping the thread 1–2 cm behind the needle.

Clips are useful for ligating vessels rapidly. Reusable or disposable clip appliers are available. Forward pressure should be maintained while applying the clip to ensure that the entire circumference of the vessel is clipped.

Stapling devices are also useful during endoscopic surgery. Tissue-approximating staples and linear staples are available. Linear staples have both a gastrointestinal load and a vascular load. Mesenteric vessels should be stapled with the vascular load. Cautery should never be used on a staple line if break-through bleeding occurs. Cauterization may cause retraction of the tissues through the staples. Suture loops are also valuable tools for controlling vessels and stumps. They are less costly than staples.

In summary, satisfactory instruments for pediatric laparoscopic can be a decisive factor in the quality of an endoscopic operation. They should be chosen with great care by the operating surgeon and individualized to the surgeon's preferences. The growing interest in microendoscopy for adults has widely expanded the availability of instruments suitable for pediatric endoscopic surgery.

CHAPTER 3

Basic Technique

A.S. Najmaldin, D. Grousseau

Introduction

Endoscopic surgery is the application of established surgical procedures in a fashion which leads to a reduction in the trauma of access, thereby reducing surgical complications, accelerating recovery, and improving cosmesis. Surgical procedures are conducted by remote manipulation within the closed confines of the peritoneal or extra-peritoneal spaces and visual control via telescopes and television screens.

The ability to perform safe and successful endoscopic surgical procedures relies greatly on the understanding and appropriate application of the equipment and instruments as well as the creation of safe access and pneumoperitoneum. Failure to do this produces unnecessary complications and puts patients at risk.

At present the application of endoscopic surgery within the extra-peritoneal space has limited use in paediatric cases. This technique is highlighted elsewhere in this volume (see Valla, "Videosurgery of the Retroperitoneal Space").

Anatomy

The principle of endoscopic anatomy is that structures and their relations are viewed across the television screen in two dimensions instead of normal three dimensions, with the quality and size altered in accordance with their distance from the telescope as well as the character of the camera, light source and monitor in use. Anatomical landmarks and colour variations are used to identify structures. Inappropriately planned and placed access cannulae and telescope, technical problems with imaging, adhesions, unexpected enlarged structures and bleeding can greatly hinder the laparoscopic access and view of the anatomical structures. It is important to recognise that in infants and small children, the surface area for access is small, the abdominal wall is thin and highly compliant, the liver margin is below the ribcage, the bladder is largely an intra-abdominal structure, the viscera is close to the anterior abdominal wall and the abdominal cavity is small (Fig. 1). In small infants a pneumoperitoneum may only require 400 ml CO_2 to establish. The so-called obliterated structures, umbilical vein and arteries, and urachus remain relatively large and partially patent in infants.

3 Basic Technique

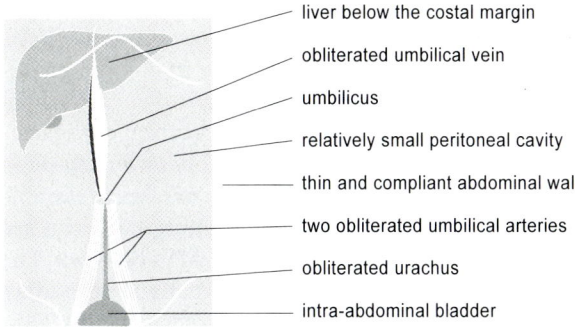

Fig. 1. Anatomy in infants and small children

These anatomical characteristics make access and manipulation in the younger age group a more demanding and difficult task when compared to grown up children or adults. On the other hand, young children have well-defined anatomical landmarks due to lack of excess fat, making recognition and dissection of structures a relatively easy task.

Patient Preparation and Theatre Layout

Before starting any endoscopic procedure:
- An informed consent must be available for both laparoscopic and conventional open approach.
- Check that all the required equipment and instruments are available, functioning and compatible. Colour coding cables/leads with input/output points on the camera video-screen facilitate quick setting up.
- The insufflator should be present for the required flow and pressure, and the display panel is visible and accessible to all surgeon, anaesthetist and technician.
- The electrocoagulation power supply must be set at the minimal effective level: in infants and small children monopolar diathermy power should start at 2.5 W and gradually increased to 50 W if and when necessary.
- A conventional set of laparotomy instruments must always be available and accessible next to the laparoscopy instruments for emergency use and when a conversion to an open technique is required.
- Inspect and palpate the abdomen for previous scar, enlarged organs such as liver or spleen, and abdominal masses.

It is important that the urinary bladder is empty before inserting the Veress needle/primary cannula and during the lower abdominal/pelvic laparoscopic procedures. Catheterisation is required only if the bladder is palpable, for monitoring renal function, and in prolonged lower abdominal procedures. In children a palpable bladder can be adequately emptied by expression. The use of a naso-gastric tube to drain the stomach is usually necessary from the anaesthetic point of view and to facilitate access to the upper abdomen. In colonic procedures a routine preoperative enema may prove advantageous.

The patient must be properly positioned to facilitate safe insertion of the cannulae, to optimise exposure and allow for the comfort of the operator. Although endoscopic surgery can be performed with only one monitor, two are preferable so that the surgeon and assistant on either side of the operating table can see along a direct 'straight' line with the target organ/operative field in between. The operator, assistant and nurse may stand on either side of the patient depending on the type of the laparoscopic procedure and surgeons preference. In upper abdominal procedures, however, the surgeon may find it more comfortable to operate standing between the patient's legs (large patients), or at the foot of the table (small children and infants) (Fig. 2). A degree of Trendelenburg position, reverse Trendelenburg or lateral tilt, often improves exposure. In renal surgery a complete lateral position may be needed. Appropriate shoulder and side supports, with or without strappings and wedge blocks, permit change of patients' position during the operation.

In paediatric patients the whole abdomen is usually prepared and draped. This is because the site of cannulae insertion are often away from the operative field, and an unplanned or additional cannula may be necessary for retraction or manipulation, or wide access may be necessary for conversion to emergency open surgery. The cables/leads are secured to the drapes in such a way that they cause no obstruction to access the patient and movement around the operating table by the surgeon, anaesthetist and the theatre staff. To prevent interference on the video screen, keep the camera cable and power point separate from that of the diathermy.

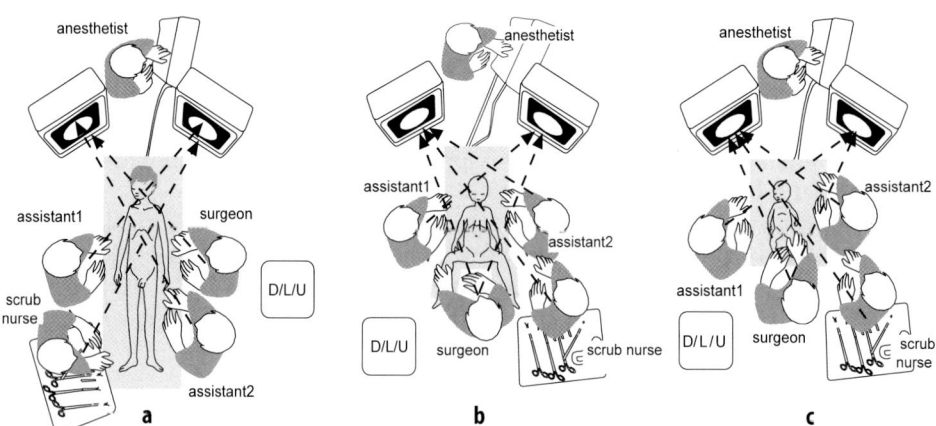

Fig. 2a–c. Position of patient and theatre layout. **a** Standard. **b** Upper abdominal surgery. **c** Infants and small children. *D*, Diathermy apparatus; *L*, laser apparatus; *U*, ultrasound apparatus

3 Basic Technique

The heat produced at the end of the fibreoptic or telescope can be sufficient to burn the drape, patient or internal organs if there is prolonged contact. Further, the high intensity light can also cause retinal damage if shone directly into the eye. Therefore, switch on the light source to the desired intensity and focus and white balance the camera, in this sequence, and only then the primary cannula is in place and the telescope is ready to enter the peritoneal cavity.

Creating a Pneumoperitoneum

A pneumoperitoneum may be created by two methods: closed method (blind) using Veress needle and/or primary cannula or the open method using Hasson's technique [1] or its modifications [2]. The gas that is usually used for insufflation is CO_2 because it is safe and rapidly cleared by the lungs, suppresses combustion during electro-coagulation, has no optical distortion, and is inexpensive. Oxygen and air support combustion and have a higher risk of embolism. Nitrous oxide has a risk of gas embolism and occupational hazards to the theatre staff.

Closed Method

The Veress needle is usually inserted at the site where the primary cannula will be placed (Fig. 3). In an unscarred abdomen an initial skin incision to fit the size of the primary cannula is made usually at the peri-umbilical region or umbilicus. A small nick on the surface of the linea alba, or rectus sheath, facilitates the subsequent passage of the primary cannula. An alternative site along the para-recti lines, usually left upper [3] or right lower, may be used especially if the umbilical region is abnormal due to previous surgical scars, patent embryonal ductus or portal hypertension, or if there is a large underlying intra-abdominal mass.

First, check the needle is patent and the spring mechanism is functioning properly. Hold the needle somewhere in the middle between your thumb and forefinger, grasp the abdominal wall by the other hand below the incision to produce counter-traction against the needle and allow the omentum/intestine to fall away from the site of insertion, and carefully insert the needle towards the middle of the pelvic cavity (Fig. 3). A definite give with a click is usually experienced as the needle passes through the peritoneum. Once the peritoneum is breached, the needle may only be advanced in parallel and on the inner surface of the parietal peritoneum and the following checks should be carried out to ensure that the needle is in the peritoneal cavity (Fig. 4)

- The tip of the needle should move freely from side to side on the inner surface of the parietal peritoneum.
- A 5- to 10-mm saline-filled syringe should aspirate no blood or fluid and there should be no resistance to the flow of saline via the needle. Once the syringe is disconnected from the needle, any saline left in the hub should disappear rapidly into the peritoneal cavity.

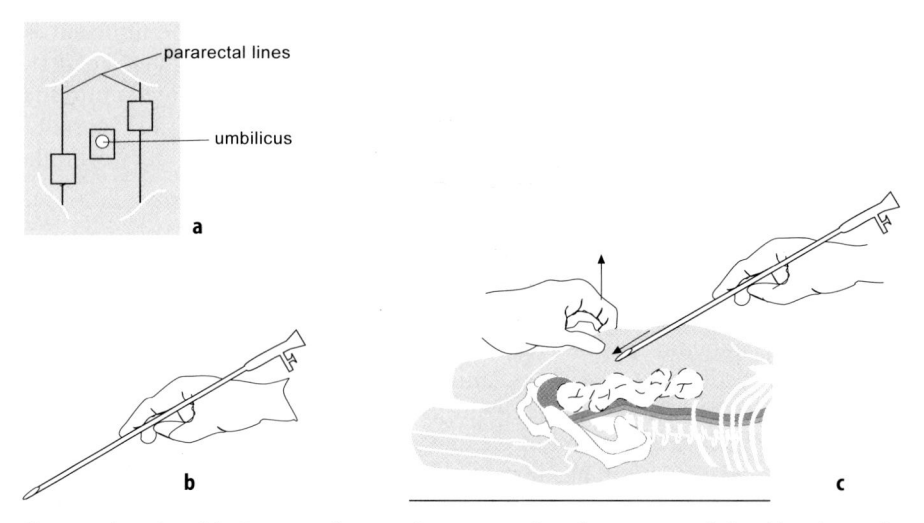

Fig. 3a–c. Insertion of the Veress needle. **a** sites for Veress needle and primary cannula. **b** Holding the needle. **c** Technique for insertion

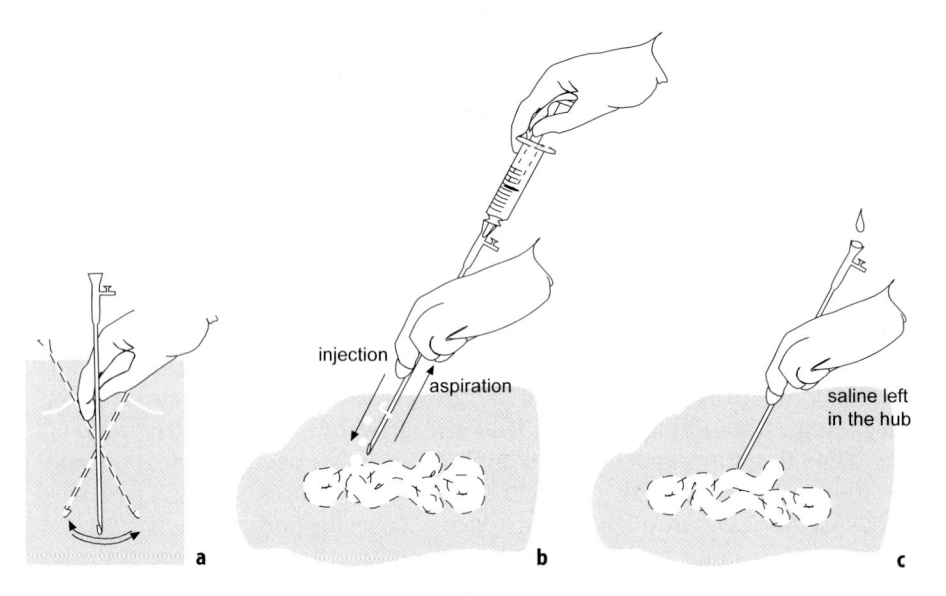

Fig. 4a–c. Safety checks to confirm that the needle is in the correct position. **a** Free movement on the inner surface of the abdominal wall. **b** Syringe aspiration and injection. **c** Saline drop test

The initial pneumoperitoneum is established gradually (gas flow 100–500 ml/min) to the required level of pressure (6–15 mmHg). The initial pressure reading should be low (less than 3 mmHg) and rise gradually. In a fully relaxed patient, an initial high pressure and low or no flow indicate an incorrectly placed insufflation needle, a kinked tube or an unopened tap. An established

Fig. 5. Insertion of the primary cannula. The index/middle finger along the shaft acts as a stop and reduces the risk of visceral injury

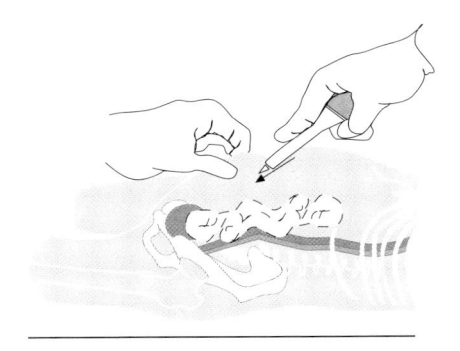

pneumoperitoneum requires 400 ml gas in infants and more than 3 l in an adolescent. Throughout the insufflation the abdomen should expand symmetrically and patients' ventilation and cardiac output are constantly monitored. In a scarred abdomen a Veress needle may be used a few/several centimetres away from the scar and particular care must be taken not to injure the viscera. A misplaced Veress needle may cause surgical emphysema of the extra-peritoneal spaces, omentum or mesentery; or a penetrating injury to the bowel or major vessels [4]. These complications are further discussed elsewhere in this volume (see Bax and van der Zee, "Complications in Laparoscopic Surgery in Children").

Once the desired pneumoperitoneum is created, the primary cannula (preferably with safety shield/device) is held in the palm of one hand and the index or middle finger is placed along the shaft to act as a stop, and introduced through the skin incision towards the middle of the pelvic cavity while the abdominal wall is stabilised/lifted anteriorally by the other hand or one or two towel clips (Fig. 5). A definite give (with an audible click if a cannula with a safety device is used) is experienced as the tip of the cannula passes through the peritoneum. The trocar is then withdrawn, and the cannula is advanced 2 cm into the abdominal cavity. For long operations a form of cannula fixation by means of grip-on devices, skin/abdominal wall sutures or towel clips, is advisable to prevent the cannula from falling out. The telescope is then inserted, and an initial laparoscopy is carried out and the sites of secondary 'working' cannulae are selected.

Open Method

Poor technique and intra-abdominal adhesions are major factors which predispose the closed method of laparoscopy to the danger of visceral and vascular injuries by the Veress needle and primary cannula. The open technique of laparoscopy provides an alternative safe method for insertion of the primary cannula and creation of a pneumoperitoneum.

In this technique the peritoneal cavity is opened and under direct vision, a blunt-tipped 'Hasson's' cannula or an ordinary disposable or re-usable cannu-

Fig. 6a–d. A method of open technique laparoscopy. **a** Periumbilical skin incision. **b** Skin is retracted and an incision is made through both fascia and peritoneum, and edges are held with mosquito forceps. **c** Purse-string including fascia and peritoneum with a single throw. **c1** Single suture as an alternative to the purse-string. **d** Cannula in position with the suture tied around the gas port leaving 1–2 cm of the cannula inside. **d1** A cuff of rubber tube may prevent the cannula from falling inside

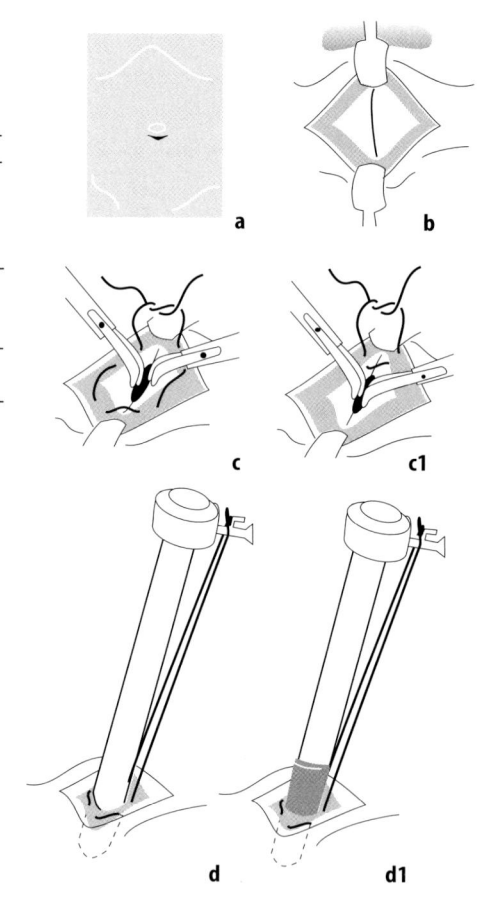

la/trocar introduced [1, 2]. For peri-umbilical primary cannula insertion, we make an adequate skin incision down to the linea alba which is picked up with mosquito forceps. An incision is then made through both the linea and peritoneum and a 2/0 or 3/0 absorbable, purse-string suture is inserted. Care must be taken to include both the linea and peritoneum with each bite. An ordinary 'primary' cannula is pushed off its trocar through the purse-string into the abdominal cavity and secured with a single throw of suture, thus allowing snug opposition of the linea to the cannula during the procedure, thereby preventing a gas leak. The suture is then secured around the gas port of the cannula, allowing 1–2 cm of the cannula to remain inside the abdominal cavity (Fig. 6). If desired, a cuff of pre-adjusted rubber tube on the cannula may be used to prevent the cannula from falling into the peritoneal cavity. Occasionally, placing a purse-string into the fascia/peritoneum is difficult, in which case a simple stitch may prove an effective alternative (Fig. 6).

3 Basic Technique

Fig. 7. Different types of abdominal wall lifters

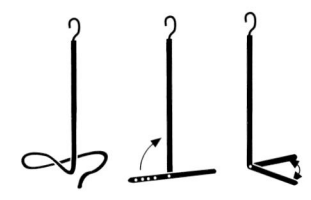

Abdominal Wall Lift

The technique of low pressure or gasless laparoscopy and creation of an operating space by mechanical traction/lift of the anterior abdominal wall has not gained popularity. Once the initial pneumoperitoneum is induced, under direct telescopic vision, multiple strong sutures through the abdominal wall or a specifically designed device (L, T or loop shaped) introduced percutaneously into the peritoneal cavity are used to lift the anterior abdominal wall with or without a low pressure pneumoperitoneum (less than 6 mmHg) (Fig. 7). The technique eliminates the risks of high pressure pneumoperitoneum and allows operating during continuous suction and gas leak.

Secondary Cannula Insertion

The position and number of secondary cannulae depends on the type of surgical procedure to be executed, the size of the patient and the presence or absence of abdominal scarring and other abdominal pathology. The cannulae which are used for the working instruments (manipulation, dissection, suturing, etc.) are best sited on either side and in front of the telescope at 45°–125° angle to allow easier eye/hand coordination and manipulation and to keep the instruments in view at all times (Fig. 8). Straight line instruments are very difficult to work, and instruments entering the abdomen against the line of view give mirror imaging and are consequently difficult to function (Fig. 8).

A small skin incision that matches exactly the diameter of the cannula and a small nick in the underlying fascia facilitate insertion of the trocar/cannula. As for insertion of the primary cannula, it is advisable to stabilise the abdominal wall anteriorally by one hand and to proceed carefully with insertion of the trocar/cannula with the index or middle finger acting as a stop, using a gentle continuous pressure and rotating movement. The direction of insertion should be towards the operative field. An oblique route of entry through the abdominal wall is slightly more difficult than the direct 'perpendicular' but has the theoretical advantages of reducing the risk of gas leak during the operation and herniation of viscera through the cannula site post-operatively. Abdominal wall vessels may be avoided by transillumination or viewing from within. As the peritoneal layer is tenting in (just before entering the cavity), keep the direction of cannula/trocar insertion in parallel to the abdominal wall, or push

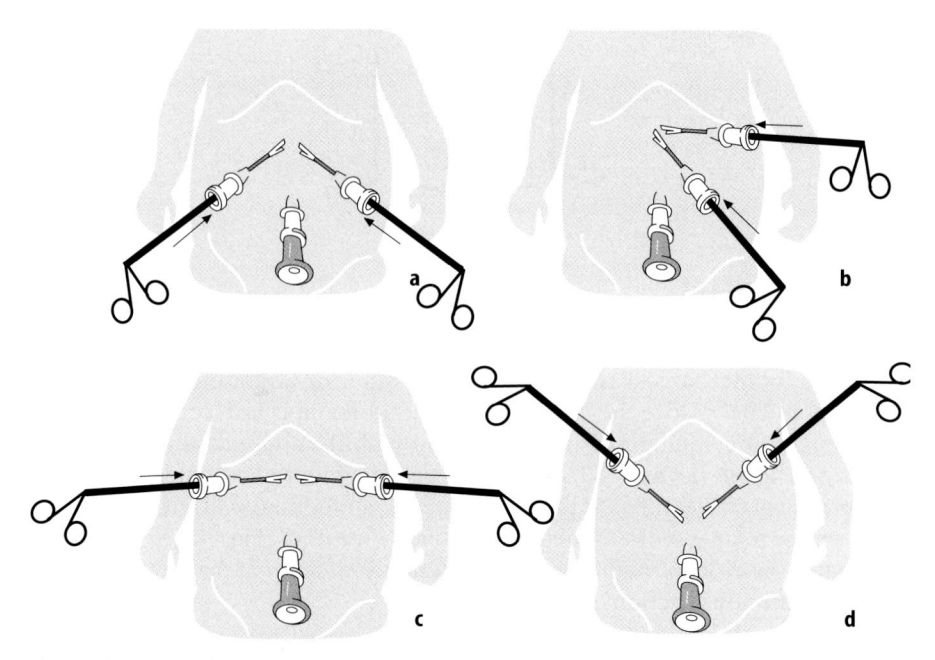

Fig. 8a–d. Position of the secondary cannulae "working cannulae". **a,b** Keep any two working instruments at 45°–125° angle and in front of the telescope if possible. **c** Straight line instruments are difficult to work. **d** Instruments against the line of view give mirror imaging

the cannula straight into the primary cannula when the telescope is withdrawn half way out (to avoid damaging the telescope) or another but empty secondary cannula. These manoeuvres help towards minimizing the risks of cannula injury to the intra-abdominal viscera. The point of entry to the peritoneal cavity should be placed under direct vision (Fig. 9). It is advisable to fix all busy secondary 'working' cannulae by means of anchoring devices or stitch through the abdominal wall. An instrument (retractor) which does not require change during the procedure, may be introduced into the abdominal cavity without a cannula.

Cannula insertion is probably the most important and potentially dangerous part of any laparoscopic procedure. It can lead to serious complications albeit very rarely [5]. The complications of cannula insertion are discussed elsewhere in this volume (see Bax and van der Zee, "Complications in Laparoscopic Surgery in Children").

Exiting the Abdomen

At the end of the procedure the areas close to the access cannulae and the operative field are thoroughly inspected for bleeding and signs of inadvertent injury.

3 Basic Technique

Fig. 9. Insertion of the secondary cannulae under viewing. Note the index finger along the shaft acts as a stop, and the camera keeps the point of entry as well as the viscera nearby under complete view

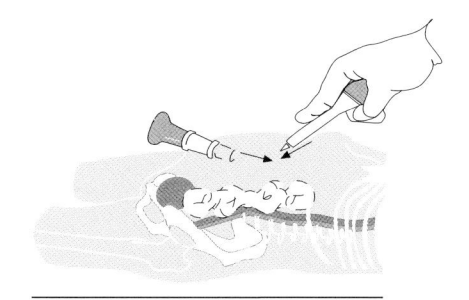

Fig. 10. Actions to stop an abdominal wall bleed: percutaneously inserted laparoscopically guided stitch, or traction on a balloon tipped catheter through the cannula site

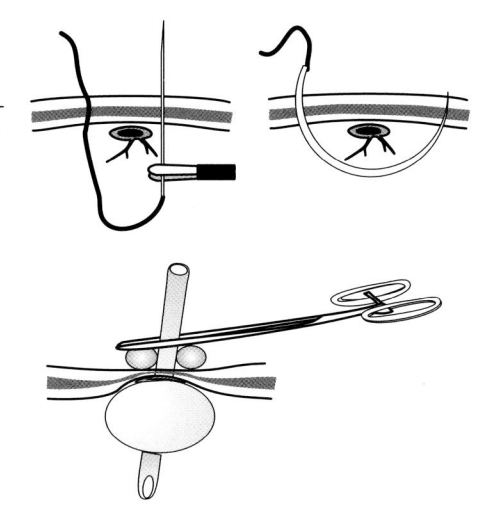

Hollow viscus perforations which are typically unrecognised at the time of operation, often present late with peritonitis, intra-abdominal abscess or cutaneous fistula [6]. Check for peri-cannulae bleeding before and after removal of cannulae. Abdominal wall bleed may be stopped by pressure from the cannula, a traction on the inflated balloon catheter through the cannula site, or a percutaneously inserted laparoscopically guided simple of square stitch (Fig. 10). Remove all instruments and secondary cannulae under vision, evacuate the pneumoperitoneum just before, or at removal of the last cannula. The fascial incisions of cannulae sites greater than 4 mm should be sutured with absorbable material. Local infiltration of the wounds with an appropriate dose of anaesthetic agents may provide adequate pain relief for a few hours post-operatively. Skin closure may be obtained using adhesive strips or sub-cutaneous fine absorbable sutures.

Fig. 11. The tip of all functioning instruments must be in view when entering the abdominal cavity and approaching, working and withdrawing from the operative field

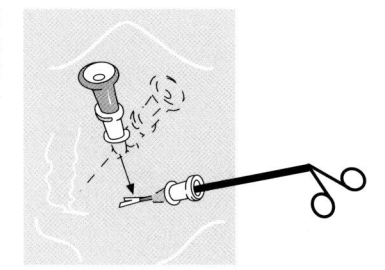

Manipulation and Dissection

Laparoscopic surgery is a combination of manipulation, retraction, sharp and blunt dissection, haemostasis and irrigation. As a rule, the tip of all instruments, particularly sharp ones, entering, moving or leaving the operative field, must be kept under vision (Fig. 11). Tissue planes and structures are exposed by careful manipulation. Access can be improved by gravity shift (change of position of the patient and/or operating table) and retraction. Sharp dissection is achieved by scissors, diathermy energy, harmonic scalpel or laser. Blunt dissection may be carried out by the tip of scissors and atraumatic grasping forceps as well as pledget swabs. Strands of tissues and minor adhesions can be disrupted by careful stripping manoeuvres using two atraumatic grasping forceps.

Electro-coagulation

Mono-polar coagulation or cutting current are used commonly, but bipolar coagulation is accepted as a safer option. This is because in the case of the monopolar diathermy, the interaction may take place anywhere in between the applied diathermy probe and the grounded pad. While in the case of the bipolar diathermy, the interaction is restricted to the small area of tissue between the two limbs of the applied forceps and the energy required is low (Fig. 12). With the monopolar system, coagulation is best achieved by grasping the vessel with a fine atraumatic and insulated forceps whilst the energy is delivered. Cutting is achieved by either touching or pulling using a fine probe (needle-curved or L-shaped) (Fig. 13). Alternatively, diathermy scissors may be used in which case the insulation sleeve of the scissors should be long enough to reach the blades in order to avoid thermal injury to the surrounding tissues (Fig. 14). Care must be taken not to injure other tissues by direct or indirect contact or capacitive coupling (Fig. 15). As a rule, power setting should be minimum, never activate before the contact with the tissue and never use a combination of metal cannula and plastic anchoring device, but instead use either all metal or all plastic. Immediately after prolonged use, the tip of the diathermy instrument remains hot and can easily burn tissue on contact.

3 Basic Technique

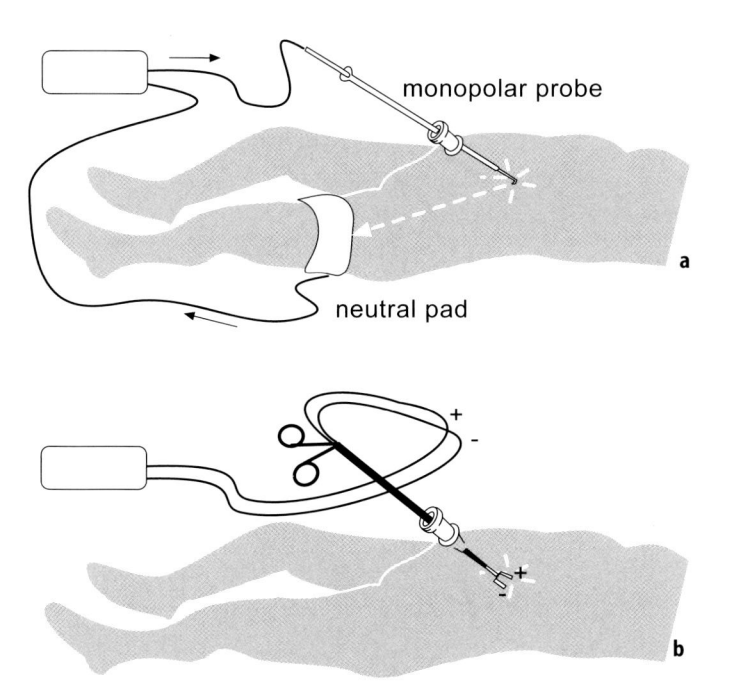

Fig. 12a,b. Principle of diathermy surgery. **a** Unipolar current applied to the tissue, travels through the body and returns to the generator via the neutral pad. **b** Bipolar current is restricted to the area between the two limbs of the applied forceps

Fig. 13a–c. Cutting with the unipolar probe. **a** Touch with needle. **b** Touch with hook. **c** Pull with hook

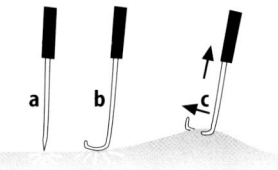

Fig. 14a,b. Diathermy scissors. **a** Note thermal injury from the non-insulated section of the instrument above the blades. **b** Insulation sleeve down to the blades gives better protection

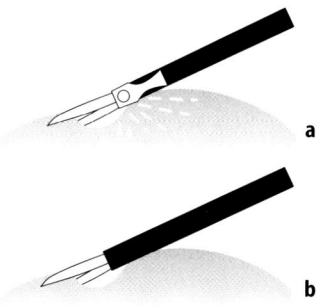

Fig. 15a–c. Diathermy injury. **a** direct contact from the tip of an active instrument or a failed insulation. **b** Indirect injury via another conductive instrument such as an un-insulated instrument or a metal cannula. **c** Capacitive coupling injury. Stray current may travel from an active instrument to un-insulated telescope or instrument, or a metal cannula anchored by a plastic anchoring device

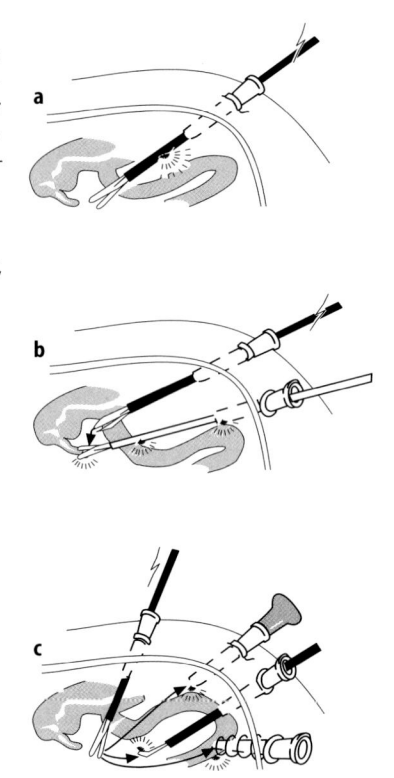

Laser

In the hands of experienced surgeons, laser energy offers safe and effective surgical cutting, coagulation and vaporization properties. CO_2, argon, KTP and YAG lasers may be used for endoscopic surgery. The use of laser has not received wide acceptance because electro-coagulation provides a safe, effective and economical cutting and coagulation modality for laparoscopic surgery.

High-Energy Ultrasound

The ultrasound activated scalpel/shears has recently been developed for use in laparoscopic surgery (Fig. 16). Its energy is delivered as 55 kHz vibration and the mechanism for coagulation is similar to that of diathermy and laser [7]. The scalpel produces cutting and coagulation by its sharp edge and flat side respectively. The shears have two blades which provide cutting and coagulation properties (coagulation of vessels less than 2 mm in diameter) [8]. This system produces a slight mist and its processes of cutting and coagulation are slower than electro-coagulation and laser. However, it has the advantages of being

Fig. 16a,b. High-energy ultrasound. **a** Scalpel. **b** Shear

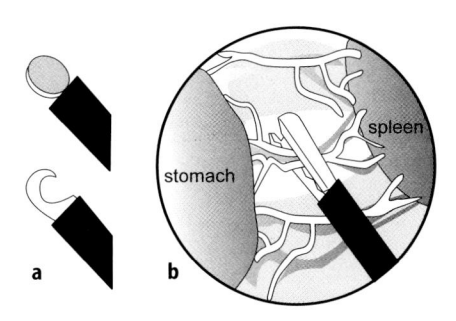

smokeless and produces no direct tissue injury beyond the point of contact. However, high energy ultrasound can cause cavitational injury along the tissue planes.

Haemostasis

During laparoscopic surgery bleeding has been the most common cause of conversion to open surgery. Therefore prevention of haemorrhage, by careful manipulation and dissection, and appropriate application of cutting and coagulation energy should remain one of the most important principles in laparoscopic surgery.

Small vessels should be coagulated by diathermy, laser or high-energy ultrasound. Large vessels are clipped, ligated or stapled. It is worth pointing out that at laparoscopy minor haemorrhage often appears major because of the magnification. Blood absorbs light and the laparoscopic viewing becomes poor. A suction irrigation system should always be available for use, and clots can be difficult to aspirate via 3–5 mm suction probes.

Suction Irrigation

A saline drip stand and conventional suction unit connected to a two-way single lumen probe which has an easy to operate hand unit, is a simple and effective way to achieve suction and irrigation during laparoscopic surgery (Fig. 17). If desired, antibiotics/antiseptics or even heparin and anaesthetic agents may be mixed with the irrigation fluid. Often omentum, mesentery and intestinal wall are sucked onto the suction probe. Care must be taken to release the attached tissues before the suction probe is withdrawn into the cannula. This may be achieved by switching off the suction, transient switch on the irrigation and a gentile manipulation of the trapped tissue. In general use a low, but adequate, suction power and to avoid rapid loss of pneumoperitoneum, keep the probe below the level of fluid to be aspirated.

Fig. 17. Saline stand irrigation and conventional suction apparatus for laparoscopic use. Keep the tip of the probe below the surface of the fluid

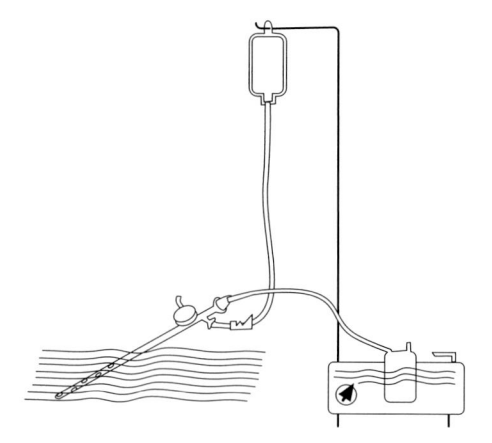

Fig. 18a,b. The application of external knotting. **a** Suture introducer, suture and Roeder Knot in place; *arrows*, direction of suture introduction. **b** Knot is delivered by a knot pusher and an instrument is placed within the loop to minimise risk of serration injury; *arrows*, direction of force

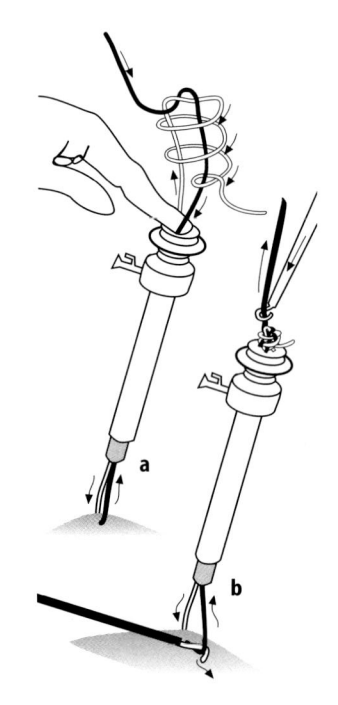

Knotting

Proper knotting is essential in laparoscopic ligation and suturing. External one way slip knots, 'Roeder', or surgeon's knots, 'Reef', are less popular than the internal knot. To tie an external knot, a suture applicator and a knot pusher are required (Fig. 18). The disadvantages of external knotting are:

Fig. 19a,b. A pre-tied loop of suture ligature. **a** The device with a suture introducer. **b** The loop in position

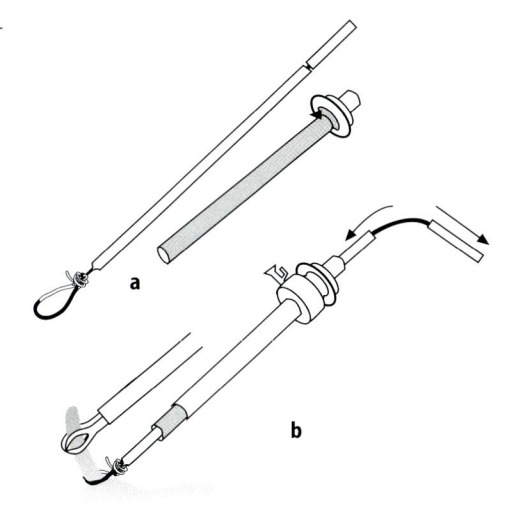

- More cumbersome to perform than internal knotting
- Unsuitable for continuous suturing
- Has the potential to damage tissue by serration
- Unreliable with certain suture materials

Catgut and, to a lesser extent, silk are the best suture materials to use for this knot. A commercially available pre-tied loop of suture material with a push-rod and introducer can be used as a single ligature around most vascular pedicles and tubular structures (Fig. 19).

For a beginner, internal knotting is one of the most difficult tasks to perform in laparoscopic surgery. With practice, however, the internal knotting can be executed easily, effectively and quickly (Fig. 20). The technique suits most suture materials and all purposes. Care must be taken not to weaken the suture by rough handling, and until experience is acquired, use a short length of suture for each individual ligature/suture.

Suturing

Laparoscopic suturing requires considerable practice and its principle is similar to that of open surgery. Straight, ski or curved needles may be used. However, the size of the curved needle to be used in laparoscopy is dictated by the diameter of the available access working cannula (10 mm or more). If desired, an ordinary curved needle may be straightened or made into a ski shape. The technique requires a needle holder to introduce the needle/suture materials and a second needle holder or curved atraumatic grasping forceps to assist. It is important

Fig. 20. Internal knotting. *1, 2,* Positioning the suture; *3, 4,* first component double throw; *5,* repositioning the ends; *6, 7,* second component single throw; *8,* re-positioning; *9,* third component single throw

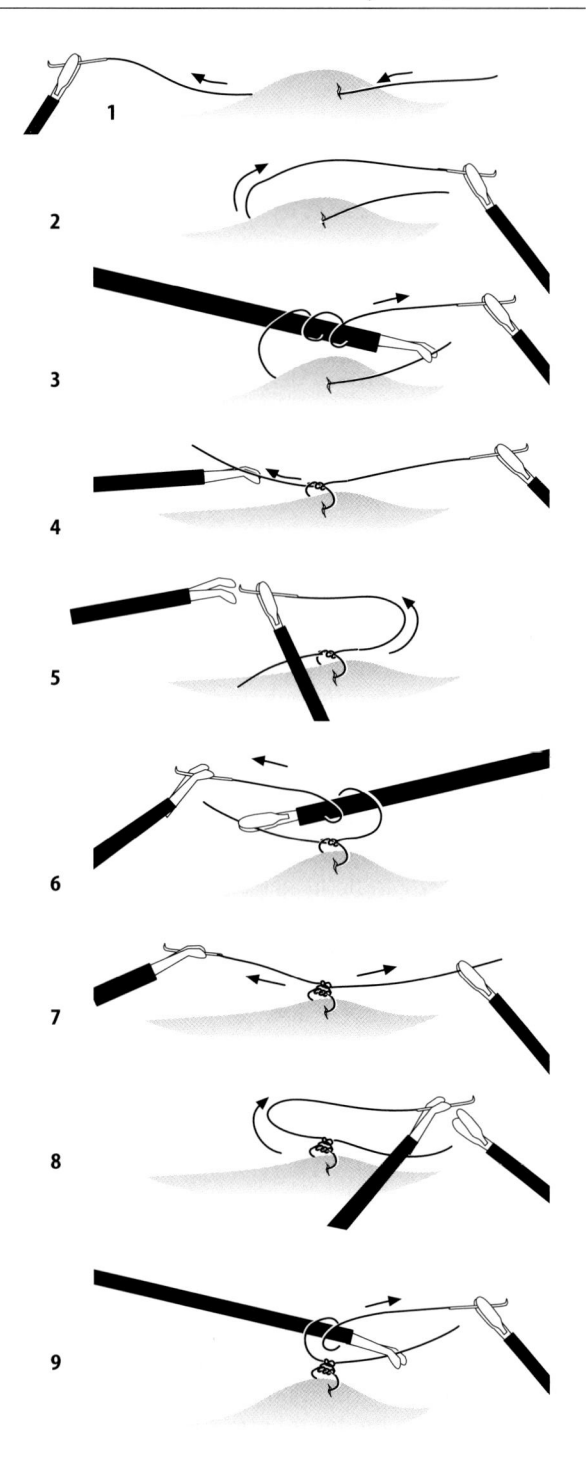

3 Basic Technique

Fig. 21a,b. Hinges of the needle holder or grasping forceps used for suturing. **a** Smooth hinge. **b** Troublesome hinge prevents the suture from a smooth glide

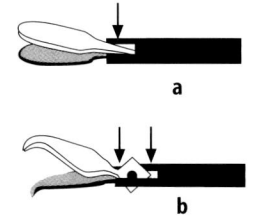

Fig. 22a–c. Introducing the needle/suture into the abdominal cavity. **a** Holding the needle – ski or curved. **b** Holding the suture attached to the needle. **c** Needle passed percutaneously into the peritoneal cavity

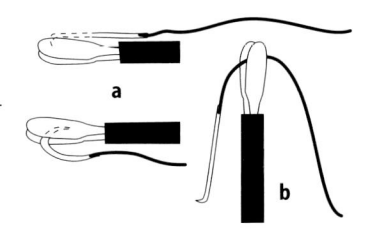

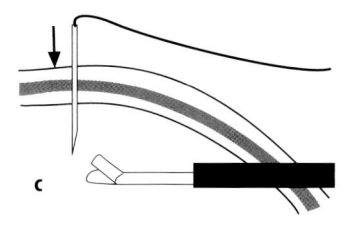

Fig. 23. Continuous suturing. A grasping forceps align tissues. A rubber-shod grasper keeps tension on the suture line without damaging the material

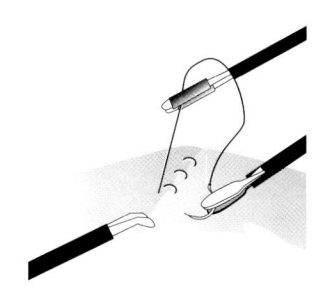

that both instruments have boxed-in hinges to allow a smooth glide over the instrument and prevent tangling at the hinge (Fig. 21).

First prepare and align the tissue; then introduce the suture by grasping either the needle in the line of the needle holder or the suture near the needle. In difficult or special circumstances, as in formation of a gastrostomy, a straight needle/suture may be passed percutaneously into the peritoneal cavity (Fig. 22). The second instrument is used to assist in introducing the suture and knotting. Care must be taken not to grasp the suture material hard thereby weakening the material. Also, an intra-corporeal needle can cause visceral, diaphragmatic or even pericardial injuries. Therefore keep the tip of the needle in laparoscopic view at all times, if possible, and care must be exercised in handling needles intracorporeally. During continuous suturing, a rubber shod grasper through a third cannula is advisable to maintain tension and stabilise the suture (Fig. 23).

Clips and Staples

The application of a metal or absorbable ligature clip is simple and effective to completely occlude small and medium-sized vessels and other ductal structures. It is important that the clip applier approaches the target structure at an angle that allows the surgeon to view the clip as it passes across the structure to be ligated, to ensure safe application and to confirm that no other tissue is trapped within the jaws of the applier. It is advisable to use two clips on the proximal side of structures. Absorbable self-locking clips are less reliable than metal because of their delicate hinge structure. Metal clips are likely to interfere with radiographic and magnetic imaging. Adequately prepare the structure to be clipped and hold it by an atraumatic grasping forceps. The loaded applier is then inserted in full laparoscopic view and placed across the structure. Gently rotate the shaft of the applier to ensure safe and correct positioning of the clip before the handles of the applier are gently squeezed. Before the grip on the handles is relaxed, move the grasping forceps and reposition to prepare for the application of the second clip (Fig. 24).

A linear stapler device with a rotatable shaft delivers four or six rows of metal staples and with a knife cuts the tissue in the middle. This device allows safe and secure occlusion and division of vascular pedicles and hollow organs such as the intestinal tract (Fig. 25).

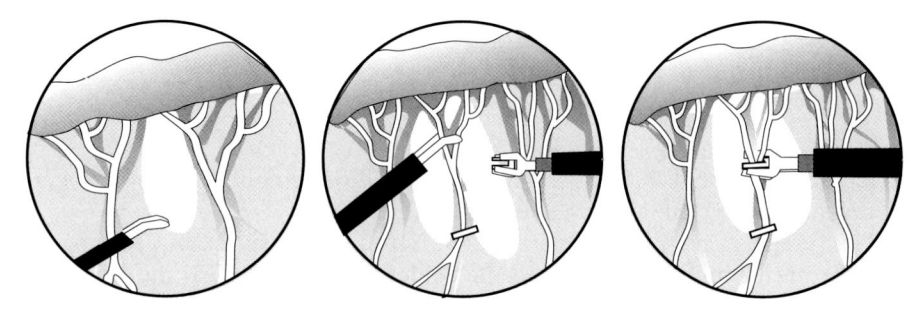

Fig. 24. The application of the clip. The tissue is prepared, the applicator inserted, and the jaws/clip placed across the structure while a grasping forceps holds the tissue

Fig. 25. Linear stapler

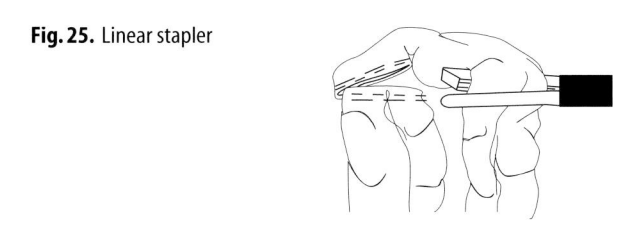

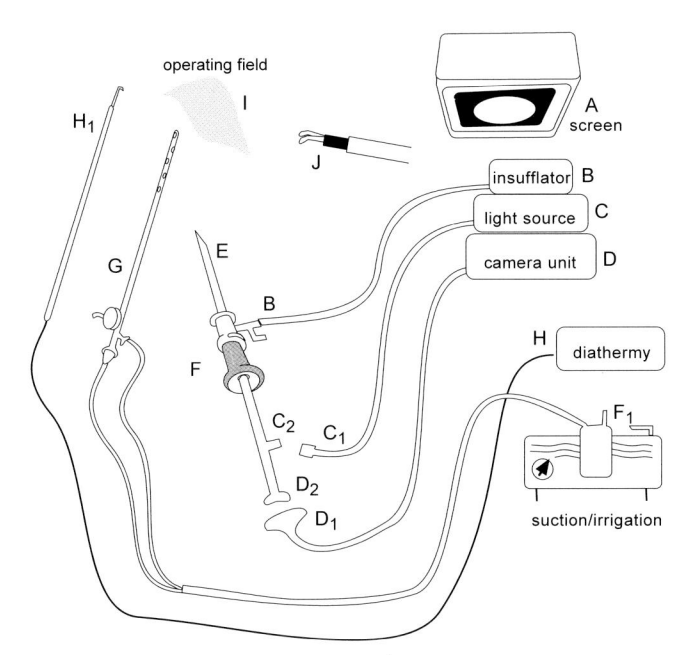

Fig. 26. Imaging problems. *A*, Screen connected and set properly; *B*, cold gas blow at the telescope cause fogging – change to another cannula if possible; *C*, light source set appropriately and connected to the cable; *C1*, cable is not broken, *C2*, interface between light cable and telescope is clean, dry and connected properly; *D*, camera unit is set and connected properly; *D1*, focus/zoom are set; *D2*, interface between camera and telescope is clean, dry and connected properly; *E*, telescope is not broken, is clean, warm and properly connected; *F*, losing pneumoperitoneum from leaking cannula; *F1*, powerful suction; *G*, irrigation fluid not splashing onto the telescope; *H*, diathermy unit is set to a minimum required power, corrected properly, and both the electricity plug and diathermy lead are not close to the camera plug/lead – these may cause interference on screen; *H1*, coagulation may cause interference on screen and snowstorm from debris and smoke – evacuate pneumoperitoneum intermittently; *I*, appropriate space (pneumoperitoneum and retraction) is necessary for laparoscopic viewing and blood absorbs light – consequently the images become dark; *J*, smooth and shiny metal (instrument/cannulae) cause light reflection which affects the camera function (iris)

Imaging Problems

High-quality imaging is critical in laparoscopy. Problems with imaging are a common occurrence and can happen at any time during the procedure. They can be dangerous, time-consuming and very frustrating. Poor imaging, total blackout and interference on screen can be caused by faulty equipment and/or connections. To minimize interference, place the diathermy cable, generator and the socket away from that of the camera system. Glare occurs as the result of disturbed balance light intensity by the camera. Dark images are usually due to low light intensity secondary to either low light output or camera reaction to high reflection of light from polished metal instruments. Blood in the peritoneal cavity absorbs light, thereby reducing the amount of reflected light which results in dark images. Blurred or 'poor' imaging is usually due to inadequate focusing of camera, light imbalance, mismatch between camera/light source and telescope, loose connections, moisture and debris at the interfaces (cables-camera-telescope) or telescope tip contaminated with peritoneal fluid and blood distort imaging. A quick wipe or rinse inside or outside the peritoneal cavity should restore proper imaging. Fogging is often due to a cold telescope and/or cold CO_2 blowing at the telescope from its cannula. Keep the telescope warm before use or use anti-fogging solutions, and change the port of gas entry from the telescope cannula to another if possible. Smoke and debris occur as the result of intraperitoneal tissue coagulation and intermittent desufflation via cannula valves clears the space (Fig. 26).

References

1. Hasson HM (1971) A modified instrument and method for laparoscopy. Am J Obstet Gynecol 110:886–887
2. Humphrey GME, Najmaldin A (1994) Modification of the hasson technique in paediatric laparoscopy. Br J Surg 81:1320–1323
3. Mouret PH (1990) La chirurgie coelioscopique. Chirurgie 116:829–833
4. Valla JS et al (1991) Laparoscopic appendicectomy in children: report of 465 cases. Surg Laparosc Endosc 1:166–172
5. Champault G, Cazacu F (1995) Chirurgie par laparoscopie: les accidents graves des trocarts. J Chir (Paris) 132(3):109–113
6. Wolfe BM et al (1991) Endoscopic cholecystectomy: an analysis of complications. Arch Surg 126:1192–1198
7. Amaral JF (1994) Experimental development of an ultrasonically activated scalpel for laparoscopic use. Surg Lap Endosc 4:92–97
8. Fowler (1994) Use of ultrasonically activated shears in laparoscopic colectomy. Chir Int 11–12:10–11

Ergonomics of Task Performance in Endoscopic Surgery

G.B. Hanna, C. Kimber, A. Cuschieri

Introduction

Ergonomics is the scientific study of people at work, in terms of workplace layout, equipment design, the work environment, safety, productivity and training. Ergonomics is based on multiple disciplines such as anatomy, physiology, psychology and engineering combined in a systems approach. The ergonomic approach has been used in industry and the military to improve the safety and productivity of the work environment. By contrast, in surgical practice, morbidity and mortality are used as an index of safety, but this approach does not address adequately the causation of surgical complications or the measures that increase efficient delivery of surgical care.

During the past decade there has been widespread use of endoscopic surgical techniques in almost all surgical specialties, and the laparoscopic approach has become the gold-standard management of many surgical disorders. Both industry and surgeons have responded positively to the new endoscopic era. The medical technology industry has developed and marketed a whole range of new endoscopic instrumentation and video equipment. On their part, surgeons have developed or modified existing techniques and, more recently, instituted measures to audit the benefit, safety and impact of the new endoscopic surgical management. This rapid advancement of endoscopic surgery has encountered and still faces some problems. Most of the endoscopic equipment and instruments in current usage are adaptations from other areas of technology and from open surgery without adequate considerations to the demands of laparoscopic techniques. The ergonomic layout of the current operating theatres, designed for conventional open practice, is not ideal for the needs of endoscopic surgery where a variety of high technology ancillary devices are necessary for the conduct of endoscopic interventions. Despite the increasing complexity of these technologies used in the operating theatre ergonomic progress and design has lacked behind these developments. Only a few surgeons maintain interest in recent advances in medical technology and in ergonomic studies.

Constraints in endoscopic surgery

In endoscopic surgery the surgeon utilises a limited access to approach the operative field. Instruments and endoscopes are passed into the body cavity via cannulae which are inserted through the body wall to provide narrow channels of fixed positions but of variable directions. This minimal access approach creates a set of mechanical and visual restrictions on the execution of surgical tasks. Some of these are considered below.

Mechanical Restrictions

These are the restrictions encountered on handling the tissues by endoscopic instruments:
- Limited number of degrees of freedom (DOF)
- Diminished tactile feedback
- Small and long endoscopic instruments
- Problems of tissue retrieval

Standard endoscopic instruments have four DOF. A degree of freedom is the potential for movement in a single independent direction, or a rotation around one axis. The surgeon can move the endoscopic instrument in and out along the Z axis, rotate the instrument in the line of Z axis, move it from side to side pivoted on a point on the Y axis and move it up and down about the X axis. By contrast, the body-limb-fingertips movements in open surgery have more than 36 DOFs. There are six DOFs for the position of the trunk, three rotations at the shoulder, one at the elbow, one in the forearm and two at the wrist. There is also a complex mobility from several types of protraction and retraction by the precision grip of the hand, as well as rotation of instruments within the fingertips. These probably constitute two DOFs at each of the five metacarpophalangeal joints and one DOF for each of the nine interphalangeal joints giving a total of 19 for the hand and a total of 32 DOFs at the finger tips (Patkin and Isabel 1995). The limited number of DOFs of endoscopic instruments makes handling of tissues in endoscopic procedures more difficult than during conventional open surgery.

In endoscopic surgery direct tactile feedback (hand to tissue) is lost, and the indirect tactile feedback (through the instrument) is markedly diminished due to the length of endoscopic instruments and the friction between the instruments and the ports. This degrades the ability of the surgeon to identify the nature of component tissues and tissue planes. It also can lead to tissue damage from excessive instrument grip, poorly appreciated, by the surgeon.

The small size of endoscopic ports dictates the size of endoscopic instruments. This causes several difficulties in the design of endoscopic instruments to perform the same function as their open counterparts. Long thin instruments have a poor mechanical advantage. The narrow end of instruments may cause tissue damage either accidentally if the instruments are not moved under direct endoscopic vision or during gripping the tissues with the small jaws. The length of endoscopic instruments exaggerates hand tremors especially in a magnified endoscopic field.

Another intrinsic problem in endoscopic surgery is tissue retrieval after detachment from adjacent tissues. This problem has two aspects: (a) the tissue must be reduced to the size of access wounds with preservation of tissue architecture, and (b) the risk of contamination including spillage of cancer cells must be eliminated.

Visual Limitations

The use of image display system as the visual interface between the surgeon and the operative field has several visual limitations compared to conventional open surgery, including:
- Loss of normal binocular vision
- Decoupling of motor and sensory spaces (monitor location)
- Reduced size of endoscopic field of view
- Disturbed endoscope-instrument-tissue relationship (port location)
- Magnification of the operative field
- Limitations of the quality of endoscopic image

These limitations of current image display systems are responsible for the degraded task performance in endoscopic surgery compared to direct normal vision (Crosthwaite et al. 1995; Tendick et al. 1993).

Standard monitors in current use in surgical practice are two-dimensional (2-D) imaging systems. They present only 2-D depth (pictorial) cues of the operative field to the surgeon. On the other hand, there are several depth cues presented to the observer by direct binocular vision:
- Pictorial cues
  - Linear perception
  - Interposition
  - Height in the plane
  - Light and shadow
  - Relative size
  - Familial size
  - Arial perspective
  - Proximity-luminance covariance
  - Texture gradients
- Kinetic cues
  - Motion parallax
  - Kinetic depth effect
- Physiological cues
  - Convergence
  - Accommodation
- Retinal disparity

For controlled endoscopic manipulations, the surgeon must reconstruct a 3-D picture from a 2-D image. This entails intense perceptual and mental processing which must be sustained by the surgeon throughout the operation.

The current ergonomic layout of operating theatres with crowding of free-standing equipment often precludes optimal placement of the viewing monitor in front of the surgeon who usually operates from one or other side of the patient. In consequence the visual axis between the surgeon's eyes and the monitor is no longer aligned with the hands and instruments. Furthermore, the monitor is often far removed from the surgeon and thus the spatial location of the display system (sensory information) is remote from the manipulation area at the hand level of the operator (motor space). These factors degrade task performance in endoscopic surgery.

Reduced field of endoscopic vision compared to ordinary unrestricted sight results in a decrease in the sensory input from the periphery of the operative field. The viewing angle of the endoscope refers to the angle formed by the two outer visual limits and determines the diameter of the field of view and the size of the objects seen. The field of view describes the area inspected by the objective of the endoscope (Berci 1976). At a given distance from the objective lens, the larger the field of view, the greater is the area that can be observed. Restricted field of endoscopic vision accounts for the incidental tissue injury when instruments move outside the field of view.

The position of the instrument ports in relation to each other and to the optical port is an important determinant of the ease of performance of an endoscopic procedure and its execution time. For bimanual tasks, manipulation, azimuth and elevation angles govern optimal port sites (Fig. 1). The manipulation angle is the angle between the active and assisting instruments, while the azimuth angle describes the angle between either instrument and the optical axis of the endoscope. The elevation angle of the instrument is defined as the angle between the instrument and the horizontal plane. These angles determine optimal port location.

As the linear magnification of an endoscope is inversely proportional to the object distance, a better resolution (smallest detail that can be resolved) is obtained when the object viewed is closer to the distal end of the endoscope (Hopkins 1976). The specification of an endoscope should include a statement of the magnification obtained for a stated object distance. On the other hand, magnification increases the apparent speed of movement and the operator must adjust the speed of movement of the manipulations to the degree of magnification.

There are three major components that determine the quality of the image: resolution, luminance and chroma (Satava et al. 1988). Resolution determines the clarity of the image; luminance measures the amount of light available in the image signal and the chroma represents the intensity or saturation of the colour. In addition to the quality of the monitor, the final image produced by the endoscopic system depends on the optical characteristics of the endoscope and quality of the camera.

Fig. 1. Angles govern port placement. *1*, Manipulation angle; *2*, azimuth angle; *3*, elevation angle

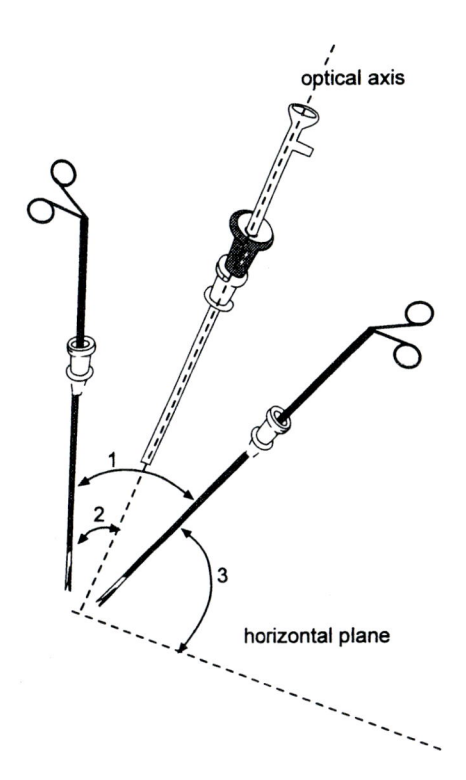

Ergonomics of the Set-Up in Endoscopic Surgery

For a particular operation the surgeon must select the appropriate endoscope and place the ports and the monitor in optimum location. The principles of the set-up of endoscopic equipment are:
- Endoscope selection
  - Optical axis-target view angle (OATV) of 90°
  - Visual field changes on rotating forward oblique endoscopes
  - Endoscopes of different directions of view have no significant effect on task performance with the same OATV angle
- Port placement
  - Manipulation angle 60°
  - Equal azimuth angles
  - Narrow manipulation angle necessitate narrow elevation angle
- Monitor location
  - In front of the surgeon
  - At the level of manipulation work space

There are some special considerations that relate to paediatric surgery since the patient's size and physiology markedly varies from standard adult surgery.

The operative work space is significantly reduced in children due to their small abdominal cavity and the minimal distension created by low pressure pneumoperitoneum. In addition, particularly in neonates, the liver is relatively larger, and the abdomen is greater transversely than it is lengthwise. Further difficulties occur in kypho-scoliotic patients, particularly those undergoing fundoplication. The equipment set-up should be discussed with the anaesthetist as the endoscopic instruments often compromises the access to the child.

Endoscope Selection

Direction of view of the endoscope describes the angle between the centre of the visual field (optical axis) and the physical axis of the endoscope. Endoscopes can be of forward viewing (0°) or forward oblique direction of view (30°, 45°). The angle between the optical axis of the endoscope and the plane of the target is referred to as the optical axis-to-target view angle (OATV) (Fig. 2).

The best task performance during endoscopic work is obtained with an OATV angle of 90° and relatively small decreases in this viewing angle are attended by a significant degradation of task performance. The error rate increases from 17% with an OATV angle of 90° to 79% with 45° angle. In addition a significant increase in the execution time and the force applied on the target with the decrease in the OATV angle were observed in this study (Hanna and Cuschieri 1998).

Endoscopes of different directions of view have no significant effect on the execution time or the quality of task performance when the optical axis of the endoscope subtends the same OATV angle (Hanna et al. 1997a). In practice, however, only oblique viewing endoscopes or ones with flexible tips (chip on stick technology) can achieve an adequate OATV angle approximating 90°. For this reason forward-oblique endoscopes are preferable despite the easier deploy-

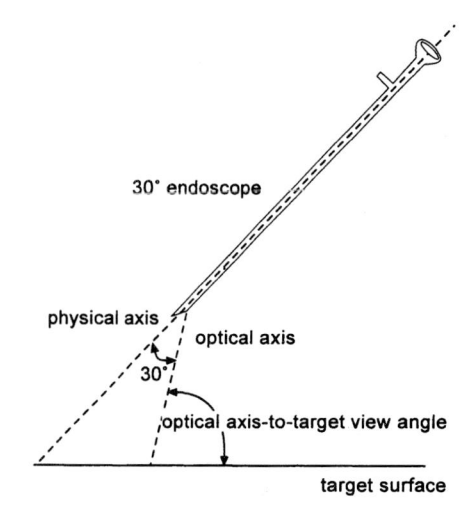

Fig. 2. Direction of view on the endoscope and target-to-endoscope distance

ment of forward viewing types. In addition, the visual field changes when the forward oblique endoscope is rotated; whereas the operative field of forward-viewing endoscope is unaltered. Different perspectives can be obtained by rotation of the forward-oblique endoscopes which provide more visual information for the execution of advanced laparoscopic procedures.

There are two factors which determine optimum OATV angle: the location of the optical port in relation to the centre of the operative field and the direction of view of the endoscope. Variations in the build of patients necessitate a careful selection of the location of the optical port in the individual patient to obtain both an optimum OATV angle and the correct target-to-endoscope distance for a specific endoscopic operation. The endoscope should be selected to obtain an OATV angle approximating 90°.

To achieve the optimal balance between light availability and endoscope diameter, 4-mm endoscopes are recommended for general paediatric use while 2.9-mm endoscopes are useful for neonatal and fetal applications. Several miniscopes (1.9 mm or less diameter) are currently being marketed for paediatric usage. The current generations of miniscopes have inadequate optical resolution for advanced procedures and the available light is easily absorbed with bleeding. In addition, these miniscopes have a small field of vision, peripheral distortion and limited focal length.

Port Placement

The maximal efficiency and quality performance of intracorporeal knotting are obtained with a manipulation angle ranging between 45° and 75° with the ideal angle being 60°. Manipulation angles below 45° or above 75° are accompanied by increased difficulty and degraded performance. Therefore on placing the operating ports for the active and assisting instruments, for example, needle drivers, these should subtend a manipulation angle within the 45°–75° range and as close to 60° as possible. A better task efficiency is also achieved with an equal than wide unequal azimuth angles on either side of the optical port. In practice, equal azimuth angles may be difficult to achieve, but wide azimuth inequality should be avoided since this degrades task efficiency irrespective of the side, right or left, of the azimuth angle predominance. When a 30° manipulation angle is imposed by the anatomy or build of the patient, the elevation angle should be also 30° as this combination carries the shortest execution and an acceptable knot quality score. Likewise with a 60° manipulation angle, the corresponding optimal elevation angle which yields the shortest execution time and optimal quality performance is 60°. Thus within the range of angles that ensure adequate task efficiency, a good rule of thumb is that the elevation angle should be equal to the manipulation angle (Hanna et al. 1997b).

On planning port location an adequate intracorporeal instrument length should be obtained. This depends on the size of the patient and the site of the operation. The intra- to extra-corporeal shaft ratio for optimal task performance is 2:1. Consequently instruments designed for adult surgery are not suitable to paediatric procedures.

Trocar length should generally be less than 6 cm. For operations that do not involve significant tissue extraction a trocar diameter of less than 5 mm is adequate. To prevent trocars advancing into the abdominal cavity and crowding the operative field they should be sutured and externally wrapped with adhesive tape. Radially expanding trocars are currently available; they are inserted via a Veress needle, and the polymer can be stretched to 12 mm with dilators. Recent developments have enabled reduction in instrument diameter to less than 3 mm without significant shaft bowing. These smaller instruments tend to tear tissues and thus the recommended diameter is 3.5 mm.

Monitor Location

The best task performance is obtained with the monitor located in front of the operator at the level of the manipulation work space (hands), permitting 'gaze-down viewing' and alignment of the visual and motor axis (Hanna et al. 1998). Gaze-down viewing by the endoscopic operator allows both sensory signals and motor control to have a close spatial location and thus bring the visual signals in correspondence with instrument manipulations, similar to the situation encountered during conventional open surgery. In practice, the location of the monitor is determined by the site of the operation. For advanced upper abdominal procedures, such as fundoplication, the child is placed in a frog-leg position with the surgeon standing between the patients knees looking at the monitor above the patient's head. During appendectomy the monitor is located over the right iliac fossa and the surgeon stands on the left side near the patient's hypochondrium.

To obtain the optimum monitor location, alterations in the design of the operating room and operating table are necessary to improve the ergonomic layout. In addition, technology which projects the image onto the manipulation work space is needed. This could be achieved by head-up display systems which project the image on collimating glass although these systems are known to cause eye accommodation problems (Edgar et al. 1994). The best technical solution would project the image back on top of the patient above but close to the 'real operative field'. The surgeon would then be looking down at the organs and instruments in the operative field much as in open surgery as if there was no intervening abdominal wall. Such a system of 'suspended imaging', still in its prototype stage, is being developed. The suspended image display technology utilises precision retro-reflector and advanced beam splitting technology for projecting an image in space (Holden et al. 1997). In the absence of these developments in image display technology, the use of flat television screens may allow better placement of the monitor in close proximity to the operative field.

Modality of the Imaging System

Over the past 5 years 3-D imaging systems have been introduced to improve depth perception during endoscopic surgery. The vast majority are based on rapid sequential imaging, alternating between the two eyes by means of optical shutters (active or passive) thus presenting two slightly different images in an alternating sequence to each of the two eyes separated by a few ms. Image fusion for 'stereopsis' is made from the *after image* in one retina (shutter closed) with *current image* in the other retina (shutter open). This is, of course, quite different from normal stereoscopic vision which requires co-instantaneous images on each retina with the image falling on different sectors of the two retinas (retinal disparity), eyeball convergence, accommodation and input from the vestibular system.

These 'quasi 3-D' systems have a major disadvantage: significant reduction in light transmitted through the optical shutters to the retina, so that the image is distinctly darker and the colour is degraded (von Pichler et al. 1996a). Nonetheless, a number of reports and reviews have suggested that these 3-D systems improve task efficiency in endoscopic manipulations (Satava 1993; Becker et al. 1993; Pietrabissa et al. 1994; von Pichleret 1996a,b; von Pichler et al. 1996b) while others did not find any superiority of the 3-D systems over 2-D systems (Chan et al. 1997). No significant difference in intracorporeal knot tying (Crosthwaite et al. 1995), endoscopic bowel suturing (Hanna and Cuschieri 1997) or the performance of laparoscopic cholecystectomy in a randomised controlled trial (Hanna et al. 1997c) between 3-D and 2-D imaging systems has been found.

There are several limitations of the current 3-D video-endoscopic systems which are not, strictly speaking, real stereoscopic displays. The 3-D display does not reconstruct the scene's pattern of light rays in three-dimensional space, and hence does not present vertical, longitudinal and horizontal parallax as the observer's viewpoint changes. If the surgeon's head moves, the two retinal images do not transform as they normally would in direct viewing of the operative field (Merritt 1987). Furthermore, the current 3-D video-endoscopic systems have a single disparity which yields different magnitudes of depth depending on the viewing distance, in contrast to the human visual system which perceptually rescales disparity information for different distances to produce valid depth, a process called stereoscopic depth constancy (Coren and Ward 1989). The depth perceived by the current 3-D systems is valid if it corresponds to the predicted depth by geometry (Cormack and Fox 1985). As a result there is a limited operational distance such that a 3-D effect is obtained but outside this range, the surgeon operates from non-valid depth information. In addition, flatness (or anticues) emanating from the monitor frame and surface reflections degrade depth perception (Yeh and Silverstein 1991).

The use of optical shuttering glasses results in a substance loss of photons transmitted to each retina causing significant degradation of the sensory input especially with respect to brightness and colour (von Pichler et al. 1996a). Therefore 2-D imaging has better sharpness and contrast than a 3-D system. Visual strain on using 3-D systems may result from a decoupled relationship between accommodation and vergence and from inter-ocular cross-talk between the two eye-views (Yeh and Silverstein 1991). Accommodation tends to remain at the screen distance while vergence follows the induced retinal disparity and thus visual strain results from the sustained force vergence effort during prolonged viewing (Tyrrell and Leibowitz 1990). The visual strain and headache may account for the surgical fatigue syndrome during endoscopic operations.

Surgeon-Instrument Interface

The use of laparoscopic instruments results in greater forearm discomfort, possibly due to the need for increased forearm flexor muscle contractions compared to conventional surgical instruments (Berguer et al. 1997a). The handling of the current generation of laparoscopic instruments during grasping motions entails flexion and ulnar deviation of the wrist which decrease maximum grip force. The handle configuration of laparoscopic instruments also requires the operator to use the opposing muscles of the thenar and hypothenar compartments for gripping rather than the more powerful grasping grip that uses the deep forearm flexors. Some reports have documented thumb paraesthesia in surgeons during laparoscopic procedures (Kano et al. 1993; Majeed et al. 1993). Furthermore, surgeons exhibit decreased mobility of the head and neck and less anteroposterior weight shifting during laparoscopic manipulations despite a more upright posture. This more restricted posture during laparoscopic surgery may induce fatigue by limiting the natural changes in body posture that occur during open surgery (Berguer et al. 1997b). Also, operating from the side of the patient results in muscle fatigue in the shoulder region.

In addition to physical fatigue, laparoscopic surgery requires more mental concentration than open surgery. The surgeon must reconstruct a 3-D picture from a 2-D image and to perform the task under several mechanical and visual restrictions. The physical, mental and visual demands of endoscopic manipulations may be responsible for surgical fatigue syndrome encountered in endoscopic surgery (Cuschieri 1995). After a variable but finite time, the surgical fatigue syndrome sets in, manifested by mental exhaustion, increased irritability, impaired surgical judgement and reduced the level of psychomotor performance.

The human-instrument interface creates a set of demands to ensure safety and efficiency of the surgical system. The influence of the surgeon-instrument relationship on muscle fatigue and joint position is currently the subject of several studies to investigate the optimum conditions for the surgeon in relation to the patient and instruments. This research is also essential to develop new generations of instruments designed to fulfil the requirements of endoscopic surgery.

Safety Considerations

Safety aspects in endoscopic surgery should include (a) control measures to regulate the introduction of new equipment into clinical practice and (b) sound principles of handling the tissues during laparoscopic procedures. It is crucial to control the rate of diffusion of new technologies into surgical practice according to the evidence related to their safety and benefits. In this respect, the Advisory Council on Science and Technology in the United Kingdom has the following recommendations:

- All new medical devices or novel applications/treatments used within the National Health Service (NHS) should be developed under controlled conditions.
- Only procedures and equipment that have been subjected to assessment and approval should be used within NHS.
- Novel surgical procedures and surgical teams practising them should be registered with a committee on the safety and efficacy of procedures.
- The NHS should adopt codes of agreed practice in deciding the most cost-effective way of introducing novel devices, applications and treatment.
- Specific centres specialising in appropriate diseases and techniques should be resourced to develop, evaluate and educate the rest of the profession.

New equipment should be the subject of ergonomic studies to evaluate the effect of such technology on task performance. There will be always a room for personal preference, but basic safety requirement is essential. Instrument design must be as "fail-safe" as possible, i.e. when the surgeon fails to use the instrument correctly it should remain in a safe, non-injurious state.

Basic endoscopic training should aim at teaching the principles required for safe surgical practice rather than the techniques of different procedures. Acquisition of skills required for generic tasks should be an essential part of training in endoscopic surgery. Accurate movements of instruments under direct endoscopic vision prevent incidental tissue injury. Controlled endoscopic manipulations require hand-to-eye coordination, two hand coordination, visuo-spatial ability, aiming ability and steadiness of the hand in a magnified field. In addition to the development of psychomotor skills, surgeons should be aware of the hazards of surgical equipment. For instance, the temperature at the end of fibreoptic light cables may reach 240°C which is enough to ignite surgical drapes or cause skin burns (Hensman et al. 1998). Finally, surgeons should be acquainted with the physics governing the function of ancillary equipment/devices used in endoscopic surgery, and this aspect should form an integral part of the surgical training programme.

Ergonomic Approach To Evaluate Surgical Techniques

Traditionally surgery uses morbidity and mortality to evaluate different surgical techniques. However, morbidity data do not provide a prescriptive method for specifying how the performance of a procedure can be improved. This requires a detailed study of the causation of complications. Analysis of the mechanisms underlying surgical complications necessitates the identification of *errors* enacted during surgical procedures. The consequences of any error are dependent on circumstances present at the time, as the same error could have a range of different consequences. For example, if a surgeon was to allow the electrosurgical hook knife to jump (follow-through effect) once it has cut through a tissue plane, the consequence of this error depends on where the hook impinges – neighbouring abdominal wall causing small burn (little consequence), hollow organ with perforation (major consequence requiring remedial action) or large vessel with major bleeding (life threatening consequence). In addition, several factors may contribute to the occurrence of the same error. In the example quoted above, the reason the surgeon caused the electrosurgical hook knife to jump could have been due to several factors: (a) misjudgement of the tension required on the instrument and its direction, (b) poor positioning of the ports limiting manual control of the instrument, (c) inadequate visual control during the step of the procedure.

An ergonomic approach can be used to evaluate surgical techniques to identify errors enacted during laparoscopic procedures. The research group in Dundee has adopted a modified human reliability analysis (HRA) approach to categorise and record errors encountered during laparoscopic cholecystectomies based on direct observation with a checklist (Joice et al. 1997). The observational analysis identified a high error rate ($n=189$ in 20 procedures) although none of the patients developed any postoperative complications. In this context, errors are of two types: execution and procedural. Execution errors (intra-step) refer to mistakes in carrying out a step, for example, cutting with the electrosurgical hook knife. Procedural errors (inter-step) refer to an adverse consequence which occurs when the surgeon does not follow the component steps of the particular task in the right order, or omits a step. A higher than expected number of procedural errors ($n=73$) was identified, of which 9% required corrective action during the operation. Of the 116 execution errors, 28% required remedial action. Errors were most frequently enacted with use of endoscopic graspers ($n=70$), clip applicators ($n=41$) and the electrosurgical hook knife ($n=40$). Errors associated with clip applicators were the result of surgeons undertaking incorrect procedural steps, suggesting the need to re-evaluate surgical training. In contrast, the nature of the errors associated with the use of graspers and electrosurgical hook knife merit further investigations into the design of these instruments.

The use of ergonomic approach to evaluate surgical techniques should improve the safety of surgical procedures and increase the efficiency of endoscopic manipulations.

References

Becker H et al (1993) 3-D video techniques in endoscopic surgery. End Surg 1:40–46
Berci G (1976) Instrument I: rigid endoscope. In: Berci G (ed) Endoscopy. Appleton-Century-Crofts, New York, pp 74–112
Berguer R, Remler M, Beckley D (1997a) Laparoscopic instruments cause increased forearm fatigue: a subjective and objective comparison of open and laparoscopic techniques. Min Invas Ther Allied Techn 6:36–40
Berguer R et al (1997b) A comparison of surgeons' posture during laparoscopic and open surgical procedures. Surg Endosc 11:139–142
Chan ACW et al (1997) Comparison of two-dimensional vs three-dimensional camera systems in laparoscopic surgery. Surg Endosc 11:438–440
Coren S, Ward LM (1989) Space. In: Coren S, Ward LM (eds) Sensation and perception, 3rd edn. Harcourt Brace Jovanovich College Publishers, Florida, pp 274–303
Cormack R, Fox R (1985) The computation of disparity and depth in stereograms. Percept Psychophys 38:375–380
Crosthwaite G et al (1995) Comparison of direct vision and electronic two- and three-dimensional display systems on surgical task efficiency in endoscopic surgery. Br J Surg 82:849–851
Cuschieri A (1995) Whither minimal access surgery: tribulations and expectations. Am J Surg 169:9–19
Edgar GK, Pope JCD, Craig IR (1994) Visual accommodation problems with head-up and helmet-mounted displays? Displays 15:68–75
Hanna GB, Cuschieri A (1997) Influence of two and three dimensional imaging on endoscopic bowel suturing. Association of Endoscopic Surgeons of Great Britain and Ireland, London
Hanna GB, Cuschieri A (1998) Influence of optical axis-to-target view angle on endoscopic task performance. Surg Endosc (in press)
Hanna GB, Shimi S, Cuschieri A (1997a) Influence of direction of view, target-to-endoscope distance and manipulation angle on endoscopic knot tying. Br J Surg 84:1460–1464
Hanna GB, Shimi S, Cuschieri A (1997b) Optimal port locations for endoscopic intracorporeal knotting. Surg Endosc 11:397–401
Hanna GB, Shimi S, Cuschieri A (1998) Randomised study of influence of two-dimensional versus three-dimensional imaging on performance of laparoscopic cholecystectomy. Lancet 351:248–251
Hanna GB, Shimi S, Cuschieri A (1998) Task performance in endoscopic work is influenced by location of the image display. Ann Surg 227:481–484
Hensman C et al (1998) Total radiated power, infra-red output and heat generation by cold light sources at the distal end of endoscopes and fibre optic bundle of light cables. Surg Endosc 12:335–337
Holden J, Frank TG, Cuschieri A (1997) Developing technology for suspended imaging for minimal access surgery. Sem Lap Surg 4:74–79
Hopkins HH (1976) Optical principle of the endoscope. In: Berci G (ed) Endoscopy. Appleton-Century-Crofts, New York, pp 3–26
Joice P, Hanna GB, Cuschieri A (1998) Errors enacted during endoscopic surgery – a human reliability analysis. Appl Ergon 29:409–414
Kano N, Yamakawa T, Kasugai H (1993) Laparoscopic surgeon's thumb. Arch Surg 128:1172
Majeed AW et al (1993) Laparoscopists's thumb: an occupational hazard. Arch Surg 128:357
Merritt JO (1987) Visual-motor realism in 3D teleoperator display systems. SPIE True Three Dimens Imaging Techn Display Technol 761:88–93
Patkin M, Isabel L (1995) Ergonomics, engineering and surgery of endosurgical dissection. J R Coll Surg Endinb 40:120–132
Pietrabissa A et al (1994) Three dimensional versus two dimensional video system for the trained endoscopic surgeon and the beginner. Surg Endosc 2:315–317

Satava RM (1993) 3-D vision technology applied to advanced minimally invasive surgery systems. Surg Endosc 7:429–431

Satava R, Roe W, Joyce G (1988) Current generation video endoscopes: a critical evaluation. Am Surg 54:73–77

Tendick F et al (1993) Sensing and manipulation problems in endoscopic surgery: experiment, analysis and observation. Presence 2:66–81

Tyrrell RA, Leibowitz HW (1990) The relation of vergence effort to reports of visual fatigue following prolonged near work. Hum Factors 32:341–357

von Pichler C, Radermacher K, Boeckman W (1996a) The influence of LCD shatter glasses on spatial perception in stereoscopic visualisation. In: Weghorst SJ, Sieburg HS, Morgan KS (eds) Medicine meets virtual reality: health care in the information age. IOS, Amsterdam, pp 523–531

von Pichler C, Radermacher K, Rau G (1996b) The state of 3-D technology and evaluation. Min Invas Ther 5:419–426

Yeh Y-Y, Silverstein LD (1991) Human factors for stereoscopic colour displays. SID Dig 91:826–829

CHAPTER 5

Training in Paediatric Endoscopic Surgery

A.S. Najmaldin

Introduction

Wickham noted that three seminal events have indelibly altered surgery: the introduction of anaesthesia, the development of antiseptics, and endoscopy [1]. In recent years endoscopic surgery has undergone a dramatic development in all surgical specialities. Surgeons are faced with increasing competition and pressure from peer, media and patients to apply this new approach in their routine clinical practice as soon as possible.

Throughout the developed world, the technique has already become the method of choice in surgical treatment of benign gall bladder disease. Patients undergoing laparoscopic cholecystectomy can expect less than 2 days of hospital stay with very little if any requirement for intravenous fluid and opiate analgesia, and return to normal life within 10 days [2]. Laparoscopic anti-reflux surgery, appendicectomy and diagnostic procedures in cryptorchidism, abdominal trauma and suspected peritoneal malignant deposits are becoming increasingly popular [3-7]. The benefits accruing from the avoidance of a thoracotomy by the established thoracoscopic procedures are even greater than those given by laparoscopic surgery [8]. Examples are thoracoscopic single port sympathectomy for the treatment of hyperhidrosis and diagnostic mediastinal and pulmonary procedures. Whilst most surgeons acknowledge the potential benefits of endoscopic surgery, and are very enthusiastic to take up the technique, only a few non-adult general and gynaecological surgeons have had the opportunity to train adequately and appropriately.

Good surgery consists of proper decision making and competent manipulative skills [9]. The craft skills of surgery are acquired by the apprentice from his or her master by watching, listening, assisting and being assisted, encouraged and corrected [10]. Basic and individual operative movements are learned first before they are coordinated effectively into complex actions and re-produced without the need to think of the basic components [11]. The acquisition of automatic surgical skills demands a repeated practice. The natural place to learn operative skills is in the operating theatre and the natural specimen to learn from is patients. However, it is becoming increasingly difficult for present and future surgeons to acquire all surgical skills in the operating room, largely because of concern about safety, time, cost, and the development of sub-specialization craftsmanship. Therefore an increasing number of basic and specialised operative skills will have to be taught outside the operating rooms. This will allow repeatedly stressing selection of the correct procedure and tactical flexibility if circumstances change away from the pressure of the operating theatre. The damaging effects of surgical mistakes of all kinds may be demonstrated and corrected by both the trainer and trainee in a cost effective fashion without the worry about the patient's safety.

In endoscopic surgery established conventional operative procedures are performed via a completely new approach [12]. It involves restricted access through the abdominal wall by trocars and cannulae, creation of an artificial space by gas such as CO_2, remote manipulation and dissection by delicate and long handled instruments, loss of tactile sense and working with two dimensional imaging instead of direct vision and hand manipulation, and problems of hand-eye coordination and depth perception. A system of training is therefore required which addresses these specific and new issues.

Bench Trainer (Phantom Model)

A variety of training devices has been designed to enable basic endoscopic surgical skills such as manipulation, cutting, clipping, stitching and removing items, to be undertaken from a distance with or without a camera in place. Using instruments through a TV image enables trainees to developed hand and eye coordination skills and learn the essentials of team work and theatre layout. This model is portable, readily available and inexpensive, and can be used outside the surgical skill centres if required.

Training in Animals

Animal models give the opportunity to apply almost all the steps of the endoscopic surgical operation under circumstances which are fairly similar to those normally encountered in clinical practice. Probably the most suitable animal for this purpose is a small pig. It is relatively expensive and requires special set up in designated skill centres. An animal exercise provides good practice for safe and successful creation of a pneumoperitoneum and insertion of cannula/trocar. It allows the trainee to become familiar with the endoscopic anatomy and tissue handling, trouble-shooting and management of endoscopic bleeding and contamination with body fluid, imaging problems, the use of energy sources such as electrocautery, ultrasound and laser, as well as the use of suction and irrigation systems.

Training Course

Training courses have become an essential part of our strive to achieve better training in both conventional and endoscopic surgical skills. It is important that training institutions and hospitals formulate there own specific needs for training. Whilst basic and principals of endoscopic anatomy, physiology, anaesthesia, and operative skills can be learned from any well structured course, essential paediatric endoscopic surgical skills can only be taught through well and specifically structured courses for paediatric surgeons by experienced and practising paediatric surgeons. The value of courses depends to a great extent on the enthusiasm of both the trainees and the appropriate and realistic simulation provided by phantoms and laboratory models. A suitable course should have three essential components: didactic sessions, video or live operating demonstrations and a laboratory training period. In the laboratory, basic courses should provide both bench trainer and animal exercises whilst an advanced course provides animal exercises.

Training of Qualified Surgeons

A fully trained, accredited, and enthusiastic paediatric surgeon may acquire his or her endoscopic surgical skills by: first attending one or more basic paediatric training courses; then visit sessions of endoscopic surgery by adult surgeons or gynaecologists in there own institutes, followed by visits to specialised paediatric centres before the setting up of very basic and simple diagnostic and therapeutic clinical procedures. It would be invaluable to have an experienced endoscopic surgeon present to assist, correct and encourage during the first one or more procedures. The acquisition of complex endoscopic surgical skills demands assiduous repeated practice. Attending advanced endoscopic training courses provide additional and essential support. The surgeon may embark on complex endoscopic procedures only in the presence of an experienced endoscopist.

Training Residents

In Europe and the United States current adult general and gynaecological surgical residents learn the principles and advanced aspects of endoscopic surgery throughout their structured training programme which usually lasts 5–8 years. The situation is different with surgical specialities including paediatric surgery. At present there are only a few centres in Europe and the United States which can provide adequate endoscopic surgical training facilities to paediatric surgical residents because so little experience is available. Outside these centres, paediatric residents may undertake endoscopic training by: first attending one or more basic courses, then attending regular sessions of diagnostic and therapeutic endoscopy performed either by adult general or gynaecological surgeons in their own institution. Finally, he or she must find a period of clinical training under the supervision of an experienced paediatric endoscopist before starting clinical endoscopic operations independently as a qualified surgeon.

Summary

Current practice in paediatric surgery demands even more than formerly to focus major emphasis on the acquisition of operative skills. Once the aspects of good basic technique are covered, the trainees need practice to refine and establish advanced skills. As opportunities to acquire structured training in paediatric endoscopic surgery is limited to a few centres world wide, present surgeons and residents must spend a period in specialised centres where there is a reasonable workload of predominantly endoscopic surgery.

Apprenticeship remains the most important element for acquiring the craft skills. However, appropriately structured paediatric training courses, basic and advanced, are valuable adjuncts for formal instruction and hands on experience. The feasibility and place of virtual reality and computer video-supported training are under investigation.

References

1. Wickham JEA (1991) Editorial. J Minim Invasive Surg 1:1–5
2. Perissat J et al (1990) Cholecystectomie par laparoscopie. La technique operatoire. Les resultats des 100 premieres observations. J Chir (Paris) 127:347–355
3. Cardiere GD et al (1994) Laparocopic Nissen fundoplication: technique and preliminary results. Br J Surg 81:400–403
4. Valla JS, Limonne B, Valla V et al (1991) Laparoscopic appendicectomy in children: report of 456 cases. Surg Laparoscopy Endosc 1:166–172
5. Najmaldin A (1994) Laparoscopy. Curr Opin Urol 4:316–320
6. Humphrey GME, Najmaldin AS (1996) Laparoscopic Nissen funodoplication in disabled children. J Pediatr Surg 31:596–599
7. Cuschieri A (1992) Diagnostic laparoscopy and laparoscopic adhesiolysis. In: Cuschieri A, Buess G, Perissat J (eds) Operative manuel of endoscopic surgery. Springer, Berlin Heidelberg New York, pp 180–193
8. Rogers BM, Talbert JL (1976) Thoracocoscopyy for diagnosis of intrathoracic lesions in children. J Pediatr Surg 11:703–708
9. Spencer FC (1978) Teaching and measuring surgical techniques – the technical evaluation of competence. Bull Am Coll Surg 63(3):9–12
10. Kirk RM (1996) Teaching the craft of operative surgery. Ann R Coll Surg Eng 78:25–28
11. Kirk RM (1994) Basic surgical techniques, 4th edn. Churchill Livingstone, Edinburgh
12. Buess G, Cuschieri A (1992) Training in endoscopic surgery. In: Cuschieri A, Buess G, Perissat J (eds) Operative manual of endoscopic surgery. Springer, Berlin Heidelberg New York, pp 64–82

CHAPTER 6

Basic Physiology and Anesthesia

M. Sfez

Introduction

Endoscopic surgery was a challenge for pediatric anesthesiologists as long as data were not available on physiological changes induced by this surgical approach. Experimental and clinical studies in adults, available since the 1970's, show that cardiorespiratory changes induced by insufflation of carbon dioxide (CO_2) are of clinical relevance only for intra-abdominal pressure (IAP) levels higher than 15 mmHg, which is not used in humans. Furthermore, there is clinical and experimental evidence that the magnitude of cardiorespiratory changes during peritoneal CO_2 insufflation is related to the IAP level in young individuals (Sfez 1994; Lister et al. 1994). Nevertheless, no clinically significant adverse effect related to IAP level lower than 15 mmHg has been reported in children older than 6 months. In young infants and neonates, some teams are reluctant to apply IAP level above 6 mmHg in order to prevent major complications, as has been reported in one case due to reduced intrathoracic compliance (Sfez 1994; Pighin et al. 1993).

The development of retroperitoneal surgery has been much slower since few data are available. The data obtained from peritoneal insufflation cannot reasonably be extrapolated as the retroperitoneal space offers an unrestricted compartment to CO_2 diffusion. As a consequence the level of retroperitoneal pressure seems to be much less clinically relevant. On the other hand, resorption of the CO_2 stored in this space may become of clinical concern (Mullet et al. 1993). Quantitative data are lacking in children, even though incidental extraperitoneal CO_2 insufflation does not lead to hypercabnic (Sfez et al. 1996). Therefore definite guidelines for this approach in children cannot be derived at the time being.

Endoscopic thoracic surgery has developed even more slowly in children. From early clinical experience it is possible to draw the main features of the physiological changes related to this particular approach.

Regardless of the body compartment submitted to endoscopic surgery, physiological changes are the basis for defining adequate anesthetic choice. In these situations the anesthesiologist must compensate for the changes in vital functions induced by the surgeon. Thus, both physicians are closely involved in patients' safety, and the surgeon must be aware of the possible limitations of the technique in a particular patient. If the anesthesiologist cannot cope with major changes in vital functions the surgeon must convert the operation to an open technique.

This chapter reviews physiological changes and anesthetic implications separately for thoracic surgery and for other procedures since CO_2 insufflation is uncommon in thoracic endoscopic surgery.

Intra- and Retroperitoneal Surgery

Most of the nonsurgical, unwanted effects result from both CO_2 insufflation and patient position (Sfez et al. 1996). These two factors induce changes in IAP responsible for cardiorespiratory changes, even though these changes can be without clinical significance. In addition, carbon dioxide resorption is responsible for the commonly reported increase in CO_2 excretion assessed by expired CO_2. The quantitation of individual effects of these factors is difficult in a clinical setting. Experimental data are therefore essential to understand the effect of factors such as IAP level, developmental changes, preoperative cardiovascular and respiratory status. Applying the conclusions of experimental studies to children improves anesthetic and surgical management.

Physiological Changes During Abdominal and Retroperitoneal Surgery

Cardiocirculatory Changes

Cardiocirculatory changes have been studied extensively during laparoscopic surgery in school-age children undergoing appendicectomy. These changes are grossly similar to those reported in adults, except for cardiac preload (Raux et al. 1995). Such discrepancy can be either age related or due to methodological differences between adult and pediatric studies. Animal studies show that some factors involved in cardiovascular changes have not been taken into account in human studies, which could explain the observed differences. These factors include the level of IAP, the level of blood CO_2, possible hypovolemia and patient position. The effect of each of these factors is described in the following sections with successive presentation of studies in animals, adult patients and children.

Effect of IAP Level

Animal Studies

Increasing IAP alters venous return and systemic vascular resistance (Ishizaki et al. 1993) and therefore alters cardiac output as shown in Table 1. Diphasic venous return changes are reported during gradual increase in IAP in the usual clinical range. When IAP is lower than 6 mmHg, venous return and cardiac output are increased owing to an autotransfusion of pooled blood from the splanchnic region. Venous return and cardiac output are reduced when IAP is higher than 8 mmHg. Inferior vena cava blood flow is dramatically reduced when IAP is gradually increased from 8 to 16 mmHg, while cardiac output is significantly re-

Table 1. Percentage changes from preinsufflation values in central hemodynamics and IAP levels (from Ishisaki et al. 1993)

	IAP (mmHg)		
	8	12	16
Inferior vena cava blood flow	−50	−63	−100
Cardiac output	−5	−9	−32
Systemic vascular resistance	4	4	65

duced only in animals submitted to IAP of 16 mmHg (Ishizaki et al. 1993). In young piglets a 15 mmHg IAP induces a reduction in inferior vena cava flow by 22%–25% in normocapnic animals while it is unchanged in hypercapnic animals (Graham et al. 1994). Although venous return is reduced, central venous, right atrial and left atrial pressures increase, paralleling IAP (Ishizaki et al. 1993). Whether this increase contributes to cardiac output changes remains unclear. Such increase may be due only to the transmission of abdominal pressure into the thorax, with reduced transmural filling pressures of the heart leading to reduced cardiac output in animals submitted to IAP levels higher than 15 mmHg, which is no longer used in clinical practice. Furthermore, the relationship between venous return and filling pressures of the heart is not linear, so that venous return cannot be reliably assessed by changes in filling pressures of the heart. Species difference in this relationship does not allow to derive threshold values of IAP reducing venous return from animal studies.

In small dogs systemic vascular resistance is unchanged when IAP is 8 or 12 mmHg but significantly increases by 50% when IAP reaches 16 mmHg, while mean arterial pressure changes are not significant (Ishizaki et al. 1993). Whether arterial pressure increases depends on the balance between increased systemic vascular resistance and reduced venous return. Nevertheless, the net effect is an increase in left ventricle afterload and work (Graham et al. 1994).

Studies in Adults

In a recent review of cardiovascular changes during adult laparoscopic cholecystectomy, a biphasic pattern is described during the first 15 min of pneumoperitoneum insufflation (Wahba et al. 1995). These include initial decrease in cardiac output while mean arterial pressure and left ventricle afterload indexes increase. Simultaneously it is unclear whether venous return is decreased, increased or unchanged (Wahba et al. 1995). When this issue is specifically addressed, a simultaneous increase in right and left ventricles filling pressures and in end-diastolic left ventricle echographic area is found when IAP level is set to 11–13 mmHg, suggesting that venous return is increased in these patients (Gannedahl et al. 1996). Whatever the changes in venous return, all parameters are corrected partly spontaneously within the first 15 min of pneumoperitoneum, although the return to normal values is obtained only 20 min after pneumoperitoneum deflation (Wahba et al. 1995).

Studies in Children

In 31 children aged 9.4±2.9 years venous return index was significantly reduced by IAP in the 7.5–9.1 mmHg range during laparoscopic appendicectomy (Raux et al. 1995). Left ventricle preload and cardiac output were reduced by 20% as systemic vascular resistance index was increased by 50%. This accounted for arterial pressure increase by 20%–25%. It is unclear why, despite a much lower IAP level, left ventricle preload is reduced in children, in contrast to adults (Gannedahl et al. 1996). First, pediatric data (Raux et al. 1995) have been obtained using bioimpedance, which is not designed for children. Second, ventricle compliance is not the same in adults as in children, which could account for the observed differences. Finally, this discrepancy is also found between different adult studies.

Simultaneously to changes in venous circulation and heart filling, increased IAP induces a significant increase in systemic vascular resistance, thus increasing arterial pressure in spite of the reduction in cardiac output (Raux et al. 1995). For the same reasons as suggested for venous return, these results are different from those obtained in animals. The simultaneous decrease in venous return together with elevated systemic vascular resistance can be of concern in children with limited cardiac reserve. Furthermore, there is a risk of underestimating the importance of cardiac reserve under these circumstances since elevated arterial pressure is a poor indicator of the adequacy of cardiac output to the individual clinical situation. It is nevertheless to be noticed that blood lactate has been reported to be within normal limits in healthy children (Raux et al. 1995). In addition, this high level of systemic vascular resistance contributes to reduced cardiac output. Pharmacological reduction in vascular resistance improves cardiac output without significantly altering arterial pressure.

Role of Humoral Factors

The persistence of cardiovascular changes in the first 20 min of pneumoperitoneum deflation suggests that factors other than mechanical vascular compression by the pneumoperitoneum are involved in these changes.

Animal Studies

In piglets submitted to CO_2 pneumoperitoneum hypercapnia increases cardiac output and prevents changes in systemic vascular resistance, while cardiac output is unchanged and systemic vascular resistance increases in normocapnic animals (Graham et al. 1994). Hypercapnia is known to have direct vasodilatory and indirect cardiovascular effects due to the stimulation of the sympathetic nervous system, which is blunted by general anesthesia. The relative magnitude of these effects have not been studied, and it is therefore difficult to assess their real importance in the clinical changes observed. Furthermore, hypercapnia and sympathetic stimulation may induce the secretion of vasoactive hormones.

Studies in Adults

The hypothesis that mechanical compression of the abdominal vessels induces the secretion of humoral vasoactive hormones such as vasopressin and norepinephrine is supported by preliminary reports. The plasma concentration time course of these hormones parallels that of the changes in cardiac output and systemic vascular resistance (Wahba et al. 1995). The relationship between these changes and the level of blood CO_2 has not been studied.

Studies in Children

There are no clinical data to support the role of humoral factors in cardiovascular changes in the pediatric patient. No statistical correlation has been found between end-tidal CO_2 and changes in arterial pressure in either retrospective or prospective studies (Sfez 1994; Sfez et al. 1996). The only study in which end-tidal CO_2 was much higher than normal values did not examine the relationship between cardiovascular changes and end-tidal CO_2 (Tobias et al. 1994). In addition, capnography is a poor estimator of arterial CO_2 during laparoscopy, as discussed below.

Effect of Patient's Position

Studies in Adults

The effects of the reverse Trendelenburg (rT) position include reduced venous return, cardiac output and arterial pressure. These are counteracted by pneumoperitoneum inflation to 11–13 mmHg in adults (Gannedahl et al. 1996).

Trendelenburg position associated with increased IAP may be of concern in patients with limited cardiac reserve. In adult patients, insufflating the pneumoperitoneum to 11–13 mmHg enhances cardiocirculatory changes due to the Trendelenburg position. Thus, filling pressures of the heart increase while cardiac output remains unchanged. Left ventricle performance is therefore reduced since higher filling pressures are necessary to keep cardiac output constant. This can be due to the reduction in myocardial diastolic compliance assessed by increased end-diastolic diameter of the left ventricle and slowing of early ventricle filling following pneumoperitoneum insufflation and Trendelenburg position (Gannedahl et al. 1996).

Studies in Children

In the rT position reduced arterial pressure occurring prior to inflation of the pneumoperitoneum does not persist when peritoneal cavity is insufflated, suggesting that the cardiocirculatory effects of elevated IAP to a mean level of 9 mmHg limit those of the operating position (Sfez et al. 1995).

Arterial pressure is increased differently following the level of IAP and the operating position in children (Sfez et al. 1996). Elevated arterial pressure is significantly more frequent when children are placed in the Trendelenburg position

Table 2. Percentage changes in regional blood flow and increasing IAP (from Masey et al. 1985; Ishisaki et al. 1993)

	IAP (mmHg)			
	8	12	15–16	20
Total liver	7.69	−7.69	−26.92	−31.25
Total portal	10.00	−10.00	−35.00	−38.89
Mesenteric artery	−6.25	−18.75	−37.50	−56.00
Kidney	N.A.	N.A.	−8.33	−19.70
Diaphragm	N.A.	N.A.	−28.57	−35.71

N.A., Not available.

when IAP is higher than 8 mmHg, while no position related difference exists when IAP is lower. In these children increased arterial pressure requires no specific therapy. Such difference with adult results can be explained by different study design or by age-related differences in left myocardial relaxation.

Effects of Hypovolemia

Physiological effects of hypovolemia are similar to those induced by the rT position. Nevertheless, there is experimental evidence for dramatic decrease in filling pressures of the heart and cardiac output in hypovolemic animals submitted to excessively high IAP levels.

Regional Circulation

In dogs the study of graded increase in IAP from 8 to 16 mmHg shows that only the highest IAP level induces a significant decrease in total hepatic blood flow (29%), portal blood flow (33%), and superior arterial mesenteric blood flow (37%; Ishizaki et al. 1993). Furthermore, at IAP 16 mmHg hepatic blood flow is still decreased as the duration of pneumoperitoneum increases. In neonatal lambs, where increased IAP was obtained by filling a peritoneal bag with saline, similar results were obtained when IAP reached 15 mmHg. Simultaneously kidney, adrenal, and diaphragmatic and various cerebral blood flows are unchanged compared to control values (Table 2). At higher IAP levels up to 25 mmHg only diaphragmatic blood flow is decreased (Masey et al. 1985).

All the cardiocirculatory effects of CO_2 insufflation have been reported following peritoneal insufflation, and therefore only little is known of the effects of retroperitoneal insufflation.

Respiratory Changes

Mechanical effects of peritoneal or retroperitoneal gas insufflation may lead to hypoventilation, while the resorption of insufflated CO_2 contributes to hypercapnia commonly reported in adults and in animals. Hypercapnia is not demonstrated in children, although end-tidal CO_2 is commonly increased during laparoscopic surgery (Sfez 1994). Intraoperative mechanical ventilation is therefore mandatory during surgery as children in spontaneous ventilation during short duration laparoscopy exhibit major increase in end-tidal CO_2 despite significant increases in minute ventilation (Tobias et al. 1994). However, postoperative respiratory function improves rapidly after laparoscopic surgery.

Intraoperative Changes

The effects of CO_2 insufflation differ during peritoneal and retroperitoneal insufflation, owing to the limited CO_2 diffusion in the restricted space of the peritoneal cavity (Mullet et al. 1993). Nevertheless, most changes have been studied during peritoneal insufflation.

Animal Studies

The difference between the mechanical effects of increased IAP and the effects of peritoneal CO_2 resorption can be made by insufflating the peritoneum with either CO_2 or helium (Lister et al. 1994). The mechanism of P_{aCO2} increase following CO_2 insufflation depends on the IAP level. When IAP is lower than 10 mmHg, P_{aCO2} and pulmonary CO_2 elimination (V_{CO2}) increase owing to peritoneal CO_2 resorption. Further increasing IAP to 25 mmHg increases P_{aCO2} and alveolar dead space (VD/Vt), while V_{CO2} plateaus. CO_2 resorption is considered as self-limited by the compression of capillary peritoneal vessels.

Studies in Adults

The time course of respiratory CO_2 elimination (V_{CO2}), P_{etCO2}, P_{aCO2} P_{vCO2}, and tissue CO_2 is characterized by a continuous increase during at least 2 h, as presented in Table 3 (Aoki 1993), although there is a trend toward plateauing in P_{etCO2}, V_{CO2} and P_{aCO2} from the 30th minute of insufflation (Mullet et al. 1993). After the first 30 min the steep increase in P_{aCO2} and P_{etCO2} may reflect the saturation of buffering capacities of the tissues, with a risk of secondary acido-

Table 3. Percentage changes in CO_2 metabolism with time following peritoneal insufflation (from Aoki 1993)

	Time (min)					
	5	10	15	30	60	120
End-tidal CO_2	11.54	19.23	23.08	34.62	34.62	57.69
Arterial CO_2	20.00	23.33	30.00	40.00	46.67	66.67
Venous CO_2	15.15	21.21	27.27	36.36	45.45	63.64
Tissue CO_2	2.56	7.69	12.82	25.64	46.15	66.67
Buffer capacity	−50.00	−60.00	−63.33	−63.33	−66.67	−66.67

sis. Acidosis is more likely to occur during CO_2 retroperitoneal insufflation as CO_2 pulmonary elimination is then time dependent (Mullet et al. 1993). This CO_2 slow elimination rate results from low blood flow in the retroperitoneal space or continued dissection of this space by insufflated CO_2.

The increase in alveolar dead space at high IAP may be due to the cephalad shift of the diaphragm and abdominal organs, leading to reduced thoracopulmonary compliance. At IAP in the 13–16 mmHg range total compliance is reduced by 33%–38% (Hirvonen et al. 1995). Patient's position does not alter the reduction in compliance, which reaches 50% of the control value in the Trendelenburg and in the rT positions (Bardoczky et al. 1993). Furthermore, increasing alveolar dead space contributes to the time-dependent increase in alveolar to end-tidal CO_2 gradient (Aoki 1993; Hirvonen et al. 1995).

Studies in Children

When IAP is lower than 8 mmHg, P_{etCO_2} is higher than 40 mmHg only in children placed in the Trendelenburg position. This suggests that in these patients a combination of increased CO_2 resorption and increased alveolar dead space contribute to increased P_{etCO_2}.

In young infants a dramatic reduction in total compliance may occur while insufflating the pneumoperitoneum and lead to major intraoperative hypoventilation (Pighin et al. 1993).

Insufflating CO_2 changes the direction of the alveolar to end-tidal CO_2 gradient in an unpredictable manner in 30% of the patients, probably in relation to the balance between alveolar dead space and cardiac output changes (Gouchet et al. 1995). P_{etCO_2} is therefore not a reliable estimator of P_{aCO_2} during laparoscopic surgery.

Postoperative Changes

Studies in Adults

Mechanical ventilation is necessary for at least 10 min following pneumoperitoneum exsufflation to remove CO_2 load and to return to baseline P_{etCO_2} values. Retroperitoneal CO_2 removal is much slower since 45 min after the end of insufflation P_{etCO_2} is higher than preinsufflation values, although the duration of insufflation is 30% lower than in patients undergoing laparoscopic cholecystectomies (Mullet et al. 1993).

Following this recovery period respiratory function is less altered than following the same operation by laparotomy as shown following cholecystectomy. Respiratory alterations are of shorter duration and reduced magnitude in the laparoscopic than in the open surgical group. Thus the laparoscopic approach leads to higher values of forced vital capacity (FVC) and forced expiratory volume in 1 s (FEV_1) from the 6th postoperative hour and higher functional residual capacity values at 72 h. FRC recovered preoperative values at 24 h in the laparoscopic group while it remained reduced in the laparotomy group. FVC recovered in less than 72 h in both groups, although the values were higher in laparoscopic patients. In neither group had FEV$_1$ recovered by 72 h (Putensen-Himmer et al. 1992).

Diaphragmatic dysfunction can partly explain early postoperative respiratory changes. It can be due to phrenic nerve inhibition secondary to the operative splanchnic nerve stimulation resulting in a reduced postoperative abdominal wall motion with an increased contribution of chest wall muscles to minute ventilation (Erice et al. 1993). In addition, postoperative diaphragmatic dysfunction is all the more altered as the operating site is close to the diaphragm (Erice et al. 1993). Furthermore, diaphragmatic dysfunction is not related to the residual pneumoperitoneum in adult patients undergoing laparoscopic diagnosis procedure under local anesthesia (Benhamou et al. 1993). Most respiratory postoperative changes are therefore likely related to the operating procedure but are of less magnitude for a given procedure than that induced by the open approach.

Studies in Children

Following laparoscopic Nissen fundoplication 25% children experience hypoxia in the first 4 h postoperatively, partly related to the residual effects of anesthesia (Sfez et al. 1995). During the following 24 h neither hypoxia nor atelectasis occurs. The laparoscopic approach might contribute to prevent early postoperative atelectasis generally related to reduced FRC, which is of particular importance in neonates and young infants due to their physiological low FRC.

Furthermore, the laparoscopic approach is considered safer for cholecystectomy in sickle cell patients for preventing the occurrence of postoperative sickling (Tagge et al. 1994). No data exist on the postoperative respiratory changes related to retroperitoneal insufflation.

Other Physiological Changes

Hypothermia, which is a particular concern in neonates and young infants, is likely to occur following long duration procedures or when large volumes of cold saline are used for peritoneal washing. Its prevention by using warm water can cloud the video lens.

The association of Trendelenburg position and increased IAP alters intracranial pressure and the cardial barrier pressure. The latter is increased by both factors, but this does not completely suppress the intraoperative risk of silent aspiration of gastric content. In the 2 pigs of 11 with the lowest control low esophageal sphincter pressure, regurgitation was reported while fasting (Tournadre et al. 1996). These data do not allow conclusions on the real aspiration risk in emergency patients with full stomach. Intracranial pressure is significantly increased when IAP is 15 mmHg while cerebral perfusion pressure is significantly increased only in the Trendenlenburg position. Nevertheless, a recent report of two pediatric cases shows that intracranial pressure increases while cerebral perfusion pressure decreases when IAP is 10 mmHg or less (Uzzo et al. 1997).

Both parameters are corrected by monitored removal of cerebrospinal fluid. It is therefore necessary to monitor intracranial pressure in patients presenting with ventriculoperitoneal shunts. The use of laparoscopic approach in emergency surgery therefore requires avoiding the Trendelenburg position and using IAP as low as possible to prevent neurological complications.

Anesthetic Considerations

Anesthetic guidelines for laparoscopic and retroperitoneal surgery result from physiopathological changes, although these guidelines are not supported by comparative studies.

Preoperative Selection and Assessment of Patients

Contraindications result from adult guidelines and from pathophysiological considerations:
- Absolute contraindications
  - Hypovolemia
  - Cardiac disease
  - Lung distension
- Relative contraindications
  - Intracranial hypertension
  - Premature babies

Absolute contraindications therefore include uncorrected hypovolemia, pulmonary distension, especially as a sequella of bronchodysplasia in the former premature newborn due to the high risk of pneumothorax, cardiac or great vessels abnormalities with or without shunt due to possible hemodynamic failure or paradoxical gas embolism. This major but uncommon accident may occur in patients presenting with a silent patent foramen ovale which is present in at least 25% children younger than 5 years. Unfortunately, its preoperative diagnosis remains unreliable by non-invasive methods (Sfez 1994). Moderate and stable intracranial hypertension is not an absolute contraindication when IAP is lower than 15 mmHg and Trendelenburg position is avoided. Patients presenting with sickle cell disease have a high incidence of cholelithiasis and circulatory and respiratory impairment secondary to multiple sickling crisis. Preoperative assessment therefore requires particular attention to the identification and quantitation of sequellae of visceral impairment by sickling, perioperative transfusion to obtain total hemoglobin higher than 100 mg/dl with less than 40% hemoglobin S, prevention of hypovolemia, hypothermia, and acidosis. In these patients the existence of a restrictive respiratory syndrome may lead to intraoperative respiratory failure that requires rapid conversion to laparotomy and may lead to major postoperative sickling crisis. Under these conditions laparoscopic cholecystectomy appears to induce less postoperative complications than laparotomy in sickle cell patients (Tagge et al. 1994).

Former preterm infants are at particular risk for such surgery. Until 6 months of age children have reduced left ventricle relaxation, reduced thoracic functional residual capacity, and reduced diaphragmatic function, leading to poor respiratory and circulatory tolerance to high IAP (Pighin et al. 1993). In addition, prematurity may induce hydrocephalus with intracranial hypertension and bronchodysplasia secondary to hyaline membrane disease. For these reasons most surgeons in Europe limit the level of IAP to 6 mmHg in this age group (Sfez 1994). In the United States much higher levels of IAP have been used without any adverse effect being reported. Thus in young infants the use of the lowest IAP level possible is to be recommended in the 0–15 mmHg range.

Emergency laparoscopy requires particular attention to the cardiocirculatory and infectious status of the patients as hypovolemia secondary to trauma, bleeding, and infection is common. Gastric emptying remains uncertain regardless of the duration of fasting, with the risk of aspiration of the gastric content. The risk of increased intracranial pressure must be considered in trauma patients as elevated IAP and Trendelenburg position increase intracranial pressure.

Irrespective of the preoperative evaluation, parents must be informed that conversion to laparotomy may occur should a problem occur.

Anesthetic Management

Mandatory in all patients are therefore general anesthesia with intratracheal intubation and ventilation to maintain end-tidal CO_2 in the physiological range and intraoperative monitoring of vital functions.

Intraoperative Monitoring

This necessarily includes an electrocardioscope, noninvasive blood pressure monitor, pulse oxymeter, and capnograph that displays both values and waveform of expired CO_2 as a function of time. Although P_{etCO_2} does not adequately reflect P_{aCO_2} during laparoscopic surgery, capnography is mandatory during laparoscopic surgery for the early detection of gas embolism. A rapid decrease in P_{etCO_2} of more than 3 mmHg is a better indicator of 0.25 ml embolisms than precordial stethoscope or external Doppler probe (Couture et al. 1994). This additional monitoring is uncommonly used continuously during laparoscopic operations, and its use is restricted to critical periods of surgery such as the initiation of pneumoperitoneum insufflation or the occurrence of vascular injury.

Invasive monitoring is restricted to the placement of an indwelling arterial catheter in high-risk patients such as cardiac, respiratory disabled, and sickle cell patients. It allows continuous arterial pressure measurement and multiple blood gas analysis during the operative and early postoperative period.

Anesthetic Technique

General anesthesia with tracheal intubation and controlled ventilation is mandatory. The increase in minute ventilation necessary to keep end-tidal CO_2 within the normal limits is 25% in the supine position and 50% in the Trendelenburg position (Hirvonen et al. 1995) and must be continued for at least 10 min following pneumoperitoneum deflation. This cannot be achieved by spontaneous mask ventilation even for procedures of duration as short as inspection of a patent processus vaginalis. When performed in children 15–80 months old, end-tidal CO_2 was higher than 50 mmHg in 15% patients despite a mean 40% increase in minute ventilation via a face mask (Tobias et al. 1994). In addition, the simultaneous use of general anesthesia with epidural/caudal anesthesia to prevent postoperative pain is hazardous in children older than 8 years. In this age group general anesthesia together with epidural blockade significantly decreases arterial pressure by pooling blood in the lower body compartment (Murat et al. 1987). This may be of concern when the IAP level induces a reduction in venous return.

When a limited level of IAP is used, the choice of the anesthetic agents does not alter the magnitude of respiratory cardiovascular changes (Sfez et al. 1996). Nevertheless, short-acting agents given by inhalation or intravenous route are to be preferred, in order to rapidly compensate for any anesthetic related untoward event and to obtain a rapid recovery after trocars removal. Profound muscle relaxation is necessary during gastroesophageal reflux surgery to avoid untoward diaphragmatic contractions. When diaphragmatic movement does not alter adequate surgical management, muscle relaxation is not necessarily profound as experimental data show that neither peak airway pressure nor abdominal eslastance is altered by neuromuscular blockade in pigs (Chassard et al. 1996). Short-acting myorelaxants by continuous infusion can be used, with monitoring of the depth of neuromuscular blockade and antagonism at the end of surgery.

The use of nitrous oxide (N_2O) is widely debated in laparoscopic surgery due its rapid diffusion into hollow organs and cavities. It therefore increases the volume of bowel, gas embolism, and pneumothoraces. It has been impossible to demonstrate that bowel distension secondary to using N_2O leads to significant disturbance to the surgeon (Taylor et al. 1992). In addition, the risk of bowel combustion during electrocautery due to N_2O diffusion is not clinically relevant. With regard to the severity of gas embolism, the increase in volume induced by N_2O does not increase the consequences of embolism. Furthermore, the volume of air embolism that reduces arterial pressure by 10 mmHg is similar regardless of whether 50% nitrous oxide is added to the respiratory gas mixture (Lossasso et al. 1992). There is therefore no rationale for limitation of N_2O use on the basis of safety considerations. The possible relationship between N_2O use and delayed postoperative effects requires additional studies.

Additional Considerations

As the risk of aspiration cannot be ruled out, it is prudent to provide an antacid premedication in children prone to gastroesophageal reflux.

Preventing organ injury during trocars placement requires gastric and bladder emptying and adaptation of trocars size to the patient's age (Sfez et al. 1996).

Warming the patient and, if possible, using warm fluids for peritoneal lavage are necessary, especially for long-lasting procedures and for younger children.

It is also necessary to prevent arterial hypotension by adequate fluid loading, and limitation of rT to 10° and of IAP level to 10 mmHg.

Postoperative Considerations

Most benefit of endoscopic surgery is anticipated during the postoperative period and include rapid restoration of bowel activity, reduced postoperative pain, and respiratory impairment. Although the delay in restoration of electrical activity of the antrum, small intestine, and sigmoid colon is half as long as after laparoscopy (Böhm et al. 1995), no significant difference in the delay for food intake is found in children undergoing appendectomy by either laparotomy or laparoscopy (Lejus et al. 1996).

The incidence and severity of postoperative pain after appendicectomy are similar in the laparoscopic and open groups. There is a 2.5 times higher incidence of scapular pain in the laparoscopic group (Lejus et al. 1996). It is nevertheless noteworthy that pain management following laparoscopic surgery does not commonly require opioids, not only after appendectomy but also after Nissen fundoplication. It is therefore necessary to have more data available to estimate the effect of the video-endoscopic surgery on postoperative pain severity.

The anticipated respiratory benefit of the laparoscopic approach is suggested by data obtained after Nissen fundoplication (Sfez et al. 1995) and cholecystectomy in sickle cell patients (Tagge et al. 1994). Nevertheless, the occurrence of early hypoxia following fundoplication despite additional oxygen delivery requires pulse oxymetry monitoring for at least 3 h postoperatively (Sfez et al. 1995). The occurrence of postoperative desaturation requires a chest X-ray to check for the absence of pneumothorax.

Thus there is some evidence that endoscopic techniques may be more beneficial to children than open techniques with regard to postoperative physiological improvement. Nevertheless, most of these advantages must be demonstrated by comparative studies.

Thoracoscopic Surgery

Physiological changes and anesthetic problems during surgery are related to both the preoperative patient's condition and the need for intraoperative one lung ventilation. As CO_2 insufflation is no longer used, its consequences are not described here.

Physiological Changes

Respiratory Changes

Thoracoscopy requires to place the patient in the lateral decubitus position (LDP) and to create an artificial pneumothorax, thereby reducing ipsilateral lung ventilation. The use of lung retractors further reduces lung expansion and leads to impaired gas exchange. The consequences of these surgical imperatives depend on both the anesthetic and airway management techniques used, as recently assessed (Horswell 1993; McGahren et al. 1995).

In sedated patients with regional anesthesia, spontaneous breathing induces lung collapse during inspiration and lung expansion during expiration. Gas exchange impairment may induce hypoxia leading to conversion to general anesthesia. In addition, lung displacement in the very limited intrathoracic space bears a major risk of great vessels injury.

In the anesthetized patient in the LDP respiratory changes depend on whether one or two lung ventilation is used. During two-lung ventilation there is a relatively good ventilation and a reduced perfusion in the upper lung owing to gravitational distribution of blood flow. On the other hand, the lower lung is relatively hypoventilated while overperfused. Thus, moderate hypoxia and postoperative atelectasis may occur. During one lung ventilation, an obligatory right-to-left transpulmonary shunt is created through the nonventilated lung. A significant increase in the ratio of alveolar to arterial P_{O_2} then develops, and higher inspired oxygen concentrations are necessary to maintain constant P_{aO_2}. The magnitude of intraoperative hypoxia can be reduced by delivering low-flow oxygen to the operated lung through a double-lumen bronchial tube or a bronchial blocker with a distal port. The occurrence of hypoxemia or hypercapnia is short lived provided a rapid reexpansion of the lung on the operating side is obtained (Lavoie et al. 1996). In children with preexisting shunt lesions, hypoxemia and hypercapnia may lead to pulmonary vasoconstriction and increased pulmonary vascular resistance, thus an increasing a right-to-left shunt or reverting a left-to-right shunt. In addition, the occurrence of pulmonary hypertension may lead to acute right ventricle failure in children with preexisting altered right ventricle function.

Postoperative atelectasis is uncommon although larger series are necessary to confirm preliminary data (Lavoie et al. 1996). Postoperative pneumothoraces after chest drain removal have also been reported, often in relation with surgical complications (Rodgers et al. 1992; Lavoie et al. 1996). It is therefore likely that thoracoscopic surgery induces few changes in the mechanics of ventilation since in 47% pediatric patients operated on for cardiac surgery, tracheal extubation was performed in the operating room (Lavoie et al. 1996).

Cardiovascular Changes

In cardiac patients most changes are secondary to respiratory changes. Furthermore, surgical stretching of the great vessels may lead to rapid changes in loading conditions of the heart and arterial hypotension. The simultaneous decrease in end-tidal CO_2 suggests that capnography helps in monitoring pulmonary blood flow. Nevertheless, when rapid cardiovascular changes are anticipated during video-assisted thoracoscopic surgery, continuous invasive monitoring of arterial pressure is necessary. It is noteworthy that no untoward cardiovascular changes have been reported in children aged 1 day–14.1 year undergoing various cardiovascular operations (Lavoie et al. 1996).

Anesthetic Considerations

Preoperative Assessment

One lung ventilation, not always easy to perform in young children, must be discussed. Conversion to two lungs ventilation during the operation occurred in 22% of 18 pediatric patients who initially had one lung ventilation. Half of these conversions was due to respiratory intolerance while thoracotomy was necessary for surgery in others (McGahren et al. 1995). These data suggest that one-lung ventilation is applicable in children older than 12 years or when surgery protection of the nonoperated lung from blood or secretions is not mandatory, as no preoperative prediction of the tolerance of one lung ventilation is possible. The need for postoperative mechanical ventilation must also be estimated on the basis of anticipated cardiovascular changes and preoperative values of lung volumes and flows.

In children scheduled for cardiac surgery no age, weight, or physical status limitations have been demonstrated provided they present with an amenable pathology (Lavoie et al. 1996).

Anesthetic Management

Although sedation with regional anesthesia has been reported in 9- to 21-year-old patients undergoing talc pleurodesis (McGahren et al. 1995), this technique is not suitable for most procedures. General anesthesia remains the standard for pediatric thoracoscopic operations. There is no particular indication for individual agents except in patients presenting with cardiopulmonary dysfunction where halogenated inhaled agents have been omitted in preliminary series (Lavoie et al. 1996).

The technique for one lung ventilation depend on the patient's age and weight (McGahren et al. 1995). In children weighing more than 30 kg standard double-lumen endotracheal tubes of the proper size are used. It is necessary to check for adequate tube placement by fiberoptic bronchoscopy following tube placement and after placing patients in the operating position since clinical signs are inaccurate to detect inadequate positioning of the tube. Fiberoptic bronchoscopy is also necessary for adequate placement of a single lumen bronchial tube, even for neonates since a 1.8-mm bronchoscope can be passed through a 2.5-mm endotracheal tube (McGahren et al. 1995). When no double-lumen tube can be placed, a bronchial blocker can be positioned under fluoroscopic or bronchoscopic guidance. A Swan-Ganz catheter is a better choice than a Fogarty catheter since it allows oxygen delivery to the nonventilated lung through its distal port. In such situation it is necessary to check that no air trapping occurs in the nonventilated lung. A persistent respiratory intolerance to one lung ventilation requires conversion to two lungs ventilation.

Postoperative Considerations

In the short series reported, the postoperative period is uneventful provided no surgical complications occurred. This suggests that respiratory tolerance of thoracoscopic procedure is good, whatever the patients' age and preoperative status. In these patients studied retrospectively, morphine requirements during the first postoperative day were four times lower than following thoracotomy (Lavoie et al. 1996). These findings make thoracoscopic operations a reasonable alternative to thoracotomy even in premature cardiac neonates, even though the need for one lung ventilation can make the anesthetic management more complicated.

Conclusion

The anesthetic management for pediatric endoscopic surgery requires adequate knowledge of the physiological changes induced by this approach. Although few comparative studies with the open techniques are available, there is some evidence that postoperative management is easier after endoscopic surgery, provided no surgical complication occurs. On the other hand, pre- and intraoperative management is more difficult in some patients. These latter may need specific preoperative assessment, as in sickle cell patients, or intraoperative control of respiratory and circulatory changes, as in neonates and young infants undergoing laparoscopic surgery or patients with myocardial dysfunction undergoing thoracoscopy. This management requires a strong cooperation between the surgical and anesthetic teams to determine the parameters on which conversion to an open technique should be decided. The parents must always be informed of the possibility of conversion.

References

Aoki A (1993) Augmented arterial to end-tidal P_{CO2} difference during laparoscopic CO_2 insufflation in man. Jpn J Physiol 43:361–369
Bardoczky GI et al (1993) Ventilatory effects of pneumoperitoneum monitored with continuous spirometry. Anaesthesia 48:309–311
Benhamou D et al (1993) Diaphragmatic function is not impaired by pneumoperitoneum after laparoscopy. Arch Surg 128:430–432
Böhm B, Milsom JW, Fazio VW (1995) Postoperative intestinal motility following conventional and laparoscopic intestinal surgery. Arch Surg 130:415–419

Chassard D et al (1996) The effects of neuromuscular block on peak airway pressure and abdominal elastance during pneumoperitoneum. Anesth Analg 82:525–527
Couture P et al (1994) Venous carbon dioxide embolism in pigs: an evaluation of end-tidal carbon dioxide, transesophageal echocardiography, pulmonary artery pressure and precordial auscultation as monitoring modalities. Anesth Analg 79:867–873
Erice F et al (1993) Diaphragmatic function before and after laparoscopic cholecystectomy. Anesthesiology 79:966–975
Gannedahl P et al (1996) Effects of posture and pneumoperitoneum during anaesthesia on the indices of left ventricular filling. Acta Anaesthesiol Scand 40:160–166
Gouchet A et al (1995) Gradient PaCO2-PetCO2 durant la coelioscopie chez l'enfant. Ann Fr Anesth Reanim 14 S:R40
Graham AJ et al (1994) Effects of intraabdominal CO_2 insufflation in the piglet. J Pediatr Surg 29:1276–1280
Hirvonen EA, Nuutinen LS, Kauko M (1995) Ventilatory effects, blood gas changes, and oxygen consumption during laparoscopic hysterectomy. Anesth Analg 80:961–966
Horswell JL (1993) Anesthetic techniques for thoracoscopy. Ann Thorac Surg 56:624–629
Ishizaki Y et al (1993) Safe intraabdominal pressure of carbon dioxide pneumoperitoneum during laparoscopic surgery. Surgery 114:549–554
Lavoie J, Burrows FA, Hansen DD (1996) Video-assisted thoracoscopic surgery for the treatment of congenital cardiac defects in the pediatric population. Anesth Analg 82:563–567
Lejus C et al (1996) Randomized single blind trial of laparoscopic versus open appendectomy in children. Effects on postoperative analgesia. Anesthesiology 84:801–806
Lister DR et al (1994) Carbon dioxide absorption is not linearly related to intraperitoneal carbon dioxide insufflation pressure in pigs. Anesthesiology 80:129–136
Lossasso TJ et al (1992) Detection and hemodynamic consequences of venous air embolism. Anesthesiology 77:148–152
Masey SA et al (1985) Effect of abdominal distension on central and regional hemodynamics in neonatal lambs. Pediatr Res 1:1244–1249
McGahren ED, Kern JA, Rodgers BM (1995) Anesthetic techniques for pediatric thoracoscopy. Ann Thor Surg 60:927–930
Mullet CE et al (1993) Pulmonary CO_2 elimination during surgical procedures using intra- or extraperitoneal CO_2 insufflation. Anesth Analg 76:622–626
Murat I et al (1987) Continuous extradural anaesthesia in children. Clinical and haemodynamic implications. Br J Anaesth 69:1441–1450
Pighin G et al (1993) Anästhesiologische Besonderheiten bei laparoskopischen Operationen im Säuglingsalter. Zentralbl Chir 118:628–630
Putensen-Himmer G et al (1992) Comparison of postoperative respiratory function after laparoscopy or open laparotomy for cholecystectomy. Anesthesiology 77:675–680
Raux O et al (1995) Hemodynamic changes associated with laparoscopic surgery in children. Anesthesiology 83:A1155
Rodgers D et al (1992) Thoracoscopy in children: an initial experience with an involving technique. J Laparosc Surg 2:7–14
Sfez M (1994) Anesthésie pour coeliochirurgie en pédiatrie. Ann Fr Anesth Reanim 13:221–232
Sfez M, Guérard A, Desruelle P (1995) Cardiorespiratory changes during laparoscopic fundoplication in children. Paediatr Anaesth 5:89–95
Sfez M et al (1996) Facteurs favorisant les incidents lors de la coeliochirurgie en pédiatrie. Cah Anesthesiol 44:101–102
Tagge EP et al (1994) Impact of laparoscopic cholecystectomy on the management of cholelithiasis in children with sickle cell disease. J Pediatr Surg 29:209–212
Taylor E et al (1992) Anesthesia for laparoscopic cholecystectomy. Is nitrous oxide contraindicated? Anesthesiology 76:541–543
Tobias JD et al (1994) General anesthesia by mask with spontaneous ventilation during brief laparoscopic inspection of the peritoneum in children. J Laparoendosc Surg 4:379–384

Tournadre JP et al (1996) Effect of pneumoperitoneum and Trendelenburg position on gastro-oesophageal reflux and lower oesophageal sphincter pressure. Br J Anaesth 76:130–132

Uzzo RG et al (1997) Laparoscopic surgery in children with ventriculoperitoneal shunts: effect of pneumoperitoneum on intracranial pressure-preliminary experience. Urology 49:753–757

Wahba RWM, Beïque F, Kleiman SJ (1995) Cardiopulmonary function and laparoscopic cholecystectomy. Can J Anaesth 42:51–63

Part II
Chest

CHAPTER 7

Thoracoscopy in Infants and Children: Basic Technique

S.S. Rothenberg

Introduction

Thoracoscopy is a technique which has been in use since the turn of the century. The first experience in humans was reported by Jacobaeus in 1910 (Jacobaeus 1921). He described a technique of using a cystoscope inserted through a rigid trocar to lyse pleural adhesions and cause complete collapse of a lung as treatment for a patient with tuberculosis. Over the next few years he amassed an experience of over one hundred cases using this primitive equipment. During the following 70 years the procedure gained some favor primarily in Europe for the biopsy of pleural based tumors and limited thoracic explorations in adults (Bloomberg 1978; Page et al. 1989). However, the limited nature of the optic system, light source, and instrumentation greatly hampered any significant application of this technique. Biopsy specimens could only be obtained using cup forceps inserted through the telescope sheath, significantly limiting the degree of manipulation and therefore the procedures which could be performed.

The first significant experience in children was reported by Rodgers et al. in the 1970's and 1980's (Rodgers et al. 1979). He used equipment modified for pediatric patients to perform small biopsies, evaluation of intrathoracic lesions, and limited pleural débridement in cases of empyema (Kern and Rodgers 1993; Ryckman and Rodgers 1982). However, it was only in the early 1990's, with the dramatic revolution in technology associated with laparoscopic surgery in adults, that more advanced diagnostic and therapeutic procedures were performed in children (Rodgers 1993; Rothenberg 1994; Rothenberg and Chang 1997). The development of high-resolution microchip cameras and smaller instrumentation has enabled pediatric surgeons perform even the most complicated intrathoracic procedures.

Indications

Today there is a wide variety of indications for thoracoscopic procedures in children and the number continues to expand with advances and refinements in technology and technique. Currently, thoracoscopy is being used extensively for lung biopsy and wedge resection in cases of interstitial lung disease (ILD) and metastatic lesions (Rodgers et al. 1992; Rothenberg et al. 1996):

Histological diagnoses of ILD lung biopsies

- Nonspecific interstitial pneumonitis
- Follicular bronchiolitis
- Diffuse alveolar damage with respiratory syncytical virus
- Lymphocytic interstitial pneumonitis
- Hypersensitivity pneumonitis
- Bronchiolitis obliterans
- Pneumocystis pneumonia
- Cytomegalovirus pneumonitis
- Respiratory syncitial virus pneumonitis
- Acute alveolar hemorrhage
- Allergic bronchopulmonary aspergillosis
- Congenital lymphangiectasia
- Large cell lymphoma
- Acute lymphocytic leukemia
- Normal lung

More extensive pulmonary resections, including segmentectomy and lobectomy have also been performed for infectious diseases, cavitary lesions, bullous disease, sequestrations, lobar emphysema, congenital adenomatoid malformations, and neoplasm (Hazelrigg 1993; McKenna 1994; Walker 1996). Thoracoscopy is also extremely useful in the evaluation and treatment of mediastinal masses (Mack 1993). Biopsy and resection of mediastinal structures such as lymph nodes, thymic and thyroid lesions, cystic hygromas, foregut duplications, ganglioneuromas, and neuroblastomas may be performed thoracoscopically. Other advanced intrathoracic procedures such as patent ductus arteriosus closure, repair of hiatal hernia defects, esophageal myotomy for achalasia, and anterior spinal fusions have also been described (Laborde et al. 1993; Mack et al. 1995; Pellegrini et al. 1992; Rothenberg et al. 1995; Sartorelli et al. 1996) and are presented elsewhere in this volume.

Preoperative Workup

The preoperative workup varies significantly depending on the procedure to be performed. Most intrathoracic lesions require routine radiographs as well as computed tomography (CT) or magnetic resonance imaging (MRI). Thin-cut high-resolution CT is especially helpful in evaluating patients with ILD as it can identify the most affected areas and help determine the site of biopsy. CT-guided needle localization can also be used to direct biopsies for focal lesions which may be deep in the parenchyma and therefore not visible on the surface of the lung during thoracoscopy. MRI may be more useful in evaluating vascular lesions or masses which arise from or encroach on the spinal canal. These studies can be extremely important in determining positioning of the patient and initial port placement.

The other major consideration for the successful completion of most thoracoscopic procedures is whether the patient will tolerate single lung ventilation thus allowing for collapse of the ipsilateral lung to ensure adequate visualization and room for manipulation. Unfortunately there is no test which yields this answer. However, most patients, even those who are ventilator dependent, can tolerate short periods of single lung ventilation which allows for adequate time to perform most diagnostic procedures such as lung biopsy. In cases where single lung ventilation cannot be tolerated other techniques may be used, and these are discussed below.

Preoperative Preparation

Anesthetic Considerations

While single lung ventilation is achieved relatively easily in adult patients using a double-lumen endotracheal tube, the process is more difficult in infants and small children. The smallest available double-lumen tube is a 28-F which can generally not be used in a patient under 30 kg. Another option is a bronchial blocker which contains an occluding balloon attached to a stylet on the side of the endotracheal tube. After intubation this stylet is advanced in the bronchus to be occluded and the balloon is inflated. Unfortunately size is, again, a limiting factor as the smallest blocker currently available is a 6.0 tube. For the majority of cases in infants and small children a selective mainstem intubation of the contralateral bronchus with a standard uncuffed endotracheal tube is effective. At times this technique does not lead to total collapse of the lung as there maybe some overflow ventilation because the endotracheal tube is not totally occlusive. If adequate visualization cannot be obtained then a low flow (1 l/min) low pressure (4 mm/Hg) CO_2 infusion can be used during the procedure to help keep the lung compressed. However, this requires the use of valved trocars rather then simple nonvalved ports. In general hemodynamic and ventilation problems have not arisen as a result of this small amount of positive intrathoracic pressure. This technique can also be used in patients who cannot tolerate single lung ventilation. By using a small tidal volume with lower peak pressures and a more rapid respiratory rate enough collapse of the lung can be achieved to allow for adequate exploration and biopsy. Whatever method is chosen it is imperative that the anesthesiologist and surgeon have a clear plan and good communication to prevent problems with hypoxia and hypercapnia, and to ensure the best chance at a successful procedure.

Positioning

The positioning depends on the site of the lesion and the type of procedure to be performed. While most open thoracotomies are performed in a lateral decubitus position, thoracoscopic procedures should be performed with the patient in a position which allows for the greatest access to the areas of interest and uses gravity to aid in keeping the uninvolved lung or other tissue out of the field of view.

For routine lung biopsies or resections the patient is placed in a standard lateral decubitus position (Fig. 1a). This position provides for excellent visualization and access to all surfaces of the lung. For anterior mediastinal masses the patient should be placed supine with the affected side elevated 20°–30° (Fig. 1b). This position allows for excellent visualization of the entire anterior mediastinum while keeping the lung posterior without the need for extra retractors. The surgical ports may then be placed in the anterior and mid axillary lines with clear access to the anterior mediastinum. For posterior mediastinal masses, esophageal lesions, and work on the esophageal hiatus the patient should be placed in a modified prone position with the affected side elevated slightly (Fig. 1c). This maneuver again allows for excellent exposure without the need for extra retractors.

Once the patient is appropriately positioned and draped, the monitors can be placed in position. For most thoracoscopic procedures it is advantageous to have two monitors one on either side of the table (Fig. 1). The monitors should be placed near the head of the table at or near the level of the patient's shoulder. For procedures primarily in the lower third of the thoracic cavity the monitors should be placed near the foot of the table. The majority of operations can be performed with the surgeon and one assistant. The surgeon should stand on the side of the table opposite the area to be addressed so that he can work in line with

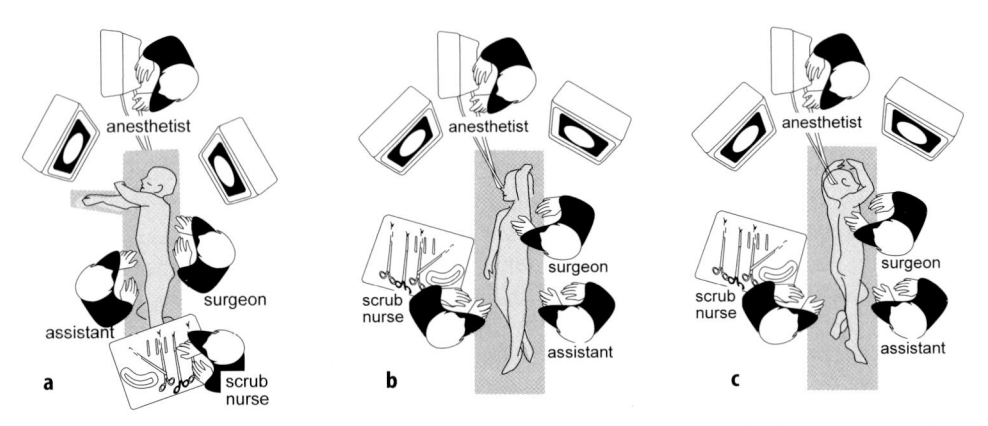

Fig. 1.a. Standard lateral decubitus position. This position provides for excellent visualization and access to all surfaces of the lung. It is advantageous to have two monitors one on either side of the table. In most lung cases such as biopsies the assistant is on the opposite side of the table and is responsible for operating the scope and providing retraction as necessary. **b** Supine position with the affected side elevated 20°–30°. This position allows for excellent visualization of the entire anterior mediastinum. In some cases where the field of dissection is primarily on one side, it is better to have the assistant on the same side as the surgeon so that both may be working in line with the field of view. **c** Modified prone position with the affected side slightly elevated. Ideal position for posterior mediastinal masses, esophageal lesions, and work on the esophageal hiatus

the camera as he performs the procedure. In most lung cases such as biopsies the assistant is on the opposite side of the table and is responsible for operating the scope and providing retraction as necessary (Fig. 1a).

In some cases where the field of dissection is primarily on one side, such as a mediastinal mass, it is better to have the assistant on the same side as the surgeon so that both may be working in line with the field of view (Fig. 1b,c).

Trocar Placement

Positioning of the trocars varies widely with the operation being performed and the site of the lesion. The most commonly performed procedures such as lung biopsy for ILD and decortication for empyema may require wide access to many areas in the thoracic cavity, and in general placement of three ports is adequate. The trocars should be placed in the anterior, middle, and posterior axillary lines between the forth and eighth interspaces (Fig. 2). The midaxillary port should be placed first to allow for modification of the other two ports once an initial survey of the chest cavity has been completed. This triangular arrangement allows for rotation of the telescope and instruments between the three ports giving excellent access to all areas. For localized lesions, such as isolated pulmonary metastasis and mediastinal masses, the trocars should be placed in such a manner as to allow the telescope and working ports to be in line with one another so that the surgeon does not find himself working against the camera, a situation which can make the simplest procedure very difficult. In these cases trocar placement can be tentatively planned based on preoperative imaging studies and then modified once the initial trocar is placed. This trocar should usually be placed across from the area of interest to allow for the widest initial survey.

Instrumentation

The equipment used for thoracoscopy is basically the same as that for laparoscopy. In general 5-mm and 3-mm instrumentation is of adequate size and therefore 5-mm and smaller trocars can be used. In most cases valved trocars are used for the reasons previously discussed. Basic equipment should include 5-mm 0°

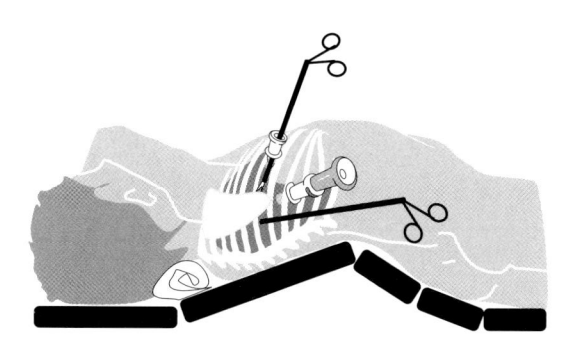

Fig. 2. The trocars should be placed in the anterior, middle, and posterior axillary lines between the forth and eighth interspaces. The midaxillary port should be placed first to allow for modification of the other two ports once an initial survey of the chest cavity has been completed. This triangular arrangement allows rotation of the telescope and instruments between the three ports giving excellent access to all areas

and 30° lenses. If procedures are being performed in smaller children and infants it is also helpful to have smaller lenses such as a short (16–18 cm) 3- or 4-mm wide angle scope and specifically designed shorter instruments. These tools enable the surgeon to perform much finer movements and dissection allowing advanced procedures to be performed in infants as small as 2 kg. A high-resolution microchip camera and light source are also extremely important to allow for adequate visualization especially when using smaller scopes which transmit less light. Basic instrumentation should include curved dissecting scissors, curved dissectors, atraumatic clamps (i.e., 5-mm atraumatic bowel clamp), fan retractor, a suction/irrigator, and needle holders. Disposable instrumentation which should be available include hemostatic clips, endoloops (pretied ligatures), and an endoscopic linear stapler. The linear stapler is a endoscopic version of the GIA used in open bowel surgery. It lays down six to eight rows of staples and divides the tissue between them, providing a air and water tight seal. This is an excellent tool for performing wedge resections of the lung, but unfortunately its current size requires placement of a 12-mm trocar precluding it use in patients weighing much under 10 kg because of the limited size of their thoracic cavity.

Technique

Lung biopsy is the most common thoracoscopic procedure performed, and it is described here to illustrate the basic techniques. The side for the biopsy is chosen based on CXR and CT findings. Under general anesthesia one lung ventilation is obtained if possible and nonvalved ports can be used. The patient is then placed in a lateral decubitus position and prepared and draped as previously described. If it is necessary to perform a mainstem intubation or if the patient cannot tolerate one lung ventilation then a low flow (1 l/min), low pressure (4 mmHg) insufflation with CO_2 can help obtain better collapse of the lung allowing for better visualization. In these cases the chest should first be pierced with a Veress needle to collapse the lung and then valved trocars should be used to help maintain the slight tension pneumothorax. In general a three-trocar technique is sufficient. The first trocar is placed in the midaxillary line in the sixth or seventh intercostal space. After the initial survey the other two trocars are placed anteriorly and posteriorly. In small children all 5-mm ports are used. In children near 10 kg or larger a 12-mm port is placed so that the stapler may be used (Fig. 3a). If a biopsy is being taken from the anterior surface of the lung, the scope should be placed in the posterior trocar, the grasper in the anterior port, and the stapler in the midaxillary site. For biopsies on the posterior surface of the lung the position of the scope and grasper are reversed. In smaller patients whose chest cavity cannot accommodate the stapler, endoloops are used to snare and ligate sections of lung. Two consecutive loops are placed at the base of the specimen and the tissue is sharply excised distal to the ligatures (Fig. 3b,c). This provides a hemostatic and air tight seal equivalent to that obtained with the stapler. Specimens 2–3 cm in size can be obtained in this manner and are more then adequate for diagnosis. Biopsies can easily be obtained from all five lobes using this technique.

For metastatic lesions trocar placement is altered depending on the site of the lesion. Although most of these nodules are peripheral, lesions less the 1 cm in diameter or deeper in the parenchyma of the lung may not be readily visible on the surface of the lung. An endoscopic ultrasound probe has been used, as has direct palpation through a trocar incision, in an attempt to identify these lesions but both have met with limited success. The best technique currently available is CT-guided localization (Mack et al. 1993). Just prior to surgery the patient undergoes CT in which the lesion is identified. A small amount of the patients own blood is then injected through a needle which has been placed in the pleura directly overlying the lesion (Fig. 4a,b). This stains the lung tissue and the visceral pleura at the site of the nodule. At surgery with the lung collapsed this area can easily be identified and if the lesion itself is not visible then the area underlying the bloodstain can be wedged out.

A frozen section is then obtained to ensure the lesion is included with the specimen. The other technique involves the placement of a localizing needle similar to that used in breast biopsies. The problem with this technique is that often the needle is placed posteriorly, making it difficult to lay the patient supine

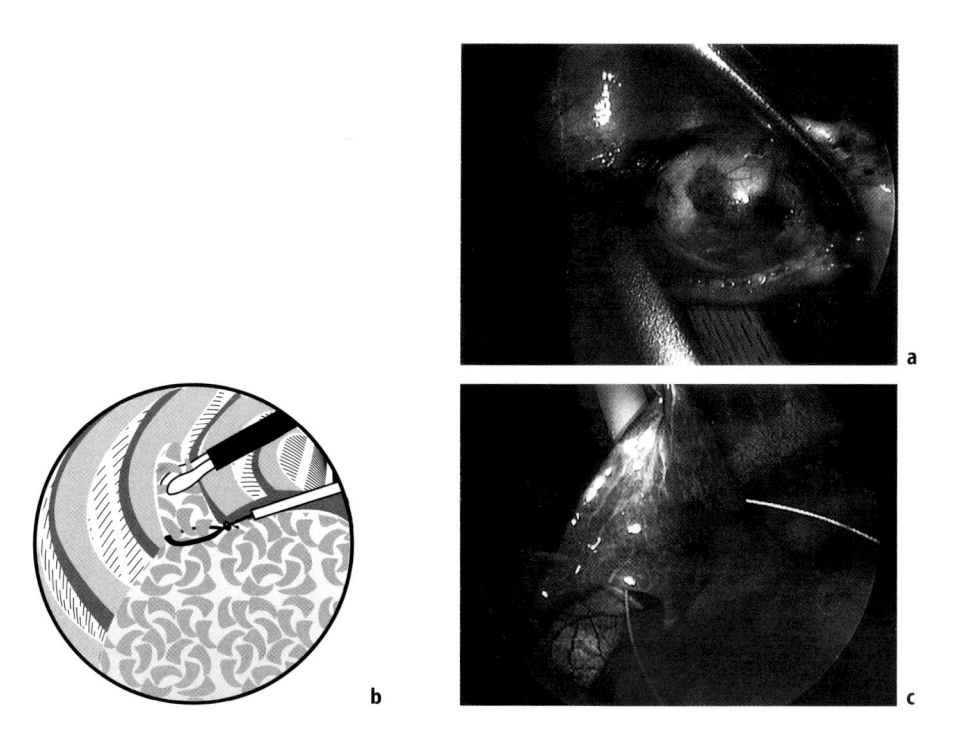

Fig. 3a. Lung biopsy. a With the linear stapler, which requires a 12-mm port and therefore a body weight of 10 kg or more. **b, c** Using pretied ligatures

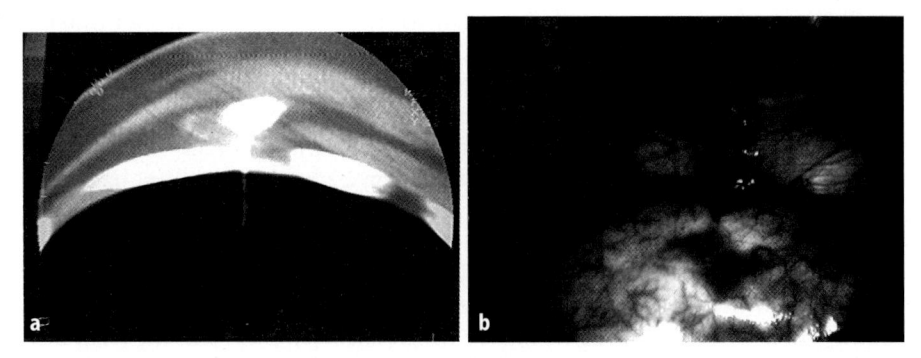

Fig. 4a. CT-guided localization of a metastasis. The patient undergoes CT in which the lesion is identified. A small amount of the patient's own blood is then injected through a needle which has been placed in the pleura directly overlying the lesion. This stains the lung tissue and the visceral pleura at the site of the nodule. **b** At surgery, with the lung collapsed, the area stained with blood can easily be identified, and if the lesion itself is not visible, the area underlying the bloodstain can be wedged out. A frozen section is then obtained to ensure that the lesion is included with the specimen

for intubation. The second difficulty is that when the lung is collapsed the needle may dislodge thus giving a false localization. Ongoing improvements in endoscopic ultrasound probes should eventually make this the technique of choice. Resection of bullae or infectious cavitary lesions can be excised using a similar technique. Any potentially malignant or infectious lesion which cannot be removed entirely through the inner channel of the trocar should be placed in an endoscopic specimen bag to prevent possible seeding.

In dealing with extrapulmonary lesions such as mediastinal masses or esophageal pathology the patient should be positioned as discussed above. The goal in trocar placement is to put the telescope in a position which allows the best direct visualization of the area to be addressed. The working ports are then placed so that the surgeon is working in-line with the camera. The trocars should not be placed too close together; otherwise the instruments and telescope will end up making the dissection much more difficult. If possible, the scope should be placed in a position superior to the working ports to avoid this problem. A 30° scope may be helpful when the working space is limited. To facilitate with identification and the dissection in posterior mediastinal masses or esophageal surgery it is useful to have a flexible gastroscope in the esophagus during the dissection. This helps in identifying the esophagus by illumination within the lumen and by palpation of the scope with the thoracoscopic instruments. It may also be useful in identifying any iatrogenic injuries to the esophagus.

Video-Assisted Thoracoscopic Surgery

Some intrathoracic operations are not amenable to a pure thoracoscopic approach through trocars alone. Either because of the size of the lesion or because of the limitations of the current equipment; certain operations such as formal lobectomies, total esophagectomies, and resection of large tumor masses require a combined approach using two or three thoracoscopic ports in addition to a minithoracotomy (5–6 cm). The thoracotomy incision can be performed using a muscle sparing technique thereby preserving the majority of the benefits of a thoracoscopic approach.

Once the intrathoracic procedure has been completed, a small chest tube is placed through one of the trocar sites and the collapsed lung is ventilated. In most cases where there is no concern over significant continued bleeding, chyle leak, or esophageal perforation the chest tube can be removed prior to extubation in the operating room if there is no evidence of any air leak. This avoids the considerable discomfort associated with the chest tube in the postoperative period. A chest X-ray is obtained in the recovery room and if the lung is fully expanded no further follow-up films should be necessary.

Postoperative Care

Postoperative care in the majority of patients is straight forward. Most patients following biopsy or limited resection can be admitted directly to the surgical ward with limited monitoring (i.e., a pulse oxymeter for 6–12 h). These patients are generally admitted as 23-h observation candidates and a number are actually ready for discharge the same evening. If a chest tube was left in it can usually be removed on the first postoperative day. Pain management has not been a significant problem. Local anesthetic is injected at each trocar site prior to insertion of the trocar and then one or two doses of intravenous narcotic is given in the immediate postoperative period. By that evening or the following morning most patients are comfortable on oral codeine or acetametaphine. It is extremely important, especially in the patients with compromised lung function, to start early and aggressive pulmonary toilet. The significant decrease in postoperative pain associated with a thoracoscopic approach results in much less splinting and allows for more effective deep breathing resulting in a decrease in postoperative pneumonias and other pulmonary complications.

Conclusions

The recent advances in technology and technique in endoscopic surgery have dramatically altered the approach to intrathoracic lesions in the pediatric patient. Most operations can now be performed using a video-assisted thoracoscopic surgery approach, with a marked decrease in the associated morbidity for the patient. This has allowed for an aggressive approach in obtaining tissue for diagnostic purposes in cases of ILD or questionable focal lesions in immunocompromised patients without the fear of significant pulmonary complications previously associated with a standard thoracotomy. In general, a lung biopsy can now be performed with little more morbidity than a transbronchial biopsy yet the tissue obtained is far superior. The same is true for mediastinal masses or foregut abnormalities. Limited biopsy can now be performed as same-day surgery, and lesions such as esophageal duplications can be excised thoracoscopically with the patient ready for discharged the following day. Even patent ductus arteriosus closures are now performed safely thoracoscopically with a hospitalization of less then 24 h. And while an thoracoscopic approach may not always result in a significant decrease in hospital days it may result in a significant decrease in the overall morbidity for the patient. Such as in the case of severe scoliosis patients in whom a thoracoscopic anterior spinal fusion results in earlier extubation, a decreased intensive care unit stay, and in general earlier mobilization. Thoracoscopic surgery has clearly shown significant benefits over standard open thoracotomy in many cases and, with continued improvement and miniaturization of the equipment the procedures we can perform and the advantages to the patient should continue to grow.

References

Bloomberg HE (1978) Thoracoscopy in perspective. Surg Gynecol Obstet 147:433–443
Hazelrigg SR (1993) Thoracoscopic management of pulmonary blebs and bullae. Semin Thorac Cardiovasc Surg 5:327–331
Jacobaeus HC (1921) The pratical importance of thoracoscopy in surgery of the chest. Surg Gynecol Obstet 4:289–296
Kern JA, Rodgers BM (1993) Thoracoscopy in the management of empyema in children. J Pediatr Surg 28:1128–1132
Laborde F et al (1993) A new video assisted technique for the interruption of patent ductus arteriosus in infants and children. J Thorac Cardiovasc Surg 105:278–280
Mack MJ (1993) Thoracoscopy and its role in mediastinal disease and sympathectomy. Semin Thorac Cardiovasc Surg 5:332–336
Mack MJ et al (1993) Techniques for localization of pulmonary nodules for thoracoscopic resection. J Cardiovasc Surg 106:550–553
Mack MJ et al (1995) Video assisted thoracic surgery for the anterior approach to the thoracic spine. Ann Thorac Surg 54:142–144
McKenna RJ (1994) Lobectomy by video-assisted thoracic surgery with mediastinal node sampling. J Thorac Cardiovasc Surg 107:879–882
Page RD, Jeffrey RR, Donelly RJ (1989) Thoracoscopy: a review of 121 consecutive surgical procedures. Ann Thorac Surg 48:66–68
Pellegrini C et al (1992) Thoracoscopic esophagomyotomy: Initial experience with a new approach for the treatment of achalasia. Ann Surg 216:291–299
Rodgers BM (1993) Pediatric thoracoscopy. Where have we come, what have we learned? Ann Thorac Surg 56:704–707
Rodgers BM, Moazam F, Talbert JL (1979) Thoracoscopy in children. Ann Surg 189:176–180
Rodgers DA, Phillippe PG, Lobe TE (1992) Thoracoscopy in children: an initial experience with an evolving technique. J Laparoend Surg 2:7–14
Rothenberg SS (1994) Thoracoscopy in infants and children. Semin Pediatr Surg 3:277–288
Rothenberg SS, Chang JHT (1997) Thoracoscopic decortication in infants and children. Surg Endosc 11:93–94
Rothenberg SS et al (1995) Thoracoscopic closure of patent ductus arteriosus: a less traumatic and more cost effective technique. J Pediatr Surg 30:1057–1060
Rothenberg SS et al (1996) The safety and efficacy of thoracoscopic lung biopsy for diagnosis and treatment in infants and children. J Pediatr Surg 31:100–104

Ryckman FC, Rodgers BM (1982) Thoracoscopy for intrathoracic neoplasia in children. J Pediatr Surg 17:521–524

Sartorelli KH et al (1996) Thoracoscopic repair of hiatal hernia following fundoplication: a new approach to an old problem. J Laparoend Surg 6:S91–S93

Walker WS (1996) Video assisted thoracic surgery: pulmonary lobectomy. Semin Laparosc Surg 3:233–244

Diagnostic Thoracoscopy in Children

B.M. Rodgers

Introduction

The initial description of thoracoscopy by Jacobaeus in 1910 was exclusively for therapeutic indications, closed intrapleural pneumolysis, in patients with pulmonary tuberculosis [1]. With an appreciation of the full capabilities of thoracoscopy, however, Jacobaeus described in 1922 its use for diagnostic purposes in patients with pulmonary carcinoma [2].

Indications

In the past three decades thoracoscopy has been used in Europe principally for the diagnosis of pleural disorders, such as malignant pleural effusions and mesotheliomas. In 1976 we described our experience with the use of thoracoscopy for pulmonary biopsy for the diagnosis of diffuse pulmonary infiltrates in immunocompromised children [3]. A review of most pediatric thoracoscopy series at this time shows that the most common indication for the procedure is for the diagnosis of mediastinal masses [4]. Thoracoscopic lung biopsy for children with diffuse pulmonary infiltrates or localized processes represents the second most common indication. The use of thoracoscopy for the diagnosis of pleural disease, such as chylothorax and pneumothorax, represents a significantly less common indication in pediatric series than in adults.

Mediastinal Masses

Thoracoscopy represents an elegant technique for the diagnosis of mediastinal masses in children. The entire mediastinal compartment, both anterior and posterior to the pulmonary hilum, can be directly visualized by thoracoscopy and the relationship of masses to vital mediastinal structures, such as the aorta and its branches and the superior vena cava, can be readily appreciated. Preoperative imaging studies are of great importance in these patients in order to plan the positioning of the patient and the best direction of access for the thoracoscopic instruments. Chest CT usually provides the information necessary. Most thoracoscopic procedures for mediastinal pathology should be performed under general anesthesia, utilizing unilateral ventilation. Manipulation of the mediastinal pleura and mediastinal structures often stimulates coughing when this procedure is performed under regional anesthesia, interfering with stable visualization of the area to be dissected. We employ contralateral mainstem intubation in most patients to achieve unilateral ventilation, although a double lumen endotracheal tube may be employed in adolescent patients. We often supplement the general anesthesia with a four-rib intercostal block to allow a lighter level of anesthesia to be used. Patients with huge mediastinal masses, with tracheal compression, may be biopsied under regional anesthesia, avoiding the substantial risk of general anesthesia in this population (Fig. 1).

After the induction of general anesthesia the patient is placed in the lateral decubitus position. Access to lymph nodes in the anterior hilar region or anterior mediastinal masses is facilitated by rolling the patient posteriorly about 45°. Access to posterior hilar nodes or cysts or paraspinous masses is facilitated by rolling the patient anteriorly about 45° (Fig. 2). The initial cannula is placed in the midaxillary line in the sixth intercostal space for most anterior mediastinal masses. Visualization of posterior lesions may be facilitated by moving the initial cannula position to the posterior axillary line. The InnerDyne expandable cannula on a Veress needle is inserted straight through the intercostal musculature into the pleural space. Tunneling this cannula, as one does for a chest tube, limits the maneuverability of the cannula in the thorax. The cannula is expanded to depending on the size of the child to 5- or 10-mm to accept a 5- or 10-mm 0° telescope. A pneumothorax is induced by opening this cannula to atmospheric pressure. We do not employ intrapleural gas insufflation but prefer to open the pleural space to atmospheric pressure through the operating cannulas to allow the lung to drop away from the chest wall.

The entire hemithorax is inspected, including the lung and pleural surfaces to search for areas of unsuspected pathology. The mediastinal lesion is then identified and its relationship to adjacent vital structures ascertained. Two 5-mm In-

Fig. 1. Frontal chest radiograph of a 10-year-old girl with large mediastinal mass. This lesion compressed the trachea and caused some respiratory symptoms. The patient underwent right thoracoscopy, performed under regional anesthesia in a semi-upright position. Biopsies of the mediastinal mass revealed non-Hodgkin's lymphoma

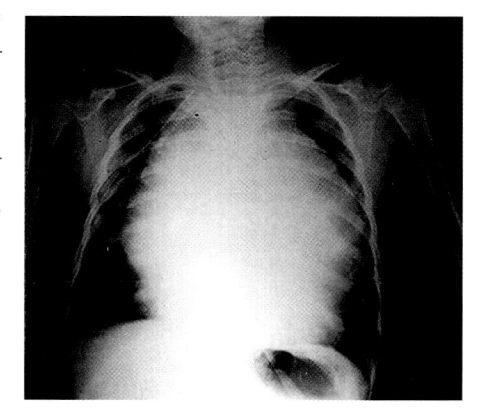

Fig. 2. Position of the patient and operating team for diagnostic thoracoscopy. The patient is placed in a full lateral decubitus position or rolled anteriorly or posteriorly, depending upon the area to be investigated. The surgeon stands on the side opposite the lesion and the assistant on the other side

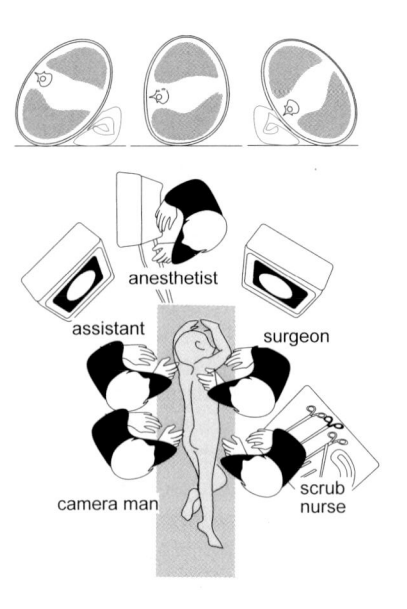

nerDyne cannulas are then inserted, usually one anterior to the telescope and one posterior. Through these cannulas grasping forceps and scissors are passed, and the mediastinal pleura overlying the mass is incised. Once the pleura is opened, extension of the incision can be carried out with the hook cautery. The mass is bluntly dissected to expose a generous portion of its surface. Enlarged lymph nodes are then biopsied using 5-mm cup biopsy forceps. Several biopsies are taken through the same site to ensure that deeper tissue is obtained in addition to superficial tissue. In the case of enlarged mediastinal lymph nodes a Trucut needle is passed transthoracically under direct vision, and deep tissue core biopsies are obtained. If purulent material is encountered as the mass is opened, this can be suctioned into a Lukens collection trap for culture and Gram stain.

Hemostasis is achieved with the electrocautery applied either through the biopsy forceps or suction. In some cases the entire mass can be resected with blunt and sharp dissection and removed. If a malignancy is suspected, the lesion should be removed in a specimen sack to prevent implantation in the cannula site. In case a 10-mm cannula has been used the 10-mm telescope is withdrawn and replaced with a 5-mm endoscope inserted through one of the 5-mm operating cannulas. The endosac is then introduced through the 10-mm cannula for removal of the tissue. The mediastinum is irrigated, and final hemostasis is achieved prior to removing the cannulas. A chest tube (14–18 F) is placed through the midaxillary cannula site and an epidural catheter is inserted through the posterior cannula site. Intrapleural marcaine (0.7 cc/kg 0.25% marcaine with epinephrine) is administered through the pleural catheter prior to leaving the operating room and every 4 h postoperatively. The remaining cannula site is closed in layers with absorbable sutures. Bronchogenic or enterogenous cysts of the mediastinum can usually be dissected free of surrounding structures with sharp dissection and removed completely. The cysts can be decompressed by passing a needle across the chest and aspirating them. Care must be exercised in the case of enterogenous cysts not to enter the lumen of the esophagus. This dissection may be facilitated by passage of a large esophageal bougie or endoscope prior to initiating the dissection.

Thoracoscopy has proven to be a safe and reliable method to achieve a tissue diagnosis in children with mediastinal masses. There has been no mortality reported with this procedure, and the diagnostic accuracy exceeds 95% [5, 6]. It is hoped that obtaining the deeper Tru-cut biopsies will reduce the false-negative biopsy rate. These patients recover quickly following thoracoscopy and chemotherapy and irradiation therapy may be started immediately.

Pulmonary Biopsy

Thoracoscopy provides an excellent method of pulmonary biopsy in carefully selected patients with either diffuse or localized pulmonary infiltrates. Patients with diffuse pulmonary infiltrates who are on high pressure mechanical ventilation at the time of biopsy are probably better served with an open pulmonary biopsy. It is often very difficult to achieve an adequate pneumothorax in these patients, and visibility at thoracoscopy is frequently limited. In addition, the high peak inspiratory pressures make postoperative bronchopleural fistulas more common. In a review of the complications of pediatric thoracoscopy in 1993 we found that virtually all of the mortality and most of the morbidity following thoracoscopy in children occur in this set of patients [6]. On the other hand, patients with diffuse pulmonary infiltrates who are not mechanically ventilated represent excellent candidates for thoracoscopic biopsy. Patients with localized infiltrates or subpleural pulmonary nodules often can be successfully diagnosed by thoracoscopy as well [7].

Preoperative posteroanterior and lateral chest roentgenograms often are sufficient to plan the thoracoscopic procedure in these patients. In patients with pulmonary nodules a chest computed tomography (CT) may help to confirm the subpleural location of these lesions. Nodules located deeper within the pulmonary parenchyma may be difficult to identify at the time of thoracoscopy because of the limitations in the ability to "palpate" the pulmonary parenchyma. Preoperative localization of such nodules with CT-guided wires has been described in adult patients but has not been reported in children. The choices of anesthesia for these procedures varies from regional anesthesia, which is quite satisfactory for biopsy of diffuse infiltrates, to general anesthesia with unilateral ventilation, which facilitates the excisional biopsy of subpleural nodules [8]. Patients with localized infiltrates are often most easily biopsied with general anesthesia with spontaneous tracheal ventilation. The use of unilateral ventilation in these patients often makes location of the area of infiltrate difficult as the entire lung becomes atelectatic. The patient is usually placed in a full lateral decubitus position, although oblique positioning may facilitate exposure of a partic-

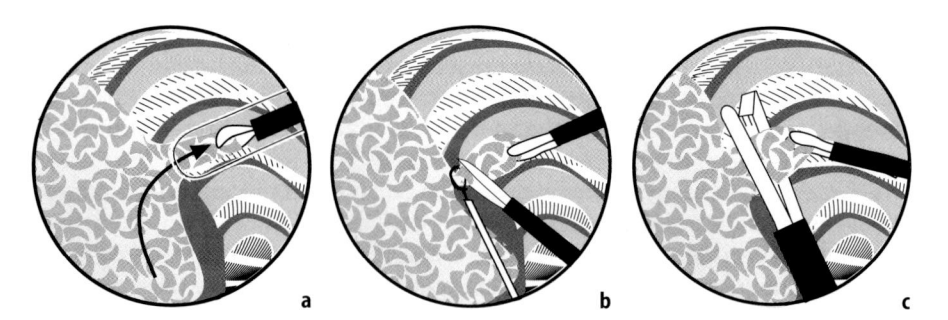

Fig. 3a-c. Methods of obtaining pulmonary parenchymal biopsy. **a** Pulmonary tissue is grasped with the biopsy forceps and shirred off by withdrawing the forceps into the thoracoscopy trocar. **b** A small tuft of pulmonary tissue is isolated with an pretied ligature and excised. **c** The endoscopic linear stapling instrument is used to excise a larger piece of pulmonary tissue

ular localized process. The chest is prepared and draped in wide fashion to facilitate placement of operating cannulas.

The initial cannula is placed in the midaxillary line, sixth intercostal space. We use a 10-mm InnerDyne expandable cannula on a Veress needle for the initial entry into the pleural space. The entire hemithorax is inspected with the initial telescope to detect other areas of pathology. In larger patients, older than 3 or 4 years, an endoscopic linear stapler may be employed for pulmonary biopsy. This instrument is passed through a 12-mm cannula, placed either anterior or posterior to the telescope through the lowest possible inner space. A second 5-mm cannula is then used for forceps to grasp the pulmonary parenchyma. Additional 5-mm cannulas may be necessary for lung retraction. The biopsy pieces are withdrawn through the 12-mm cannula with large grasping forceps. Suspected malignant lesions should be placed in a specimen sack for removal to avoid contamination of the tissues of the chest wall. In smaller patients, in whom an endoscopic linear stapler is too long to employ, biopsy specimens may be obtained either by shearing the parenchyma off with cup biopsy forceps or placing an endoloop on a tuft of pulmonary tissue and sharply excising the tissue distal to the ligature (Fig. 3). Additional hemostasis is achieved with the electrocautery. An epidural catheter is left through the posterior most cannula site for intrapleural analgesia postoperatively, and a small chest tube (12–14 F) is placed through the midaxillary cannula site. Any remaining cannula tract is closed in layers with absorbable sutures.

Thoracoscopy has proven to be a very accurate method for achieving a specific diagnosis in patients with diffuse pulmonary infiltrates. The diagnostic accuracy of these biopsies has approached 100% [6]. Likewise, patients with localized processes are accurately diagnosed by thoracoscopy with very little morbidity.

Pleural Disorders

Thoracoscopy has proven useful in the diagnosis and treatment of several pleural disorders in children, although the frequency of its reported use is less than in the adult population.

Spontaneous Pneumothorax

Thoracoscopy has been used to diagnose and treat the causes of spontaneous pneumothorax in children. In the management of pneumothorax in children it has been uniformly successful, with no mortality or morbidity encountered.

Chylothorax

Thoracoscopy has also been proven uniformly valuable in managing spontaneous and posttraumatic chylothorax, where it is associated neither with mortality nor with morbidity. Patients with chylothorax who have not responded to 5–10 days of closed pleural drainage are considered candidates for thoracoscopic evaluation [9]. Patients in whom the etiology is thought to be congenital or posttraumatic, where there is likely to be an isolated source of lymph leakage, are ideal candidates for this procedure. Children with postoperative chylothorax, in whom a wide area of the mediastinum has been opened, may not be good candidates for this technique as there may be a more diffuse lymph leakage. Preoperative imaging studies are limited to posteroanterior and lateral chest roentgenograms. If the patient has an indwelling chest tube in place this tube is clamped for a variable period of time before thoracoscopy to allow accumulation of some pleural fluid. Thoracoscopy in these patients should be performed under general anesthesia with unilateral ventilation to allow complete collapse of the ipsilateral lung and thorough mediastinal exploration.

The patient is placed in the full lateral decubitus position, and the chest is prepared and draped widely. The initial InnerDyne expandable cannula is placed in the sixth intercostal space, midaxillary line. The cannula is expanded, and a 10-mm 0° telescope is placed. A 5-mm expandable cannula is placed posteriorly in the 5th intercostal space for a suction apparatus. The residual pleural fluid is suctioned from the chest and cultured if appropriate. The mediastinal pleura is then carefully examined from the apex of the chest to the diaphragmatic surface to detect areas of lymphatic leakage. A second 5-mm expandable cannula may be placed anterior to the telescope for a retractor to facilitate this exposure. In cases of congenital and posttraumatic chylothorax an area of pleural disruption is usually identified in the mediastinum. This area is then obliterated either with deep nonabsorbable sutures or with metallic clips placed through one of the 5-mm cannulas. If necessary, one of the 5-mm cannulas can be expanded to a 10-mm sheath to allow placement of a larger clip applier.

Fig. 4a.b. Thoracoscopic approach to the thoracic duct. The duct is identified just above the diaphragm between the azygos vein and the esophagus, which may be retracted anteriorly for exposure. The duct is occluded at this point with multiple clips

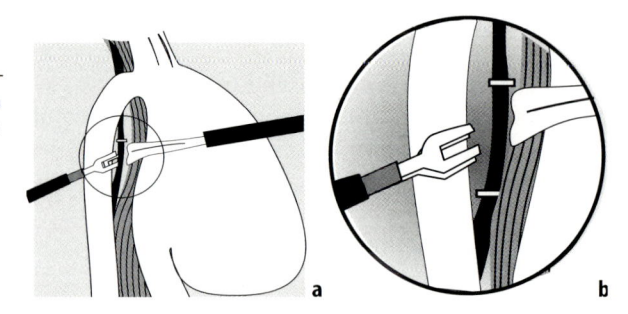

The area of lymphatic leakage is then flooded with fibrin glue to achieve a complete seal of the pleura in this region. If a specific area of lymphatic leakage cannot be identified, or if there appears to be a generalized weeping of lymphatic fluid, the thoracic duct can be occluded as it enters the chest on the right side through the aortic hiatus [10]. The right inferior pulmonary ligament is divided with the hook cautery, and the mediastinal pleura over the inferior vena cava is opened with the cautery or scissors. The thoracic duct lies in the tissue between the inferior vena cava and the azygous vein, to the right of the esophagus. In some cases the duct can be identified discretely and occluded with metallic clips. In other cases the duct cannot be specifically identified and clips are applied to all of the tissue in this region (Fig. 4). A chest tube (16–20 F) is placed through the largest cannula site, and an epidural catheter is placed through the most posterior site. The other cannula tracts are closed in layers. Postoperatively the patient is administered intrapleural marcaine through the epidural catheter.

Conclusion

The value of thoracoscopy has been confirmed in the diagnosis of various intrathoracic disorders in children. The procedure is well tolerated, with acceptable levels of mortality and morbidity. Serious complications may be minimized by careful patient selection. The diagnostic accuracy of thoracoscopy is equivalent to that of open thoracotomy. Postoperative pain is significantly reduced. In the absence of a thoracotomy incision chemotherapy and radiation therapy may be instituted immediately, if required. With greater experience and better instruments new diagnostic uses for this technique will undoubtedly be developed.

References

1. Jacobaeus HC (1910) Ueber die Moglichkeit die Zystoskopie bei Untersuchung seröser Höhlungen anzuwenden. Munch Med Wochenschr 57:2090–2092
2. Jacobaeus HC (1922) The practical importance of thoracoscopy in surgery of the chest. SGO 34:289–296

3. Rodgers BM, Talbert JL (1976) Thoracoscopy for diagnosis of intrathoracic lesions in children. J Pediatr Surg 11:703–708
4. Rodgers BM (1993) Thoracoscopic procedures in children. Semin Pediatr Surg 2 (3):182–189
5. Kern JA et al (1993) Thoracoscopic diagnosis and treatment of mediastinal masses. Ann Thorac Surg 56:92–96
6. Rodgers BM (1993) Pediatric thoracoscopy: where have we come and what have we learned? Ann Thorac Surg 56:704–707
7. Landreneau RJ et al (1992) Thoracoscopic resection of 85 pulmonary lesions. Ann Thorac Surg 54:415–419
8. McGahren ED, Kern JA, Rodgers BM (1995) Anesthetic techniques for pediatric thoracoscopy. Ann Thorac Surg 60:927–930
9. Graham DD et al (1994) Use of video-assisted thoracic surgery in the treatment of chylothorax. Ann Thorac Surg 57:1507–1511
10. Kent RB, Pinson TW (1993) Thoracoscopic ligation of the thoracic duct. Surg Endosc 7:52–53

Thoracoscopy in the Treatment of Empyema in Children

B.M. Rodgers

Introduction

Pleural empyema represents an infection of the pleural space caused either by direct introduction of bacteria, as in cases of surgery or trauma, or by indirect contamination from infections in adjacent organs, as in cases of pneumonia or subphrenic abscesses. In children the most common source of empyema is pneumonia, while postoperative infection represents the second most common etiology. Our understanding of the pathophysiology of empyema was advanced by the conclusions of the Graham Commission in 1918. The recommendations for treatment of empyema made by this group still form the basis of our treatment strategies today:
- The infected fluid within the pleural space must be completely drained. This should be performed early in the development of empyema using closed techniques, while in late stage empyema, open drainage may be more effective.
- Chronic empyema should be avoided by early therapy of the infected pleural space.
- Careful attention should be paid to the nutritional status of the patient [1].

The pathological progression of empyema has been divided into three stages. The initial stage, the exudative stage, represents the accumulation of a thin pleural effusion containing white blood cells, protein and occasionally bacteria. It is thought that this effusion develops from a capillary leak of the visceral pleura adjacent to an inflammatory process. The exudative stage lasts 3–5 days and progresses into the fibrinopurulent stage of empyema. This stage is characterized by the accumulation of more pleural fluid containing white blood cells and numerous bacteria. Fibrinous material is deposited on both the visceral and parietal pleural surfaces. As more fibrin forms, the fluid becomes loculated by fibrinous septae, joining the visceral and parietal pleural surfaces. The fibrinopurulent stage of empyema may last for several weeks. The final stage of the infection, the organization stage, occurs with the proliferation of fibroblasts on the pleural surfaces, forming an inelastic covering which prevents full lung expansion. Successful management of empyema requires treatment in the exudative or fibrinopurulent stages, before the development of chronic pulmonary entrapment.

Empyema in children is usually monomicrobial in nature. *Staphylococcus aureus* represents the most common offending organism with *Streptococcus pneumoniae* and *Hemophilus influenzae* being the next most common. With the routine use of vaccination for *S. pneumoniae* and *H. influenzae* infections in children the incidence of *Staphylococcus empyema* seems to be increasing. Anaerobic pleural infections are unusual in children. No pathogen can be cultured from the empyema fluid in 5%–25% of cases [2].

Indications

The appropriate treatment for empyema in children remains controversial. Effective therapy requires control of the infection, drainage of the infected fluid from the pleural space, and full expansion of the lung, as suggested by the Graham Commission. Antibiotic therapy is based upon cultures obtained either by sputum collection or thoracentesis. The critical clinical decision involves the timing of pleural drainage. Many patients in the exudative stage, with small pleural effusions, resorb the effusion with effective antibiotic therapy alone, while others require closed tube drainage. Light has suggested basing this decision on the characteristics of the empyema fluid obtained by thoracentesis [3].

Patients with any one of the following characteristics require tube thoracostomy: (a) the pleural fluid is grossly purulent; (b) the Gram strain of the pleural fluid is positive; (c) the pleural fluid glucose is less than 40 mg/dl; or (d) the pleural fluid pH is less than 7.00. Hoff has suggested an Empyema Severity Score using these characteristics as well as radiological signs as a method of making this treatment decision [4]. We use somewhat more aggressive and clinically based criteria in treating empyema in children. Any patient with gross purulence in the pleural space on thoracentesis should have a tube thoracostomy; otherwise tube drainage is reserved for those patients with large pleural effusions (greater than 3 cm from the chest wall) or in whom the pleural effusions fails to improve within 48–72 h of appropriate antibiotic therapy. Prior to tube thoracostomy patients should undergo transthoracic ultrasound study to determine the presence of loculation of the pleural fluid. Patients in whom loculation is demonstrated are considered candidates for more extensive pleural débridement (so-called "decortication"). Traditionally an open thoracotomy has been the method of choice for pleural débridement [5, 6]. The magnitude of this procedure, however, often caused delayed referral of children until late in the course of empyema. In 1985 Braimbridge reported the use of thoracoscopy with pleural débridement and subsequent pleural irrigation for the treatment of adults with empyema [7]. We first reported our experience with thoracoscopy in the management of empyema in children in 1993 [8]. There have been several subsequent papers that confirm its utility in this clinical situation [9–11].

Preoperative Workup

The child with suspected empyema, unresponsive to antibiotic therapy, based on clinical presentation and standard chest radiography (Fig. 1a), should undergo transthoracic ultrasound. This study can reliably demonstrate the presence of pleural fluid and can identify fibrinous septae with loculation (Fig. 1b) Patients with loculated fluid or persistent fluid and symptoms after antibiotic therapy and closed tube drainage are considered candidates for a thoracoscopic pleural débridement. The radiologist is requested to mark the center of the largest locule of pleural fluid during the ultrasound study. If there is a question of whether the fluid represents an empyema or a lung abscess a chest computed tomography may be helpful.

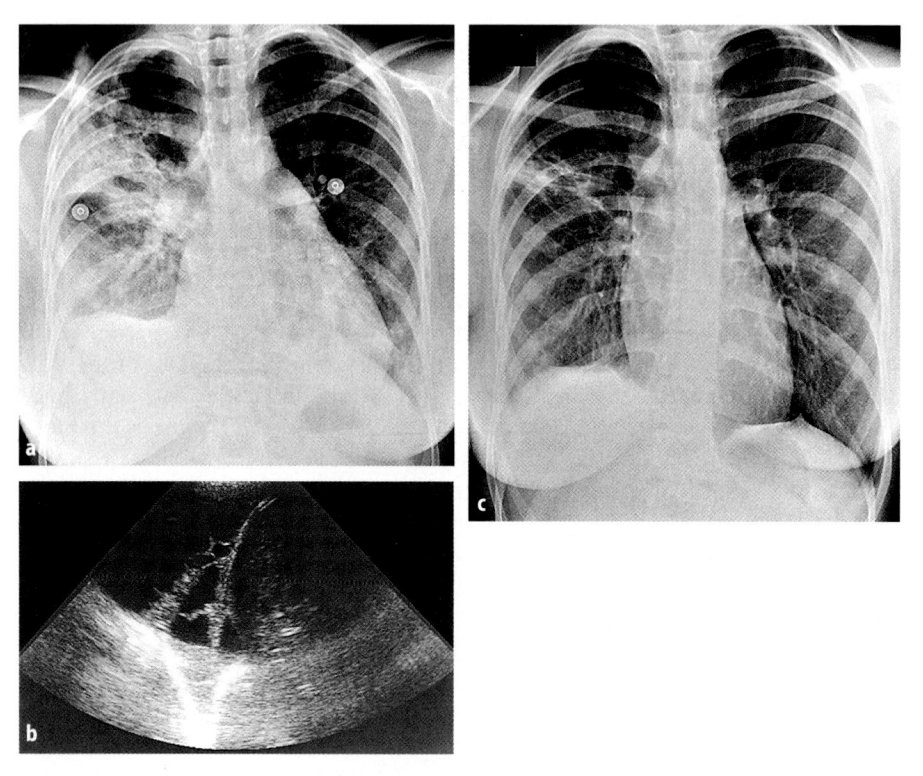

Fig. 1a-c. a Frontal chest radiograph of a 16-year-old girl with right upper lobe pneumonia. A right pleural effusion had developed while she received antibiotics and she remained febrile. **b** Transthoracic ultrasound demonstrated pleural fluid with multiple locules. **c** Frontal radiograph 3 weeks following thoracoscopic pleural débridement demonstrated a resolving process. The patient was asymptomatic at this time

Preoperative Preparation

The thoracoscopy procedure is performed under general anesthesia. Vigorous pleural débridement is painful and difficult to accomplish using regional anesthetic techniques. Bronchoscopy should be performed prior to intubation if there is a question of airway obstruction complicating the empyema, or if cultures of tracheal aspirates are required. The procedure is facilitated by unilateral ventilation, although it may be successfully performed with tracheal ventilation. We attempt to perform a contralateral mainstem intubation in these patients to achieve unilateral ventilation.

Technique

The patient is placed in the lateral decubitus position on the operating table with the area marked by the radiologist in an uppermost position (Fig. 2). The chest is prepared and draped widely to allow flexibility in placement of the operating trocars. We often use a four-rib intercostal block with 0.25% marcaine and epinephrine to encompass the region of trocar insertions to supplement the general anesthesia and to provide some postoperative analgesia. The surgeon stands at the front of the patient as most locules are located posteriorly. The initial trocar, a 10-mm expandable InnerDyne cannula, is placed at the point marked by the radiologist, into the center of the largest locule. Fluid can be aspirated through the Veress needle as it enters the pleural space if cultures have not already been obtained. A 10-mm 0° telescope is placed through this cannula to visualize the pleural space. Thin pleural adhesions may be broken down with the tip of the telescope to create a substantial pleural locule, into which may be placed other trocars. InnerDyne cannulas (5-mm) are placed under direct vision for a cautery-suction instrument and scissors. The remainder of the pleural adhesions are divided under direct visualization with either blunt or sharp dissection.

Fig. 2. Position of the patient and operating team for thoracoscopic débridement of a right-sided empyema. The patient is positioned with the chest wall mark, placed by the radiologist, uppermost. The surgeon stands to the patient's front with the assistant and camera operator to the patient's back. Monitors are placed on both sides of the operating table

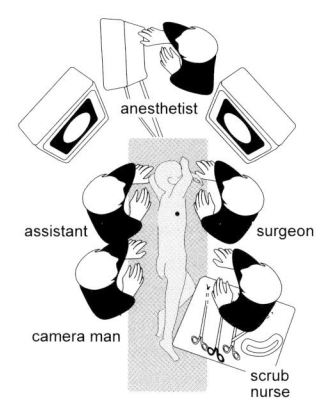

The cautery may be used for more vascular appearing adhesions, seen in the later stage empyemas. It is important that the entire pleural space be opened from paravertebral gutter to anterior mediastinum and from the apex of the chest to the diaphragmatic surface to be confident that there are no residual locules of purulent fluid. Familiar anatomic landmarks should be used to determine the completion of the pleural dissection. The residual pleural fluid is aspirated, and the fibrinous material is débrided from the pleural surface using the suction and biopsy forceps. A thorough débridement of both the visceral and parietal pleura should be performed. Forceful irrigation of the pleural space with saline through the suction instrument may facilitate this process. In patients in whom considerable pleural debris is present, one of the 5-mm cannulas may be expanded to 10 mm and a large suction instrument inserted. After completion of the débridement the anesthesiologist is asked to expand the ipsilateral lung under direct observation. If less than complete expansion is achieved, further attempts at débridement of the visceral pleural surface should be attempted. A relatively large chest tube (20–24 F) is placed through the posterior cannula site and guided to the apex of the chest under direct vision. The remaining cannula sites are closed in two layers with absorbable sutures.

Postoperative Care

If less than a complete pleural débridement can be achieved thoracoscopically, a small epidural catheter is left in the pleural space and urokinase (250,000 U in 60 ml saline) is instilled daily postoperatively for 3–4 days. Intravenous antibiotics are continued postoperatively until the patient is afebrile and the initiating infection is controlled. The chest tube is removed when 24-h drainage is less than 60 cc and the chest radiography demonstrates clearing of the pleural space (Fig. 1c).

Personal Experience

Over the past 15 years we have treated 22 children with empyema by thoracoscopic débridement. There has been one death in this series, an 11-year-old boy in whom an unsuspected pulmonary relapse of acute leukemia was diagnosed at the time of thoracoscopic pleural débridement. This patient died of pneumonia which developed at a time when he was on chemotherapy, 2 months following successful treatment of the empyema. One patient required a second thoracoscopic débridement for a persistent pleural locule, 3 days following the first procedure. In all other cases the procedure was successful in eliminating the infection. The mean time of postoperative chest tube drainage was 5 days.

Conclusion

Thoracoscopy provides an effective and minimally invasive method of pleural débridement in children with complicated empyema. It should be applied in the early stages of empyema, prior to the development of a fibrothorax. Thoracoscopy has the advantages over open thoracotomy in providing a wide view of the entire hemithorax and less postoperative pain [12].

References

1. Bryant RE, Salmon CJ (1996) Pleural empyema. Clin Infect Dis 22:747–764
2. Campbell PW (1995) New developments in pediatric pneumonia and empyema. Curr Opin Pediatr 7:278–282
3. Light RW (1992) Management of empyema. Semin Respir Med 13:167–176
4. Hoff SJ et al (1989) Postpneumonic empyema in childhood: selecting appropriate therapy. J Pediatr Surg 24:659–664
5. Hoff SJ et al (1990) Parapneumonic empyema in children: decortication hastens recovery in patients with severe pleural infections. Pediatr Infect Dis J 10:194–199
6. Eren N et al (1995) Early decortication for postpneumonic empyema in children. Scand J Thor Cardiovasc Surg 29:125–130
7. Hutter JA, Harari D, Braimbridge MV (1985) The management of empyema thoracis by thoracoscopy and irrigation. Ann Thor Surg 39:517–520
8. Kern JA, Rodgers BM (1993) Thoracoscopy in the management of empyema in children. J Pediatr Surg 28:1128–1132
9. Silen ML, Weber TR (1995) Thoracoscopic debridement of loculated empyema thoracis in children. Ann Thor Surg 59:1166–1168
10. Stovroff M et al (1995) Thoracoscopy in the management of pediatric empyema. J Pediatr Surg 30:1211–1215
11. Davidoff AM et al (1996) Thoracoscopic management of empyema in children. J Laparendosco Surg 6 [Suppl 1]:S51–S54
12. Mackinlay TA et al (1996) VATS debridement versus thoracotomy in the treatment of loculated postpneumonia empyema. Ann Thorac Surg 61:1626–1630

Therapeutic Thoracoscopic Procedures in Children: Indications and Surgical Applications in Lung and Mediastinum

J-L. Michel, Y. Revillon

Introduction

Lung and mediastinal biopsies performed thoracoscopically were initially described by Rodgers et al. in 1976 [8]. Since these early reports advances in instrumentation techniques (endoclip, endostapler, microchip camera, miniaturization) and improved surgical expertise have enabled thoracoscopy to be used in a wide variety of diagnostic and therapeutic procedures. Surgical education is improved because the surgical field can be watched by the entire team on a television monitor.

Mediastinal dissection and resection, vascular interruption, segmental and lobar lung resection can be performed. These procedures are generally more difficult in children than in adults, particularly in small children because selective ventilation is not well tolerated, and the size of some instruments is not convenient, and some procedures require minithoracotomy.

There is no contraindication to thoracoscopy. This procedure is impossible only where there is an inability to create a "pleural window" through which the telescope and operating instruments can be introduced. Pleural adhesions may make induction of the initial pneumothorax and separation of the visceral and parietal pleura impossible, but this is extremely uncommon in children. There are no age or weight restrictions when performing thoracoscopic procedures, which can be performed under the same circumstances as an open procedure. Interventions in premature infants less than 1.5 kg of weight have been reported [5].

Thoracoscopic surgery in children is still a new technique for many pathologies and procedures as lung resection. The definitive indications will be specified during the next few years.

Indication for Therapeutic Procedure in Lung and Mediastinum

Mediastinal Cysts: Bronchogenic Cysts, Esophageal Duplications, Pleuropericardial Cysts. These are the main indications for therapeutic thoracoscopic procedures in children (17 cases in our own experience). Pleuropericardial cysts are located in the anterior and inferior mediastinum as a liquid translucent pouch with poor vascularization and without pericystic adhesion. Bronchogenic cysts and esophageal duplications are located in the middle or in the posterior mediastinum at variable level: paratracheal, paraesophageal, hilar, under the carina. Dissection and resection of these are generally straightforward. In cases of infection, large size, or localization under the carina, thoracoscopic removal can be difficult and must be discussed.

Lung Masses. When they are small sized and peripheral, and removable by wedge resection, lung masses can be operated on by thoracoscopy. Evaluation of lung masses may be diagnostic (cancer primary lesion or metastasis), prognostic (active cells, necrotic tissue, or fibrous scars), or curative by complete resection. The main indication is the evaluation and the resection of lung masses in osteogenic sarcoma [4]. Large masses which require segmental or lobar resection are exceptional cases in pediatric surgery. In cases of malignant disease the necessity of a complete exploration and palpation of the lung and mediastinum nodes make a thoracoscopic procedure questionable.

Pulmonary Sequestrations, Cystic Adenomatoid Malformations, Giant Lobar Emphysema. Few cases of treatment by thoracoscopy have been reported in these diseases. These are often difficult procedures due to distension of affected parenchyma, absence of cleavage plane, infection, problems of pneumostasis and hemostasis and inexperienced surgeons. All these arguments make the indications questionable. Pulmonary sequestration can be removed in its extralobar form [10], while intralobar forms can be treated by systemic vascular occlusion by clips (our own experience). If a pulmonary lobe is completely affected, lobar resection can be performed [6]. Cystic adenomatoid malformations can be resected if small and in a peripheral location. Giant lobar emphysema is too large and not deflated in spite of pneumothorax or insufflation; thus thoracoscopic procedures should be avoided.

Recurrence of Spontaneous Pneumothorax. Recurrence of spontaneous pneumothorax is a good indication for thoracoscopy. It allows visualization of all the lung and pleural cavity from the bottom to the top. The aim is to search for responsible subpleural blebs, to resect them, and then to perform a pleurodesis. The most frequent cases are in cystic fibrosis. Particularly in this disease this procedure should be limited to untolerated recurrence of spontaneous pneumothorax because a history of pleural and pulmonary surgery may prevent pneumonectomy and lung transplantation.

Bronchiectasis. When only the middle lobe is affected, fissure and pedicular dissection can be performed and the entire middle lobe resected by thoracoscopy [1]. Lower and upper lobe resection is very difficult in bronchiectasis because there are many lymph nodes and inflammatory tissue around the hilum, and the fissure is difficult to dissect.

Hydatid Cysts. The original technique described by Becmeur et al. allows treatment of hydatid cysts by thoracoscopy [2].

Neurogenic Tumors, Myasthenia and Thymoma. Resection of neurogenic tumor such as ganglioneuroma can be performed by thoracoscopic surgery after controlling by computed tomography or magnetic resonance imaging the absence of intraspinal extension [7]. In myasthenia and thymoma thoracoscopic resection has been reported [11]. These disease are rare in pediatric patients, and the indication of thoracoscopic procedure are questionable in regard of cervicomanubriotomy. Cervicomanubriotomy is in fact minimally invasive surgery and allows a good control of complete resection of thymus.

Preoperative Preparation

Children are placed in the lateral decubitus position. Preoperative planning for patient positioning and cannula placement is essential. Gravity can be used to help retracting the lung from the line of vision. For anterior mediastinal masses, the patient is placed in a 45° lateral decubitus position, and for posterior mediastinal lesions, the patient is rotated into an exaggerated lateral decubitus position (Fig. 1). The arm is elevated for interventions involving the upper part of the hemithorax but dropped for interventions in the lower part, a padding is placed under the contralateral hemithorax. Classical incision of thoracotomy is drawn with dermographic pencil. The entire chest is prepared and draped.

The surgeon usually stands on the side of the patient opposite the lesion and maintain line of sight in the same axis as the thoracoscope. The instrument assistant is in front of the surgeon. The assistant is in front of the surgeon for manipulation of thoracoscope and lung retractor in upper or lower procedures, or beside the surgeon for avoidance of mirror image manipulation in the middle hemithorax procedures. The monitor must be placed in front of the surgeon in the line of working, at the top of the patient for upper thoracic procedures, at the bottom for lower procedures. Two monitors are preferable: one in front of the surgeon, and the other in the front of the assistant. A bridge table with the

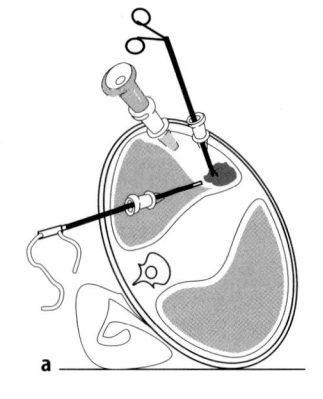

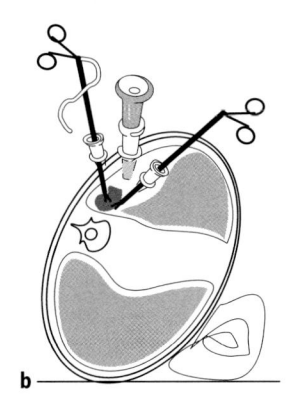

Fig. 1a,b. Orientation of patient for resection of mediastinal cysts. **a** Anterior mediastinal cyst. The patient is placed in a 45° lateral decubitus position, allowing the lung to fall posteriorly. **b** Posterior mediastinal cyst. The patient is placed in an exaggerated lateral decubitus position, allowing the lung to fall forward. The cyst is emptied after fine needle aspiration and dissected with electrocautery scissors. In both cases the instruments are placed using the basic principles of triangulation most used instruments is placed at the level of the patient's legs. Two instruments bags are placed at the level of pelvis in the front and the back for thoracoscope, dissector, suction cannula. Others instruments such as bistoury, suture, and thoracotomy instruments are placed on a table near the instrument assistant.

A three-trocar technique is used for most cases. The first port site for thoracoscope introduction depends on the procedure performed. The usual position is in the fifth, sixth, or seventh intercostal space on the posterior axillary line. The optimal position of other access sites for the trocars for the retracting and operating instruments depends on the precise localization of the lesion, and must be placed into the chest cavity under thoracoscopic visualization using the basic principles of triangulation. If possible, access ports are placed along the site of a proposed thoracotomy incision and chest tube exit site to limit the number of incisions in case of associated thoracotomy.

The classic instruments used are:
- Rigid endoscope 0° or 30°: 5-mm diameter is used in younger children, 10-mm in patients over the age of 4–6 years. Angle telescope allows a better view than 0° in parietal and apical disease.
- 3- or 5-mm diameter graspers, scissors, biopsy forceps, hook, aspiration cannula.
- Clip applier (5 or 10 mm).
- Endoscopic linear stapler lays down six rows of staples and divides the tissue between them providing an air- and water-tight seal. For its use a 12-mm port is required. This port must be placed low in the chest because the distal 5 cm of the stapler must be in the thorax before the anvil can be fully opened. It is awkward to use in patients younger than 4–6 years of age.
- Monopolar or bipolar electrocautery hook or dissecting scissors.
- Lung retractors (5- or 10-mm).
- Palmer or Veress needle insufflation. In rare cases of insufficient collapsed lung and a small "pleural window" avoiding a good vision and instrument manipulation, insufflation can be used with a low-flow (1 l/min) and low-pressure (4 mmHg) CO_2 infusion.
- Thoracoscopic ports (3, 5, 10, 12 mm). In rare cases of insufflation thoracoscope and instruments are introduced through valved ports identical to those used for laparoscopy. In the majority of cases without insufflation unvalved ports are used. In some cases the instruments can be introduced through the thoracic wall without port, allowing tools of various diameters to be used without changing port.

Several manufacturers have introduced shorter instruments that are easier to manipulate in small patients.

The choice of instrumentation depends on the anticipated goals of the technique, and are most similar to the type of instruments that they would use for a comparable open procedure.

Fig. 2. Resection of subpleural apical blebs in the left lung. The thoracoscope is placed in the sixth intercostal space in the midaxillary line. A grasper is placed in the fourth intercostal space in the posterior axillary line, and an endostapler in the fourth intercostal space in the anterior axillary line

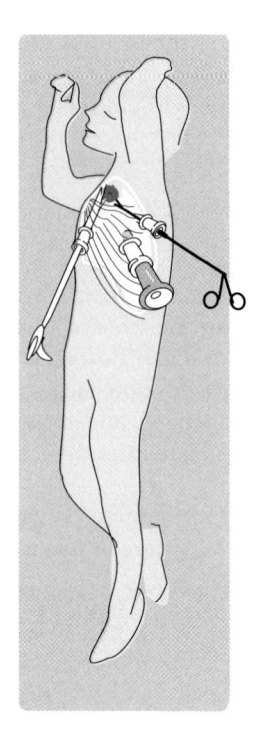

Instruments for thoracotomy in case of conversion must be in the operating room near the instrument assistant.

Trocar sites depend on the precise location of the pathology.

Anterior and Superior Lesions (Thymic Disease, Nodes, Apical Subpleural Blebs). The thoracoscope is placed in the midaxillary line in the sixth intercostal space (Fig. 2). Other trocar sites depend on the location of the lesion. Usually placed in the fourth or fifth intercostal space, one in the anterior and one in the posterior axillary line. It may be helpful to place an additional trocar for lung retraction in the midaxillary line in the third intercostal space.

Posterior Lesions (Mediastinal Cysts, Neurogenic Tumors, Pulmonary Sequestration). The thoracoscope is placed in the posterior axillary line in the fifth or sixth intercostal space (Fig. 3). Other trocar sites depend on the location of the lesion. Usually one in the sixth intercostal space posteriorly, and one in the midaxillary line in the fourth or fifth intercostal space (for superior lesions) or in the midaxillary line in the seventh intercostal space (for inferior lesions). It may be helpful to place an additional trocar for lung retraction in the posterior axillary line in the third intercostal space (for superior lesions) or in the eighth intercostal space (for inferior lesions).

Anterior and Inferior Lesions (Pleuropericardial Cysts, Pericardial Window). The thoracoscope is placed in the midaxillary line in the fifth or sixth intercostal

Fig. 3. Resection of esophageal duplication in the left posterior mediastinum. The thoracoscope is placed in the sixth intercostal space in the posterior axillary line. A lung retractor is placed in the third intercostal space in the midaxillary line, a grasper in the fifth intercostal space in the midaxillary line, and an electrocautery hook in the posterior part of the sixth intercostal space

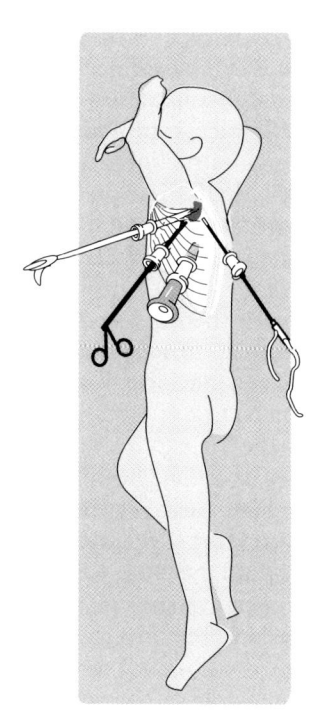

space. Other trocar sites depend on the precise location of the lesion. Usually one is placed in the posterior axillary line in the seventh intercostal space, and one in the anterior axillary line in the fourth or fifth intercostal space. It may be helpful to place an additional trocar for lung retraction in the midaxillary line in the eighth intercostal space.

Technique

Excision of Mediastinal Cysts or Masses

Precise localization of the lesion by preoperative computed tomography or magnetic resonance imaging is very important because patient positioning depends on the localization of the lesions. For superior lesions, the arm must be elevated for axillary access. For an anterior mediastinal lesion the patient is placed in a 45° lateral decubitus position, which allows the lung to drop posteriorly (Fig. 1a). For posterior mediastinal lesions, the patient is rotated into an exaggerated lateral decubitus position, which allows the lung to fall anteriorly (Fig. 1b). Trocar sites depend on the precise location of the pathology. The principle of triangulation must be respected, avoiding mirror image manipulation.

Almost the entire anterior and posterior mediastinum is visible by thoracoscopy. Posterior lesions in the region of the inferior pulmonary vein are difficult to access without dividing the inferior pulmonary ligament.

For cysts, (bronchogenic cyst, esophageal duplication, pleuropericardial cysts) dissection is often easier after fine needle aspiration, especially in very large cysts avoiding introduction and manipulation of the instruments. Three trocars are usually used: one for the thoracoscope and two for the other instruments. A fourth can be necessary for lung retraction. The principles of dissection are the same as those in open surgery. Mediastinal pleura must be incised. The lesion is grasped and pulled with an instrument and dissection and separation of other mediastinal tissue is performed with an electrocautery hook or dissecting scissors. Resection is generally easy with a combination of blunt and sharp dissection, and without hemorrhage. If there is any question of the lesion being cystic or vascular, a long needle is passed through one of the operating trocars and the lesion is aspirated. Aspiration of a mucous material suggests a bronchogenic cyst or esophageal duplication. Dissection is difficult in cases of infection, very large cysts and localization under the carina. In situations in which the cyst shares a common wall with the trachea or esophagus this portion of the cyst wall may be left attached, and the mucosa in this area may be stripped or destroyed with electrocautery. After resection the cysts are removed through the trocar aperture.

Solid masses are dissected until the pararachidian area for the neurogenic tumors. After resection they are removed in a plastic bag through one of the trocar aperture. The trocar aperture must be converted to a very small thoracotomy for removing the largest lesions.

One or two chest tubes are inserted under vision control through trocar sites guided with a grasper, and removed after 1 or 2 days.

Wedge Resection of Lung Masses

The site of the trocars depends on the localization of the lesion. Three trocars are inserted: one in the anterior axillary line in approximately the fourth intercostal space, one in the midaxillary line in the seventh or eighth intercostal space, and one in the posterior axillary line at the fourth or fifth space. In children older than 4–6 years a 12-mm port is located at the anterior site to provide access for the endo-stapler. The best site for the thoracoscope depends on the localization of the lesion: inferior for upper lobe lesions, posterior for anterior and inferior lesions, and anterior for posterior lesions. The lesion site is exposed with the grasper, and the last trocar site for ligature or stapling is chosen according to the lesion site (ideally with 90° angle with traction axis of grasper).

In younger children a ligature is used with preformed endoloop or extracorporal knot, and placed at the base of the lesion. An endo-stapler is used in older children, whose larger intercostal space allows the introduction of a 12-mm trocar, and pleural cavity large enough to allow the opening and manipulation.

One or two chest tubes are inserted under vision control through trocar sites guided with a grasper, and removed after 1 or 2 days.

Pulmonary Sequestration

In cases of pulmonary sequestration located in the inferior part of the hemithorax, the trocars are placed as described previously for posterior and inferior lesions. The lung is retracted in the front, and systemic vessels are exposed in the lower posterior mediastinum, and closed by clipping or stapling. Sequestrated lung parenchyma can be separated from normal lung and resected in cases of extralobar form. The sequestrated lung tissue is grasped and pulled with an atraumatic forceps, and dissection and separation of normal lung is performed with electrocautery dissecting scissors. After resection the lesion is removed through a trocar aperture. One or two chest tubes are inserted under vision control through trocar sites guided with a grasper, and removed after 2 or 3 days. A history of infection can make this dissection difficult. In cases of intralobar sequestration, affected parenchyma can be left in place after ligation of the systemic artery (our own experience). Indeed the absence of a cleavage plane prevents the possibility of separation with good hemostasis and pneumostasis by thoracoscopy. Resection of the right lower lobe in case of an intralobar sequestration has been described after introduction of a 5-mm trocar in the fifth intercostal space in the midaxillary line, and two 12-mm trocars in the sixth intercostal space in the posterior axillary line and in the eighth intercostal space in the midaxillary line [6]. The fissure is dissected, and the vessels are sectioned with a vascular endo-stapler. The lower bronchus is dissected and sectioned with a parenchyma endo-stapler.

Recurrence of Spontaneous Pneumothorax

In these cases resection of subpleural blebs and pleurodesis is performed. Children are usually older than 10 years. The subpleural blebs are usually located in the apical region. The patient is placed in lateral decubitus position, arm elevated. The surgeon is behind the patient, the assistant is placed in front. Three access sites are necessary (Fig. 2). The thoracoscope is placed in the sixth or seventh intercostal space in the midaxillary line, and two ports are placed in the fourth or fifth intercostal space in the anterior and in the posterior axillary line. Trocars used are 10 mm (5 mm in smaller children), and one of them is to be changed for a 12-mm trocar for introducing the stapler in the best place. The pleural cavity is explored, adhesives bands are cut, and subpleural blebs located in the lung. Exploration of the apex of the lung is facilitated by a 30° thoracoscope. The area of air leakage is located by instillation of saline on the slightly ventilated lung. This area and the subpleural blebs are exposed with a grasper and resected by endo-stapling. Pediculized subpleural blebs can be ligated. Then pleurodesis can be accomplished by mechanical abrasion. Pleural abrasion is performed by using a piece of knitted polypropylene (Marlex) attached to a forceps. Abrasion of the entire parietal pleural surface can be achieved in this manner, ideally with a curved instrument thus avoiding dead angles. Some authors report using talc for the pleurodesis [9].

Two chest tubes are inserted under vision control through trocar sites guided with a grasper, and removed after 3 or 4 days.

Pulmonary Lobectomy

Middle Lobectomy in Bronchiectasis. The patient is placed in the lateral decubitus position, with padding under the contralateral hemithorax. The surgeon is behind the patient, and the assistant is placed in front. Three or four access sites are necessary: one is placed in the fifth intercostal space in the posterior axillary line, one in the seventh intercostal space in the midaxillary line, and the third in the fifth or sixth intercostal space in the anterior axillary line. Trocars used are 10 mm (5 mm in younger children), and one of them is replaced by a 12-mm trocar for introducing the endo-stapler in the best place. The affected middle lobe is pulled with an atraumatic forceps to open the fissure. Fissure is dissected with an electrocautery hook and dissecting scissors, and the hilum of middle lobe is exposed. Vessels are dissected and closed with ligature or clip then cut. The middle lobe bronchus is closed by ligature or endo-stapling. Pneumostasis is controlled with perfusion of saline on the bronchial stump. Two chest tubes are inserted under vision control through trocar sites guided with a grasper, and removed after 2 or 3 days.

Other Lobectomies. Right lower lobectomy has been performed as previously reported in pulmonary sequestration [6]. Upper and lower lobectomy remain very difficult in pediatric patients. However, these procedures can be performed using video-assisted techniques. A minithoracotomy achieved by a muscle-sparing technique is associated with the use of two or three thoracoscopic ports.

Hydatid Cysts

Thoracoscopic treatment of hydatid cysts was reported by Becmeur et al. [2]. In their procedure the children received albendazole perioperatively. They were selectively intubed. The pleural cavity was explored, and filled with hypertonic solution. The cyst was punctured, washed with hypertonic solution and evacuated by suction. The dome of the cyst was incised and the membrane was removed. Fistulas in cystic cavity were sutured, and finally the cystic and pleural cavities were drained.

Thymectomy

The patient is placed in a 45° left lateral decubitus position. Four access sites are necessary. The mediastinal pleura is incised using scissors just in front of the superior vena cava to expose the thymus. Dissection is then carried out behind the sternum toward the contralateral side. The thymus is dissected by gentle traction and blunt dissection and separated from pericardium, aorta, and brachiocephalic vein. Thymic vessels are divided using electrocautery or clipping. The thymus is removed in a plastic bag through one of the trocar apertures. Complete resection must be confirmed by examination of the thymic bed and resected specimen [11]. One chest tube is inserted under vision control through one of the trocar site guided with a grasper, and removed after 1 or 2 days.

Results

There is no specific difference in postoperative care compared with open surgery. Most mediastinal cysts (bronchogenic cyst, esophageal duplication, pleuropericardial cyst) can be resected completely with thoracoscopic techniques. In our series this procedure was successful in 15 of 17 cases. The failures were related to previous infection or to location under the carina.

Resections of lung masses (active metastasis, necrotic or fibrous tissue) in cancer (osteosarcoma, Wilms' tumor, Ewing's tumor, rhabdomyosarcoma, hepatoblastoma) are performed successfully in the majority of cases because they are found in peripherally and subpleurally [4, 12]. However, this procedure performed by thoracoscopy is controversial. The only merit of surgical resection for metastatic disease is the ability to resect all metastases. The reported recurrence rates after thoracoscopic surgery suggest that thoracoscopic resection of pulmonary metastasis is inadequate [12]. Complete bimanual palpation of the lung through the open technique can identify more occult metastatic nodules that may not be identified with the thoracoscopic approach. However, there is no evidence that resection of occult nodules is associated with improved survival [3].

Recurrent pneumothorax is eliminated in nearly 100% of the patients, but there is some concern about using this modality in patients who may be candidates for lung transplantation because the density of the pleural sclerosis achieved can preclude pneumonectomy.

Cystic adenomatoid malformations, and pulmonary sequestrations are often difficult to resect by thoracoscopic procedure due to difficulties in exposure and cleavage plane, and must be associated with short thoracotomy.

Lung resection in giant lobar emphysema seems to be difficult or impossible because of distension of affected parenchyma.

Reported results of treating middle lobe bronchiectasis and hydatid cysts by thoracoscopy are comparable to those in open surgery.

Thymectomy by thoracoscopic procedure is questionable in regard of cervicomanubriotomy. Indeed cervicomanubriotomy is really a minimal invasive surgery and allows a good control of complete resection of thymus. Long-term follow-up will clarify the role of thoracoscopic thymectomy in treatment of myasthenia gravis and thymoma.

Conclusion

The advantages of thoracoscopic procedures for treating thoracic diseases are obvious. The pain and morbidity compared with open surgery are almost nonexistent. Most of the mediastinal masses and cysts can be removed successfully as in open surgery with uneventful follow-up. In these lesions the place of open surgery becomes restricted. For lung surgery thoracoscopic procedures are always limited by the inability to palpate and resect small masses, by difficulty to dissect hilum and fissure in case of infection, and by the large size of endo-staplers. For these reasons only lung biopsy, wedge resection of peripheral masses, cysts or blebs may be performed routinely by thoracoscopy. For the other indications such as segmental or lobar resection individual cases should be considered and performed by an experienced team.

In the future the improvement of surgical expertise, instrumentation, and anesthetic techniques in selective ventilation will allow to do most of the lung resections and esophageal surgery endoscopially.

References

1. Balquet P et al (1994) La chirurgie video endoscopique dans le traitement des dilatations des bronches de l'enfant. Proceedings of the 51st congress of the Société Francaise de Chirurgie Pédiatrique, September, Paris
2. Becmeur F et al (1994) La chirurgie thoracique vidéo-assistée des kystes hydatiques du poumon chez l'enfant. J Chir 131:541–543
3. Dowling RD et al (1993) Video assisted thoracoscopic resection of pulmonary metastases. Ann Thorac Surg 56:772–775
4. Holcomb GW et al (1995) Minimally invasive surgery in children with cancer. Cancer 76:121–128
5. Laborde F et al (1995) Video-assisted thoracoscopic surgical interruption: the technique of choice for patent ductus arteriosus. J Thorac Cardiovasc Surg 110:1681–1684
6. Mezzeti M et al (1996) Video-assisted thoracoscopic resection of pulmonary sequestation in an infant. Ann Thorac Surg 61:1836–1838
7. Riquet M et al (1995) Videothoracoscopic excision of thoracic neurogenic tumors. Ann Thorac Surg 60:943–946
8. Rodgers BM, Talbert JL (1976) Thoracoscopy for diagnosis of intrathoracic lesions in children. J Pediatr Surg 11:703–708
9. Tribble CG, Selden RF, Rodgers BM (1986) Talc poudrage in the treatment of spontaneous pneumothoraces in patients with cystic fibrosis. Ann Surg 204; 677–680
10. Watine O et al (1994) Pulmonary sequestration treated by video-assisted thoracoscopic resection. J Cardio Thorac Surg 8:155–156
11. Yim APC, Kay RLC, Ho JKS (1995) Video-assisted thoracoscopic thymectomy for myasthenia gravis. Chest 108:1440–1443
12. Yim APC et al (1995) Video-assisted thoracoscopic wedge resections of pulmonary metastatic osteosarcoma: should it be performed. Aust N Z J Surg 65:737–739

CHAPTER 11

Thoracoscopic Repair of Hiatal Hernia in Children

S.S. Rothenberg

Introduction

The incidence of a pure paraesophageal hiatus hernia in infants and children is relative rare, but the development of one following a fundoplication is a more common event. In fact the incidence of hiatal hernia following fundoplication has been reported at between 2% and 17% [1–4]. This can result in symptoms of dysphagia, failure to thrive, pain or colic, or recurrence of severe reflux. Typically this problem has been dealt with by abdominal exploration, reduction in the fundoplication back into the abdomen, and repair of the esophageal hiatus. This approach can often be extremely difficult because of the previous surgery and resultant scarring making the risk of esophageal injury high. To avoid the necessity of re-entering a previously operated field the esophageal hiatus can be approached using a thoracic approach and thoracoscopic techniques [5]. This same approach can be used for other lower esophageal lesions such as achalasia and foregut duplications. The basic technique is described below.

Indications and Preoperative Workup

The thoracic approach to the repair of a paraesophageal hiatus hernia can be used in any patient whether the hernia is associated with a previous fundoplication or has occurred spontaneously. However, since repair of most spontaneous hiatal hernias also require an antireflux procedure, these are usually best approached using an abdominal or laparoscopic approach. This technique is best utilized in the patient who has undergone a previous fundoplication but whose wrap has since herniated into the chest. If the wrap is intact then reduction in the herniated contents, and repair of the hiatal defect is all that is necessary; this can be easily achieved through a thoracic approach, thereby avoiding the previously operated field. These patients usually present with complaints of dysphagia, or in infants as a sudden decrease in oral intake. The workup should consist of a barium swallow to diagnose the hiatal hernia and to evaluate the integrity of the wrap. If necessary, upper flexible endoscopy and or a pH probe may be performed to complete the evaluation. If total disruption of the fundoplication is present then a intrathoracic wrap (i.e., Belsey Mark IV), or a repeat fundoplication through an abdominal approach can be performed. If the wrap is intact, a thoracoscopic approach is appropriate.

Preoperative Preparation

Positioning

After the patient is anesthetized, single-lung ventilation should be obtained to allow for collapse of the left lung. The patient is then placed in a modified prone position with the left side elevated 30°. The surgeon and assistant are positioned to the patient's left, and the monitor is placed to the patient's right near the foot of the bed (Fig. 1). Prior to the start of the procedure a flexible gastroscope is passed into the midesophagus and left in place throughout the procedure. This is used to help identify the esophagus and to evaluate the success of the repair. If an endoscope is not available, a bougie should be placed to help define the esophagus and ensure that the crural repair is not too tight.

Positioning of Trocars

Four trocars (5 mm) are generally sufficient to perform the procedure. The chest is first pierced with a Veress needle in the posterior axillary line at approximately the 7th intercostal space and a low flow low pressure of CO_2 is infused to help collapse the left lung. A 5-mm port is then inserted and a 5-mm 0° or 30° telescope is placed in this port. The two working ports are then placed in approximately the midaxillary line between the 7th and 10th interspaces to perform the dissection (Fig. 2). An attempt should be made to have these two ports spread far enough apart so that a 30° angle exists between them otherwise the suturing becomes to cumbersome. The forth port is placed in line with the tip of the scapula

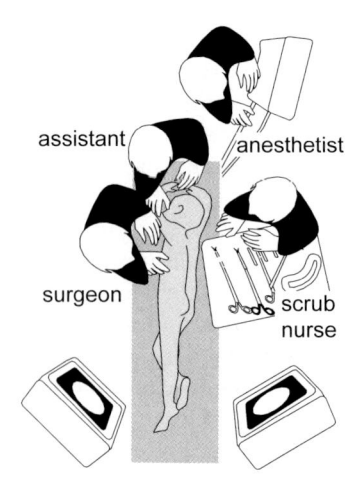

Fig. 1. Position of the patient, crew, and equipment

Fig. 2. Position of the trocars

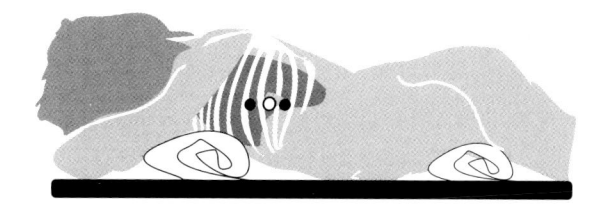

at approximately the 6th or 7th interspaces and is used to retract the lower lobe superiorly, thereby exposing the hiatus. Occasionally a fifth port is necessary to retract the diaphragm inferiorly to better show the hernia defect and crura.

Instrumentation

Depending on the size of the child 3-mm or 5-mm standard laparoscopic instruments are adequate. Instruments needed include dissecting scissors, curved dissectors, babcock clamps in order to safely reduce the stomach and grasp the crura, needle holders, and a fan retractor to retract the lung or diaphragm.

Once the left lung has been collapsed, and the trocars are in place, the first step is to take down the inferior pulmonary ligament, thus mobilizing the left lower lobe. There is usually a small vessel running through the ligament, and care should be taken to cauterize or clip it as otherwise it can create troublesome bleeding which may obscure the field. The lower lobe is retracted superiorly with the fan retractor and this exposes the esophageal hiatus. The gastroscope light source is now turned on to provide illumination of the esophagus to help in its identification. The pleura overlying the hiatal defect is incised and the hernia sac wrap is reduced into the abdominal cavity (the CO_2 insufflation aids in this), and the crural repair is performed. The crura are reapproximated behind the esophagus using a heavy-gauge braided suture. If the hiatal defect is extremely large, partial closure anterior to the esophagus may be indicated. The most medial stitch should also include a bite through the wall of the esophagus helping to further prevent herniation of the wrap (Fig. 3). At completion of the crural closure the gastroscope is used to access the adequacy of the repair, and air is insufflated in the esophagus to check for any esophageal injury. The lung is reexpanded and a chest drain is placed through one of the trocar sites to aid in this process. If no air leak is present, the drain can be removed with the lung under positive pressure prior to extubation in the operating room.

Postoperative Care

If no esophageal injury has been incurred, the patient can be admitted to the general ward for observation. A nasogastric tube is not necessary as there should be little postoperative ileus and feedings are resumed 6–8 h postoperatively. The patients are generally ready for discharge by the second postoperative day. A

Fig. 3. Crural repair with incorporation of the wall of the esophagus to prevent further herniation

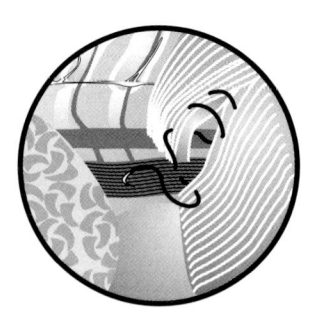

barium swallow should be obtained after 2–4 weeks to access the adequacy of the repair and to ensure the integrity of the fundoplication.

Results

We have used this technique in five patients who have presented with post-fundoplication paraesophageal hernias (three Toupet and two Nissen fundoplications all performed open). The average operative time has been 80 min (range 45–120 min). All children resumed oral or g-tube feeds on the first postoperative day and were on full feeds by day 2. The average hospital stay was 2.2 days. There were no operative or postoperative complications. Follow-up barium studies in each case showed the hernia repair and the fundoplication to be intact. Mean follow-up is 26 months.

Discussion

The development of a hiatal hernia following a standard open abdominal fundoplication is not an uncommon event. The incidence in the pediatric population has been recorded as high as 17% and has been documented following Nissen, Toupet, and Thal fundoplications. Attempts to revise the fundoplication and repair the paraesophageal hernia through an abdominal approach can be associated with significant morbidity because of the necessity of going through a previously operated and scarred field. Complication rates as high as 43% have been documented for these repeat operations, and these procedures are often associated with long operative times and prolonged hospital stays. A thoracoscopic approach in these cases allows the surgeon to avoid the previously operated field, with its difficult exposure and significant risk of esophageal, gastric or splenic injury.

In our series all of the patients presented with an acute onset of gastrointestinal symptoms which in the infants presented as poor feeding and in the older patients as dysphagia and epigastric pain. In each case the preoperative workup identified the paraesophageal hernia but suggested that the fundoplication was still intact. Since there was no evidence of recurrent reflux, a thoracoscopic approach which avoided the risks of approaching the hiatus from the abdomen seemed an appropriate choice. Following repair the preoperative symptoms resolved and further surgical correction was not necessary.

This approach provides excellent visualization of the lower thoracic esophagus and esophageal hiatus. It is an excellent approach not only for paraesophageal hernias but also for myotomies for achalasia, and for the resection of lower esophageal lesions such as duplications or leiomyomas.

References

1. Alrabeeah A, Giacomamanio M, Gillis DA (1988) Paraesophageal hernia after Nissen fundoplication in pediatric patients. J Pediatr Surg 23:766–768
2. Ashcraft KW et al (1984) The Thal fundoplication for gastroesophageal reflux. J Pediatr Surg 19:480–483
3. Festen C (1981) Paraesophageal hernia: a major complication of Nissen fundoplication. J Pediatr Surg 16:496–499
4. Caniano DA, Ginn-pease M, King DR (1990) The failed antireflux procedure: analysis of the risk factors and morbidity. J Pediatr Surg 25:1022–1026
5. Sartorelli KH et al (1996) Thoracoscopic repair of hiatal hernia following fundoplication: a new approach to an old problem. J Laproend Surg 6 [Suppl 1]:S91–S93

Closure of Patent Ductus Arteriosus

F. Laborde, T. Folliguet

Introduction

Pediatric video-assisted thoracic surgery (VATS) applications have been limited by a lack of equipment and techniques adapted to small infants. However, recently the introduction of a small video-camera has allowed the development of surgical operations in children. Pediatric VATS was initially reported for patent ductus arteriosus (PDA), followed by vascular ring divison, collateral interruption (arterial and venous), pericardial drainage, thoracic ductus interruption and diagnostic VATS (location of aberrant coronary artery) [1-4]. We started performing VATS in the pediatric population for patent ductus arteriosus closure in 1991, and since then we have performed over 300 cases.

Indications

All children presenting either an isolated PDA or PDA associated with a more complex congenital lesion can undergo the procedure. Age itself is not a contraindication since this technique has been performed in premature infants. The only contraindications are if the diameter of the ductus is greater than the size of the clip (9 mm), or if the ductus is calcified. Both of these situations can be encountered in older children or adults. In children the only contraindication would be a previous thoracotomy with pleural adhesions.

In our institution all children sent for PDA closure had VATS closure, unless PDA was part of a more complex cardiac anomaly requiring treatment with cardiopulmonary bypass. We have operated on 374 consecutive patients with this technique. Of these 8 weighed less than 2.5 kg, 329 weighed 2.5-15 kg, and 37 weighed more than 15 kg. They included three cases of atrial septal defect, six of ventricular septal defect, one of ventricular septal defect with pulmonary artery, two of anomalous pulmonary venous return, and one of aortic insufficiency. Three had undergone previous cardiac surgery and one had participated in an indomethacin trial.

12 Closure of Patent Ductus Arteriosus

Preoperative Workup

All patients undergo transechocardiography, routine chest X-ray, and routine preoperative blood work.

Anesthesia: Preparation

General anesthesia is performed with pentothal at a dose of 5-10 mg/kg, vecuronium at a dose of 0.1 mg/kg, fentanyl at a dose of 0.5–1 mg/kg, and 1%–2% enflurane. A central line is placed via a jugular vein, no arterial line is placed. ECG monitoring, oxymetry, and capnography are routine.

Procedure

After induction of general anesthesia and intubation the patient is positioned on the right side, as for a posterolateral thoracotomy. The skin is prepared with two Betadine scrubs, a regular vi-drape is placed including a steridrape. The surgeon and the scrub nurse are to the left of the patient, and the assistant is to the right (Fig. 1).

Two small incisions with an 11 blade are made in the left hemithorax, each corresponding in size to the appropriate instruments for that position (Fig. 2). The first incision is made just posterior on the left axillary line in the third intercostal space, for the videoscope (4 mm) introduced via a 5-mm trocar. A second incision is performed in the third intercostal space middle axillary line and two or three 60° right-angle hooks, 1 mm in diameter, are introduced directly through the incision without any trocar, for lung retraction. A third incision is made in the 4th intercostal space below the inferior angle of the scapula, for the electrocautery hook introduced via a 5-mm trocar (Fig. 2). The same incision is used for insertion of the clip applier, introduced without a trocar.

Fig. 1. Position of the patients, crew and equipment

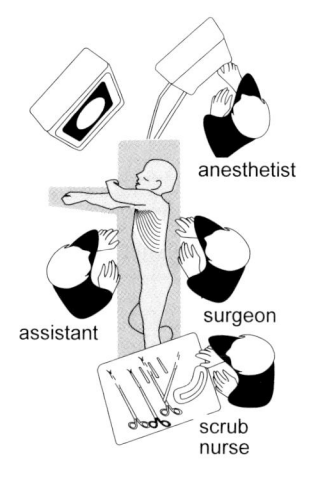

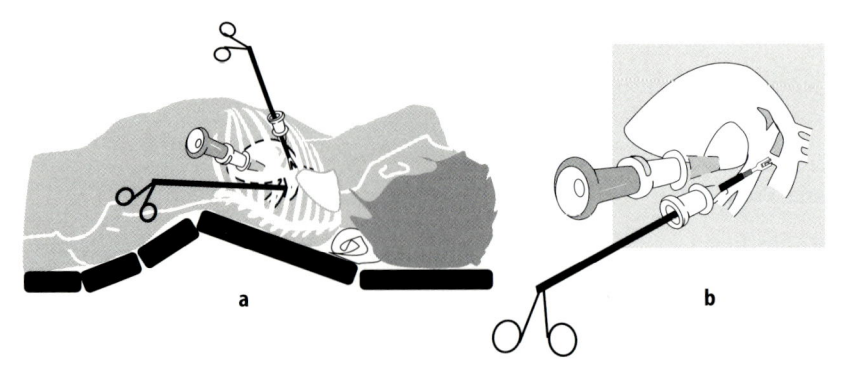

Fig. 2.a. Position of the trocars. **b** Overview of the local anatomy

Fig. 3. The PDA has been dissected from the surrounding tissues. The recurrent laryngeal nerve has been identified. A clip is being placed onto the PDA

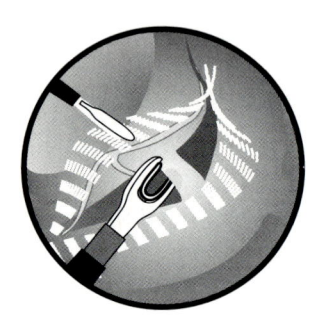

Instruments are:
- 4-mm scope
- 5-mm trocars, 2×
- Right-angle hooks, 3×
- Electrocautery hook
- Suction device
- 8-mm clip applier
- Needle holder

The monitor is placed to the right of the patient facing the surgeon; the cables also come from the right side and are clamped to the drape.

The upper lobe of the left lung is retracted inferomedially; the PDA is identified, and the mediastinal pleura is opened with cautery nerve hook (Fig. 3). The PDA is dissected from surrounding tissues, and the aorta is dissected at the junction from the PDA. The pericardium is dissected on the pulmonary side to protect the recurrent laryngeal nerve form a traumatic injury. It is essential to dissect on both sides of the PDA to place the clip adequately. The clip applier is then introduced through the posterior thoracostomy after removal of the trocar. A first titanium clip (8 mm) is placed as distal as possible from the aortic junction and a second titanium clip is applied on the side close to the aorta. After visual confirmation that both clips are well in place, the lung is inflated, and a 2-mm diameter pleural suction catheter is placed before closure of the skin incision.

Postoperative Care

For all children transechocardiography is performed in the operating room. If complete interruption of the PDA is seen, extubation is performed. Otherwise the clip is replaced. For children weighing less than 5 kg extubation is performed 4–6 h following surgery in the intensive care unit. Their stay here depends on their state and age and varies between 24 and 48 h, before being transferred to a regular room.

The pleural suction catheter is removed a few hours after extubation, a routine chest X-ray is obtained, and a transechocardiogram is performed before discharge. The average hospital stay is 72 h.

Results

Six patients had a patent ductus following VATS related to insufficient dissection resulting in inadequate clip placement (Table 1). Five patients had successful immediate clip repositioning (three by VATS, two by thoracotomy). Subsequent echocardiography revealed persistent closure in these patients. A persistent PDA with minimal flow was discovered in one asymptomatic patient following discharge. Recurrent laryngeal nerve dysfunction was noted in six patients (1.6%; five transient, one persistent). There was no mortality or transfusion requirement in this series. Mean operating time for the last 300 patients was 20±15 mm, and hospital stay averaged 48 h in those aged under 6 months and 72 h in those aged under 6 months.

Discussion

Surgical closure of PDA is now well standardized and provides excellent results, with low mortality and morbidity. Most older patients have division of the ductus through a thoracotomy, where as infants undergo closure with a clip. Surgical closure of the PDA in the neonatal intensive care unit has been described, with excellent results [5–10]. The procedure consists of placement of two clips through a thoracotomy, with an extrapleural approach. The advantages are its low morbidity, lack of mortality, and reliable PDA closure. The application of metal clips near the aorta reduces the risk of recurrent laryngeal nerve injury and does not require complete mobilization of the ductus, reducing the risk of surgical bleeding.

Table 1. Results of VATS (n=374)

Mortality	0
Reoperation for bleeding	0
Reoperation for inadequate ligation	5 (1.3%)
Conversion to thoracotomy	2 (0.5%)
Reoperation by VATS	3 (0.8%)
Persistent shunt	1 (0.26%)
Recurrent laryngeal nerve dysfunction[a]	6 (1.6%)
Other complications	6 (1.6%)
Pneumothoraces[b]	2
Unexplained fever	2
Reintubation for stridor	1
Chylothorax[c]	1
Total complications rate	12 (4.8%)
Extubation in operating rroom	237 (63.3%)
Length of stay (h)	
More than 6 months	48±24
Less than 6 months	72±24
Procedure time (min)	20±15

[a] All resolved except one.
[b] Postoperative pneumothorax did not occur after the use of small silastic drain.
[c] Chylothorax resolved spontaneously after 48 h.

Our technique of PDA closure by VATS [2, 3] provides the same results without a thoracotomy (Fig. 3). This technique is simple and safe, and it becomes very easy with good practice. Although six patients in our series had a persistent shunt after VATS, none occurred in our last 300 patients. It is extremely important to dissect both sides of the ductus adequately to place the clips.

The main complication is transient paralysis of the left vocal cord (1.6%). This can also be seen after open surgical interruption of the ductus [11]. Risks factors generally given are low weight (less than 1500 g) and extensive dissection around the ductus. We believe that minimal dissection around the ductus should be performed to avoid this complication, associated with generous retraction of the mediastinal pleura in order to visualize the nerve.

Percutaneous catheter closure of PDA has been described elsewhere [12–14]. The disadvantage remains persistent shunting, on the order of 27% at 6-week follow-up, which generally decreases to 10%–20% at 6 months. Persistent shunting increases with the size of the ductus. Possible migration or embolization of the device may necessitate surgical removal. Also reported are hemolysis and the problem of prophylaxis against bacterial endocarditis in residual shunts. In addition, this technique is applicable only in patients weighing more than 10 kg because the size of these small vessels makes the use of the device difficult. In addition, recent results have shown superiority of surgical versus transcatheter closure due to outcome and cost, and we feel that VATS probably can reduce the hospital cost even further [15]. Only a prospective trial comparing all alternatives can clarify the issue.

The technique of VATS can also be performed in premature infants (eight patients), as we and others have demonstrated with excellent results and no morbidity. The procedure is rapidly performed, with an average of 15–20 min and can also be performed in the neonatal intensive care unit if necessary. No complications related to the procedure have been reported in this age group as yet. We therefore believe that this technique can be safely applied to premature infants.

The only contraindication to this procedure is if the diameter of the ductus is greater than the size of the clip (9 mm) or if the ductus is calcified. Both of these situations can be encountered in older children or adults.

In our series we had no cases of, hemorrhage, blood loss, phrenic nerve injury, or in-hospital infection. There were no deaths related to the procedure. Prospective efforts must be made to demonstrate reductions in cost, pulmonary injury, and hospital stay. We conclude that the technique described here is safe and rapid, can be practiced with little morbidity, and can be learned easily.

References

1. Laborde F et al (1993) A new video-assisted thoracoscopic surgical technique for interruption of patent ductus arteriosus in infants and children. J Thorac Cardiovasc Surg 105:278–280
2. Laborde F et al (1995) Video-assisted thoracoscopic surgical interruption: the technique of choice for patent ductus arteriosus. Routine experience in 300 pediatric cases. J Thorac Cardiovasc Surg 110:1681–1685
3. Burke RP et al (1995) Video-assisted thoracoscopic surgery for congenital heart disease. J Thorac Cardiovasc Surg 109:499–508
4. Förster R (1993) Thoracoscopic clipping of patent ductus arteriosus in premature infants. Ann Thorac Surg 56:1418–1420
5. Taylor RL et al (1986) Operative closure of patent ductus arteriosus in premature infants in the neonatal intensive care unit. Am J Surg 152:704–708
6. Palder SB et al(1987) Management of patent ductus arteriosus: a comparison of operative versus pharmacologic treatment. J Pediatr Surg 22:1171–1174
7. Dasmahapatra BS, Dethia B, Pollock JC (1986) Surgical closure of persistent ductus arteriosus in infants before 30 weeks of gestation. J Cardiovasc Surg 27:675–678
8. Eggert LD et al(1982) Surgical treatment of patent ductus arteriosus in preferm infants: four-year experience with ligation in the newborn intensive care unit. Pediatr Cardiol 2:15–18
9. Coster DD et al (1989) Surgical closure of the patent ductus arterious in the neonatal intensive care unit. Ann Thorac Surg 48:386–389
10. Miles RH et al (1995) Safety of patent ductus arteriosus closure in premature infants without tube thoracostomy. Ann Thorac Surg 59:668–670
11. Fan LL et al (1989) Paralyzed left vocal cord associated with ligation of patent ductus arteriosus. J Thorac Cardiovasc Surg 98:611–613

12. Porstmann W et al (1971) Catheter closure of patent ductus arteriosus; 62 cases treated without thoracostomy. Radiol Clin North Am 9:203–218
13. Hosking MC et al (1991) Transcatheter occlusion of the persistently patent ductus arteriosus: forty-month follow-up and prevalence of residual shunting. Circulation 84:2313–2317
14. Khan AA et al (1992) Experience with 205 procedures of transcatheter closure of ductus arteriosus in 182 patients, with special reference to residual shunts and long-term follow-up. J Thorac Cardiovasc Surg 104:1721–1727
15. Gray DT et al (1993) Clinical outcomes and costs of transcatheter as compared with surgical closure of patent ductus arteriosus. N Engl J Med 329:1517–1523

Vascular Access

N.M.A. Bax, D.C. van der Zee

Introduction

Vascular access is very important in modern medicine in general and in the care of sick children in particular (Coran 1992; Gauderer 1992). Some children are very dependent on long-term vascular access, for example, in the case of hemodialysis for endstage renal disease, total parenteral nutrition for short bowel syndrome, and ventriculoatrial shunting. When the classical access sites have become exhausted, vascular access becomes a major problem. Procedures such as lumbar venous access to the inferior vena cava through a lumbotomy (Boddie 1989), access of the vena azygos through a thoracotomy (Malt and Kempster 1983; Redo et al. 1992), and direct right atrial cannulation after sternotomy (Hayden et al. 1981) have been described, but such procedures are very invasive, and there is a continuous search to make these procedures less invasive. Percutaneous ultrasound-guided catherization of the inferior vena cava either through the lumbar region or though the liver is an example of this (Azizkhan et al. 1992; Robertson et al. 1990). Another possibility is to cannulate the azygos vein by percutaneous punction under thoracoscopic vision (Bax and van der Zee 1996).

Technique

The child is placed in a left lateral decubitus position on the operating table, which is tilted in a slight anti-Trendelenburg position. The videomonitor stands to the left of the patient's head. The surgeon stands to the right of the patient, the scrub nurse to the right of the surgeon, and the assistant to the left of the patient (Fig. 1).

A 6-mm cannula is inserted just below the tip of the scapula in the midaxillary line and is used for a 5-mm scope. A second 6-mm cannula is inserted in the anterior axillary line at the level of the third intercostal space and is used for a retractor for the lung (Fig. 2). When the lung is to much in the way a pneumothorax with CO_2 may be created. Pressure should be limited to 3–5 mmHg and flow adjusted according to the needs.

The azygos vein with its feeding intercostal veins is visualized (Fig. 3a). From the back between the spine and the medial edge of the scapula a needle is introduced into the extrapleural space. The optimal intercostal space is chosen under

Fig. 1. Position of the patient, equipment and crew

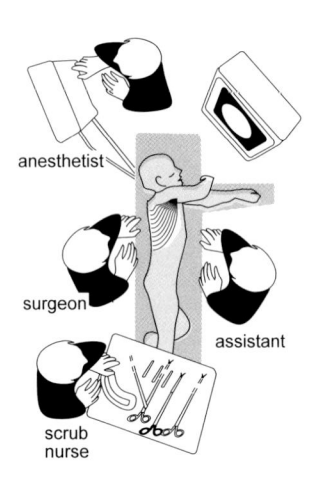

Fig. 2. Position of the cannulae and needle

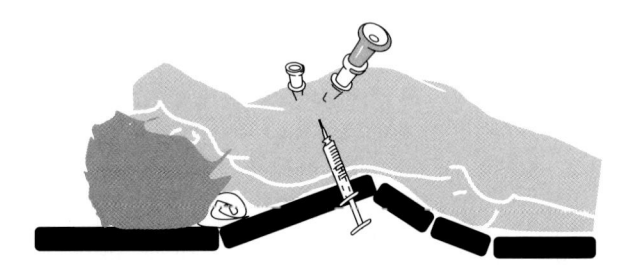

thoracoscopic control by exerting external pressure onto adjacent intercostal spaces. The needle is then advanced extrapleurally either into a large intercostal vein or directly into the azygos vein (Fig. 3b). The tip of the needle can be seen into the particular vein, and blood is easily aspirated. Next a guide wire is inserted into the vessel, and the needle is withdrawn. The position of the tip of the guide wire is positioned fluoroscopically. An appropriate plastic dilatator with peel-away sheath is then introduced over the guide wire. After tunneling of the appropriate catheter from the lower anterior chest wall to the place of insertion of the peel-away system, the catheter length is adjusted, and the catheter introduced into the peel-away sheath and further pushed into place. The place of the tip of the catheter is checked fluoroscopically. The catheter is than fixed to the chest wall. Finally the cannulae are removed, and the holes closed after aspirating the remaining CO_2. The chest is fluoroscoped a last time.

Results

This technique was used in an 8-year-old boy with severe combined immunodeficiency and chronic diarrhea from birth. He had multiple central venous lines

Fig. 3a,b. Intrathoracic view during the procedure

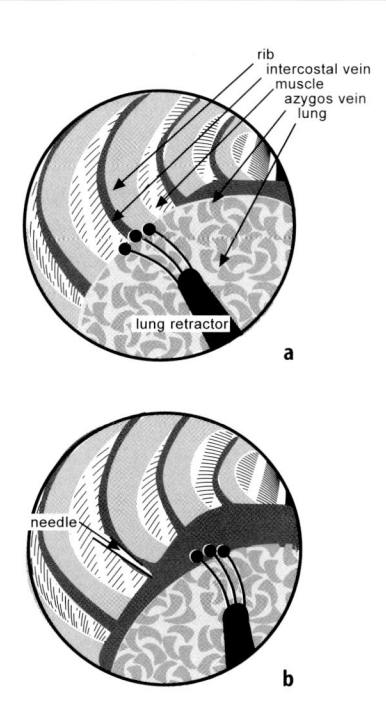

over the years, but both the upper and lower caval vein became occluded. Cannulation of the azygos vein as described proved easy, and no complications in direct relationship with the insertion occurred. As a result of repetitive septicemia with xanthomonas maltophilia, however, the catheter had to be removed 3 months later. Fortunately, the patient has not required a new central line since then.

Discussion

The technique presented here is simple and safe. The advantage is obvious: one sees what one is doing. Although we have no experience with thoracoscopic controlled cannulations of other vessels in the chest, for example, the distal part of the superior vena cava in case of thrombosis of the upper part, thoracoscopic controlled cannulation of this vessel must be feasible as well. By keeping the needle extrapleurally, there is no danger of CO_2 embolus.

References

Azizkhan RG et al (1992) Percutaneous translumbar and transhepatic inferior vena cava catheters for prolonged vascular access in children. J Pediatr Surg 27:165–169

Bax NMA, van der Zee DC (1996) Percutaneous cannulation of the azygos vein. Surg Endosc 10:863–864

Boddie AW Jr (1989) Translumbar catheterization of the inferior vena cava longterm angioaccess. Surg Gynecol Obstet 168:55–56

Coran AG (1992) Vascular access and infusion therapy. Semin Pediatr Surg 1:173–24

Gauderer MWL (1992) Vascular access techniques and devices in the pediatric patient. Surg Clin North Am 71:1267–1284

Hayden L et al (1981) Transthoracic right atrial cannulation for parenteral nutition. Anaesth Intens Care 9:53–57

Malt RA, Kempster M (1983) Direct azygos vein and superior vena cava cannulation for parenteral nutrition. J Parenter Enter Nutr 7:580–581

Redo SF et al (1992) Ventriculoatrial shunt utilizing the azygos vein. J Pediatr Surg 27:642–644

Robertson LJ et al (1990) Percutaneous inferior vena cava placement of tunneled Silastic catheters for prolonged vascular access in children. J Pediatr Surg 25:596–598

CHAPTER 14

Endoscopic Transthoracic Sympathectomy in the Treatment of Primary Palmar Hyperhidrosis in Children

G. Lotan, I. Vinograd

Introduction

Palmar hyperhidrosis is a disabling condition for a significant number of young children of early primary school age [1]. Its etiology is unknown, and excessive sweating usually affects the palms, axillae, and soles and in some cases the face, groin and legs. It has been reported as a symptom of central nervous system disorders with irritative lesions of the hypothalamus, and in hyperpituitarism [2]. Children with hyperhidrosis, especially palmar, are loath to shake hands, and suffer serious psychological, social, and occupational disabilities.

Before identifying the patient as suffering from idiopathic primary palmar hyperhidrosis one should remember that some chronic diseases, such as tuberculosis, lymphomas, and brucellosis, are associated with severe sweating. Also, secondary hyperhidrosis has been noted in diabetes, hypoglycemia, thyrotoxicosis, pheochromocytoma, and carcinoid. It is important to differentiate between primary and secondary hyperhidrosis [3].

The nonsurgical treatment, in mild cases, includes drug therapy, biofeedback, iontophoresis, and percutaneous phenol block [4–7]. Surgery is indicated in severe cases. Various surgical approaches are used, all aimed at ablating the sympathetic supply to the palms and axillae. They include the supraclavicular, the posterior thoracic and transaxillary approaches. Although all achieve the desired result of anhydrosis, they are unacceptable cosmetically, and are associated with more complications than the minimally invasive thoracoscopic approach [8].

Kux et al. [3] and Malone et al. [9] have revived interest in endoscopic thoracic sympathectomy (ETS) because of its high success and low complication rates. There are many reports in adults, but few in children. Experience gained with minimally invasive surgery and the procedure of thoracoscopic sympathectomy now allow us to offer the operation at an earlier stage, preventing many years of suffering from hyperhidrosis. Today the procedure can be offered to any young patient suffering from primary hyperhidrosis.

Technique

The surgical procedure is performed under general anesthesia, starting in the supine position, using a single-lumen endotracheal tube. During the procedure the patient's blood pressure, heart rate, electrocardiogram, pulse oximetry, and end-tidal carbon dioxide concentration are monitored continuously.

Prior to surgery the hands are abducted at 90° and the patient is brought to a sitting position.

The surgeon stands on the operative side of the chest. The monitor is situated to the patient's right (Fig. 1). A 10-mm incision is made over the 5th rib in the midaxillary line and a Veress needle is inserted over the rib; respiration is suspended while the needle is inserted. At that point a pneumothorax is created, maintaining the pressure at 6 mmHg. The volume of CO_2 insufflated depends largely on age, ranging from 200 cc in a small child to 800 cc in an adult. A 10-mm, single-use, protected trocar is inserted, and the angulated optic inserted while the pneumothorax is maintained at a constant pressure of 6 mmHg (Fig. 2a,b).

After identifying the nerve close to the costovertebral junction at the posterolateral aspect of the spine, beneath the pleura, and identifying ribs 2, 3 and 4, the operating hook is inserted. The hook is 5 mm wide and 43 cm long, with the distal 3 cm narrowing to 1 mm wide. The unprotected end is angulated at 120°.

The nerve is picked up by the hook, and the parietal pleura opened by a very short burst of coagulation near the nerve over the rib. The subsequent dissection and elevation of the sympathetic nerve is performed without coagulation.

After freeing the sympathetic nerve for a length of about 1 cm, it is held away from the chest wall over the hook, and coagulated (Fig. 3). The area is examined to make sure that there are no more sympathetic fibers before proceeding to the next rib.

The sympathetic chain is cut over the second and third ribs while monitoring changes in the amplitude of the electrocardiogram on the operative side. If the amplitude increases significantly, no further ablation is carried out on that side; if there is little change, the sympathetic chain is also cut over the fourth rib.

Fig. 1. The position of the patient, crew and equipment. Note that the monitor, insufflator and camera are permanently positioned to one side of the patient during the entire procedure (both sides)

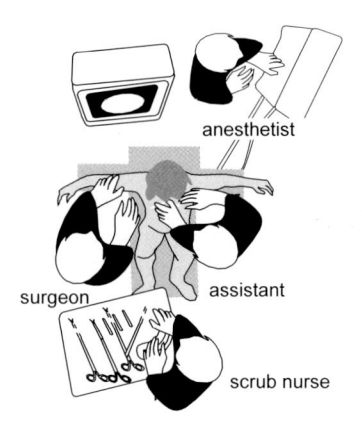

14 Endoscopic Transthoracic Sympathectomy

Fig. 2a,b. The procedure. Incision between 4th and 5th rib, midaxillary line. The sympathectic chain is identified near the costovertebral junction, at the posterolateral aspect of the spine beneath the pleura. By separating the pleura its identification is verified

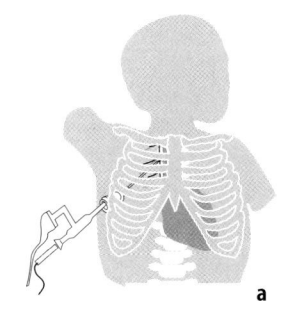

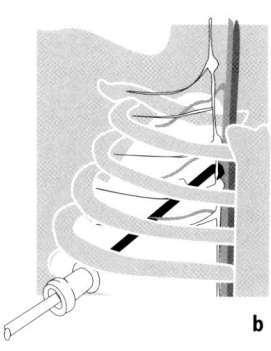

Fig. 3. The nerve is held away from the chest wall over the hook prior to coagulation

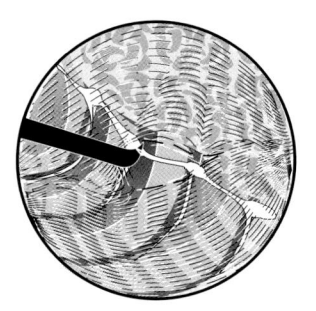

Towards the end of the operation, a no. 14 Neletone tube is inserted through the trocar until the end of the procedure, and the incision is closed by a U-shaped 3-0 nylon stitch. The same is carried out on the opposite side of the thorax.

The small tube is left in place under water until the patient is almost awake, and is removed after no more air bubbles emerge. This prevents pneumothorax and obviates the need to reinsert an intercostal tube.

Following the surgical procedure, a chest X-ray is performed in the recovery room to exclude pneumothorax or incomplete lung expansion. Three hours after the operation the patient is allowed to drink, and 4 h following surgery he may leave his bed and eat. The patient is discharged from hospital on the first postoperative day and the stitches are removed 1 week later in the outpatient clinic. Two routine examinations are performed 1 and 6 months after the operation.

Results

Over a period of 4 years we have performed 60 ETS procedures in 60 patients (age range 7–16 years). All the operations were performed using the same technique and each took 15–40 min. Complications were very minor – one patient had a transient 48-h postoperative pneumothorax; the other patients were discharged after 24 h. We did not see any of the other complications described in the literature (such as Horner syndrome or intercostal neuralgia).

In the early postoperative follow-up of 17 patients we found "compensatory hyperhidrosis" in other places, such as the abdomen, back, and feet. This condition resolved in all but three patients within 3 months. All the patients were very satisfied with the operation. Following the procedure they were recommended to keep their hands moist to prevent drying of the skin.

Discussion

Palmar hyperhidrosis is a disabling condition that affects the quality of life. The development of minimally invasive surgery paved the way for the treatment of hyperhidrosis by thoracoscopic sympathectomy, almost as an outpatient procedure, using a very small incision, with extremely good results and almost no complications. Gaining experience with the procedure, performing it on both sides at the same time, and using regular, and not selective intubation, allows one to perform the operation in early childhood, preventing years of unnecessary suffering from hyperhidrosis. The use of the hook prevents several disadvantages of the technique that arise when using cautery against the ribs. Opening the pleura along the ribs using electrocoagulation results in a pneumomediastinum that in turn causes a great deal of postoperative pain and intercostal neuralgia. We detach the sympathetic nerve from the rib using a very short burst of cautery.

Postoperatively, compensatory hyperhidrosis occurs in about 70% of patients when the sympathetic chain is cut at T_2–T_4. However, by cutting the chain while monitoring the ECG, we can reduce the incidence of this side effect to 30% or less. Horner's syndrome, although rare following the thoracoscopic procedure, can appear transiently or permanently. It is easy to identify the stellate ganglion, but prolonged use of coagulation can transmit heat to the ganglion; in our technique coagulation is used for only a very brief period.

Brachial palsy, winged scapula, and damage to the recurrent laryngeal and phrenic nerves have been reported in this procedure. One should never start cutting before ensuring that the operating field is well visualized, and one should use coagulation very sparingly so as to prevent damage.

Towards the end of the operation we leave a small tube in place within the trocar, which is left under water till the patient is almost awake. This technique prevents the development of even a small pneumothorax, compared to other techniques where the lung can be seen expanding through the trocar.

Minimally invasive surgery in general, and thoracoscopic sympathectomy in particular, requires considerable experience, in order to be able to perform the operation quickly – within 10–15 min each side – and to prevent complications. Nevertheless, this procedure for treating a very distressing situation has considerable advantages – extremely good cosmetic results, a very low complication rate, and low cost – making it worthwhile to master the technique.

References

1. Kurchin A, Zweig A, Mozes M (1977) Palmar hyperhidrosis and its surgical treatment. Ann Surg 186:34–41
2. Edmondson RA, Banerjee AK, Rennie JA (1992) Endoscopic transthoracic sympathectomy in the treatment of hyperhidrosis. Ann Surg 215(3):289–293
3. Kux M (1978) Thoracic endoscopic sympathectomy in palmar and axillary hyperhidrosis. Arch Surg 113:264–266
4. Simpson N (1988) Treating hyperhidrosis. BMJ 296:1345
5. Duller P, Gentry WD (1980) Use of biofeedback in treating chronic hyperhidrosis: a preliminary report. Br J Dermatol 103:143–146
6. Levit F (1968) Simple device for treatment of hyperhidrosis by iontophoresis. Arch Dermatol 98:505–507
7. Dondelinger RF, Rurdeziel JC (1987) Percutaneous phenol block of the upper thoracic sympathetic chain with computed tomography guidance. A new technique. Acta Radiol 28:511–515
8. Mares AJ et al (1994) Transaxillary upper thoracic sympathectomy for primary palmar hyperdydrosis in children and adolescents. Pediatr Surg 29:382–386
9. Malone PS, Cameron AEP, Rennie JA (1986) Endoscopic thoracic sympathectomy in the treatment of upper limb hyperhidrosis. Ann R Coll Surg Engl 68:93–94

Video-Asssisted Repair of Esophageal Atresia

M. Robert, H. Lardy

Introduction

Surgical repair of an esophageal atresia remains challenging because of the confined surgical space, accessed through a small incision. Moreover the size of the esophagus and surrounding anatomical structures is small, and magnification for the dissection is required to preserve these structures. The current possibilities of modern endoscopic surgery, for example, scopes with chip-camera and special instruments, can also be used to approach the esophagus as has been proposed experimentally (Kellnar et al. 1997). We started to use this approach in newborns in 1994 and share our experiences in this chapter.

Indication

In principle all esophageal atresias that are classically operated on in the newborn period can be approached. This approach can also be used in type 1 esophageal atresia, but in these patients the repair of the esophagus is often postponed for 3–4 months.

Preoperative Workup

Immediately before the actual surgical repair of the atresia, each patient should have an endoscopy of trachea and upper esophagus in order to:
- Confirm the diagnosis
- Determine the level of the tracheo-esophageal fistula(e)
- Detect associated anomalies, for example, laryngo-tracheo-esophageal cleft, tracheomalacia, aberrant crossing arteries
- Document the degree of tracheobronchial irritation

Preoperative Preparation

The patient is positioned in a left lateral decubitus position with a small cushion beneath the chest. The arm is anteverted to elevate the scapula. The position of

15 Video-Asssisted Repair of Esophageal Atresia

Fig. 1. Position of the patient, equipment and crew

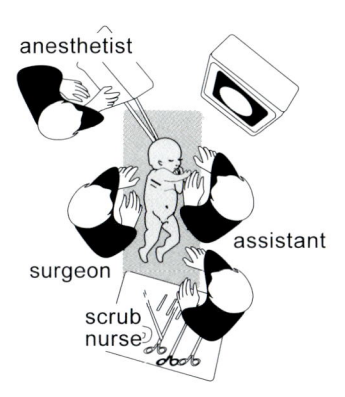

Fig. 2. Minithoracotomy with scope and instruments in situ

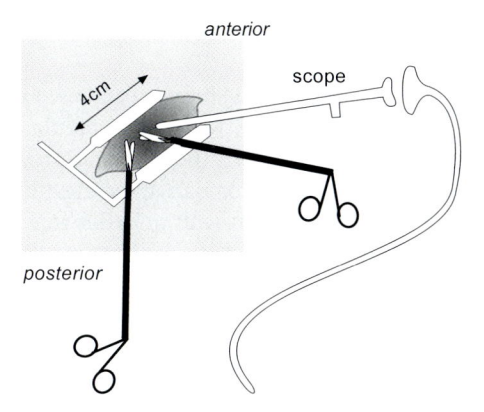

the patient, crew and equipment is depicted in Fig. 1. Specific instruments to be used are:
- 4-mm optic with camera, enveloped in a sterile bag
- 3-mm laparoscopic instruments
- Small rib spreader
- Classical neonatal instruments

Technique

This is a posterolateral, muscle-sparing minithoracotomy (maximum 4 cm; Jawad 1997). The posterior border of the latissimus dorsi muscle is lifted anteriorly, while the anterior border of the trapezoid muscle is retracted posteriorly. The thorax is entered through the 4th intercostal space, and the esophagus is approached extrapleurally. A small rib spreader is inserted.

A 4-mm scope and laparoscopic or classical instruments are introduced through the anterior part of the incision. The scope is held by the assistant or scrub nurse (Fig. 2).

A classical repair is now performed but under constant video control: the lower esophagus is identified and encircled with a vessel loop. The azygos vein is only severed between ligatures when this is necessary. The fistula is ligated with a 6 or 7-0 absorbable monofilament ligature and is then transected. Next the upper pouch is dissected way up into the neck. The distal part is opened and anastomosed with the distal esophagus using separate 5-0 absorbable monofilament stitches. A silicone nasogastric tube is inserted through the anastomosis.

The operative field is irrigated, an extrapleural drain inserted, and the two adjacent ribs are approximated with one absorbable suture. The parietal muscles are not sutured, and the skin is approximated with an intradermic running suture.

Personal Experience

Since 1994 we have operated on 13 babies (9 boys, 4 girls) in this way. All but two babies has an esophageal atresia with distal fistula, one had no fistula, and one had two fistulae, which were identified during preoperative tracheoscopy. One baby had a retroesophageal subclavian artery. In this child the aortic arch needed the be suspended to the chest wall in order to relieve the tracheal compression. None of the babies had life-threatening associated anomalies.

Discussion

The proposed approach allows for an excellent view of the operative field for all members of the team: surgeon, assistant, scrub nurse, and anesthetist (Fig. 3). It allows a very neat dissection preserving most of the branches of the vagal nerve. Because of the muscle sparing minithoracotomy the procedure is less traumatic and cosmetically more acceptable. The video-assisted approach prolongs the duration of the operation only little, to about 1.5 h. It allows perfect teaching not only during the actual operative procedure but also later on by using the videotape.

Fig. 3. Endoscopic view of the atresia

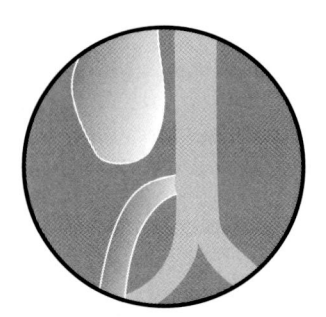

Surgical repair of an esophageal atresia by a pure thoracoscopic approach is certainly feasible. It does, however, necessitate a transthoracic approach and may require more operative time.

Conclusion

The video-assisted approach is recommended for repair of esophageal atresia. One should consider the video-assisted approach more frequently in thoracic and abdominal surgery.

References

Jawad AJ (1997) Experience with modified muscle-sparing thoracotomy in neonates, infants, and children. Pediatr Surg Int 12:337–339

Kellnar S, Till H, Böhm R (1997) Thoracoscopic surgery of the esophagus in rats: a training concept for the treatment of tracheo-oesophageal malformations in preterm infants. Pediatr Surg Int 12:116–117

**Part III
Abdomen**

Diagnostic Laparoscopy

CHAPTER 16

Diagnostic Laparoscopy

J. Waldschmidt, N.M.A. Bax

Introduction

As early as 1901 Kelling (1902) recommended laparoscopy for the assessment of intra-abdominal organs. In the 1950's, internists and gynecologists developed the technique into a routine tool. Another 20 years passed before the first reports appeared on diagnostic laparoscopy in newborns and infants (Frangenheim 1974; Gans and Berci 1971; Gazzanagia et al. 1976; Karamehmedovic et al. 1977; Leape and Ramenofsky 1977; Selmair and Wildhirt 1973; Wildhirt and Selmair 1970), but reports criticizing this soon followed (Burdelski 1979; Cadranel et al. 1979; Coleman et al. 1976; Rodgers et al. 1978; Schwöbel and Stauffer 1980; Stauffer and Hirsig 1979). With the improvement in imaging techniques and especially the development of noninvasive diagnostic imaging techniques, the interest in diagnostic laparoscopy faded. Interest was rekindled, however, with the introduction of endoscopic cholecystectomy, converting laparoscopy from a diagnostic into a therapeutic tool.

Indications

In regard to general indications, the statement of Gans and Austin (1983) that laparoscopy is indicated for diagnosis only when simpler studies are not adequate, and when exploratory laparotomy would therefore be considered still holds today, and it should be remembered that diagnostic laparoscopy is an invasive procedure. There is, however, one big difference with the past; laparoscopy, which began as a diagnostic procedure, is today often converted into a therapeutic one, for example, with the removal of an inflamed appendix in cases of acute abdominal pain and clipping of the testicular vessels as a first-stage Fowler-Stephens in the case of an intra-abdominal testis.

The specific indications are:
- Acute abdominal pain
- Chronic abdominal pain
- Regional enteritis
- Unclear gastrointestinal bleeding
- Liver-biliary tree pathology
- Oncology

- Traumatology
- Ascites
- Contralateral open processus vaginalis in unilateral inguinal hernia
- Dysfunction of ventriculo-peritoneal or peritoneal dialysis drains
- Andrology, gynecology, and intersex

Acute Abdominal Pain

The use of diagnostic laparoscopy in the event of an acute abdomen was described as early as 1937 by Ruddock (1937) and has been repeatedly recommended again in the late 1960's, early 1970's (Baerlocher et al. 1973; Fahrländer 1969; Frangenheim 1974; Sugarbaker et al. 1975).

Acute abdominal symptoms may be caused by inflammation, and obstruction, or strangulation. The pain may be colicky in cases of obstruction or strangulation or continuous, either poorly defined in the absence of peritonitis or more clearly defined in the case of peritonitis. The pain may have a sudden onset or a slower one.

Differential diagnosis for acute abdominal pain includes:
- Common
  - Constipation
  - Gastroenteritis
  - Acute appendicitis
  - Urinary tract infection
- Less common
  - Intussusception
  - Pneumonia
  - Obstruction, adhesive or congenital
  - Strangulated inguinal hernia
  - Meckel's diverticulitis
  - Salpingitis
  - Cholelithiasis
  - Nephrolithiasis
- Rare
  - Torsion of the ovary or ovarial appendix
  - Rupture of an ovarian cyst
  - Torsion of an epiploic appendix
  - Pancreatitis
  - Henoch-Schönlein purpura
  - Diabetic ketoacidosis
  - Porphyria
  - Sickle cell crisis
  - Retroperitoneal hematoma due to hemophilia

There are many other causes of abdominal pain in children, but discussion of these is beyond the scope of this chapter.

Indications for Diagnostic Laparoscopy

With a good history, clinical examination, and a limited number of additional laboratory and imaging investigations most of the above diagnoses can be made without laparoscopy. Laparoscopy only comes into view when a speedy diagnosis cannot be made otherwise but should be made.

Diagnostic laparoscopy is especially rewarding when the possibility of acute appendicitis is raised. Even today this diagnosis may be difficult. The history and clinical presentation may be doubtful, as ultrasound examination may be, while results of laboratory investigations such as the serum blood C-reactive protein level or the total and relative number of leukocytes are often not conclusive in early appendicitis. A wait-and-see policy can be adopted, but it is frustrating to experience hours later that the appendix after all was heavily inflamed. The frustration of finding a so-called negative appendix is not less, and especially when a MacBurney incision has been used, a struggle to see what usually cannot be seen through a small hole starts. Judicious application of laparoscopy to patients with equivocal findings of appendicitis significantly reduces the negative appendectomy rate (Laepe and Ramenofsky 1980; see also Valla and Steyaert: "Laparoscopic Appendicectomy in Children", this volume).

In the septic intensive care patient it may be difficult to rule out intra-abdominal pathology, and here too diagnostic laparoscopy may be very helpful (Almeida et al. 1995; Bender and Talami 1992; Brandt et al. 1993, 1994). The same applies for the child with abdominal pain and severe underlying disease such as congenital or acquired immunopathy, nephrotic syndrome, or diabetes mellitus. In such instance laparoscopy may rapidly exclude intra-abdominal disease. In case of Henoch-Schönlein purpura it may be very difficult to exclude small bowel intussusception except by laparoscopy.

In the patient with colicky abdominal pain and possible intestinal obstruction, diagnostic laparoscopy may be able to furnish a rapid precise diagnosis. If a cause is revealed, diagnostic laparoscopy may become therapeutic. The cause may be congenital, for example, internal herniation or volvulus around an omphaloenteric duct remnant, or acquired due to adhesions from previous surgery.

Technique

All diagnostic laparoscopies in children should be carried out under general anesthesia and optimal muscle relaxation. There is no absolute need to insert a urine catheter or a nasogastric tube in all patients, although this may be necessary for other reasons. The bladder can be manually emptied before surgery, and a nasogastric tube is only inserted when there is an indication for this, for example, upper abdominal laparoscopy or in case of intestinal obstruction.

If a specific diagnosis in a localized intra-abdominal area is suspected, the positioning of the patient, monitor and crew is simple: the surgeon's eyes, area to be inspected, and monitor should be in a single line, and the area to be inspected should be elevated (Fig. 1).

Fig. 1. When the diagnosis concerns a localized intra-abdominal area: monitor, target area, and surgeon should be in line

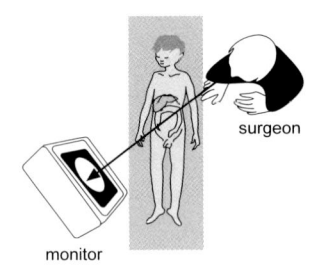

Fig. 2. The first cannula is inserted at the umbilicus; secondary cannulae, if needed, are inserted preferably so as to respect the triangle principle

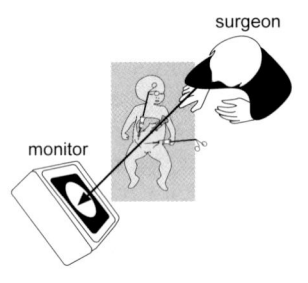

Fig. 3. When it unclear in which quadrant the pathology is, at least two monitors are needed

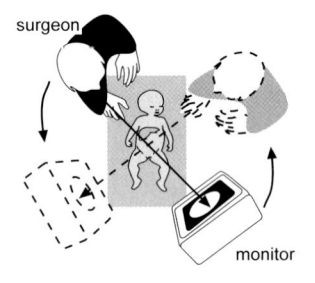

The first cannula is usually inserted at the umbilicus. An open method is preferable, especially when previous surgery has been carried out, or when the bowel is distended due to obstruction. Secondary cannulae are inserted, when needed, preferably respecting the triangle principle, which means: scope closest to the surgeon at the inverted tip of the triangle, working instruments closer to the monitor at the ends of the basis of the triangle (Fig. 2). Also in diagnostic laparoscopy one should not hesitate to introduce two or even three working cannulae for proper inspection by retraction and manipulation. Especially in diagnostic laparoscopy small-caliber instruments may be rewarding. Some of these can even be introduced through an intravenous cannula, avoiding the need for classical cannulae insertion. In obstructive syndromes, however, one should be very careful with such small-diameter instruments as inadvertent perforation of the bowel may easily occur.

When it is less clear in which quadrant the pathology may be, at least two monitors are required, one for the left site of the abdomen and one for the right

16 Diagnostic Laparoscopy

Fig. 4. When it is unclear in which quadrant the pathology is, the working cannulae should be introduced at each side of the umbilicus to allow for subsequent search in both upper and lower abdomen

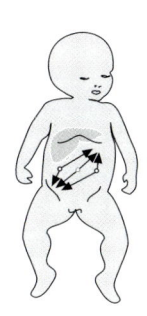

side (Fig. 3). Such a second monitor should have a long interconnecting cable with the first monitor to allow for easy relocation. Under such condition it may be wise to introduce the working cannulae at each site of the umbilicus to allow both upper and lower abdominal inspection (Fig. 4), but one should not hesitate to insert another cannula, when required

A conclusion that nothing is found can only be drawn after a thorough inspection of the whole abdomen, which is time consuming, and includes:
- Liver, bile ducts, duodenum (peptic ulcer), right colon
- Spleen, left colon
- Duodeno-jejunal flexure, broadness and fixation of the mesentery
- Small bowel
- Ileocecal region (omphaloenteric remnants; Perry 1990)
- Internal genitalia (varicoceles, also in girls, and endometriosis)

Personal Experience

Table 1 summarizes laparoscopic findings in children with acute abdominal pain (n=225, August 1979–July 1997, Department of Pediatric Surgery, University Medical Center Benjamin Franklin, Berlin)

Chronic Abdominal Pain

Indications

Laparoscopy is only one of the many diagnostic possibilities in children with chronic abdominal pain. At no means should laparoscopy replace a careful history, clinical examination, and selective additional laboratory investigations and or imaging studies.

The diagnostic laparoscopic yield in chronic abdominal pain varies considerably from study to study. Leape and Ramenofsky (1977) in their initial series found no pathology in 11 out of 14 children, while subsequently (1980) they found pathology in 16 out of 33 patients. Waldschmidt subjected 46% of the children with chronic abdominal pain to laparoscopy and found pathology in more than 99% of the cases. In contrast, in Utrecht laparoscopy for chronic abdominal pain is seldom performed. In adolescent girls with chronic pelvic pain Goldstein et al. (1979) found pathology in more than 90% of the cases, and Ozaksit et al. 1995 had a similar experience.

Table 1. Laparoscopic findings in children with acute abdominal pain (n=225)

	Age			
	<1 month ($n=29$)	<1 year ($n=37$)	>1 year ($n=158$)	Total ($n=225$)
Acute appendicitis	–	–	88	88
Ileus[a]	3	20	19	42
Ovarian pathology	24	–	–	24
Peritonitis	–	3	18	21
Salpingitis	–	–	10	10
Abscess	–	3	6	9
Mesenteric lymphadenitis	–	3	3	6
Hemoperitoneum[b]	1	2	3	6
Pancreatitis	–	–	5	5
Meckel's diverticulitis	–	3	–	3
Appendix epiploica	–	1	2	3
Intestinal perforation	–	1	1	2
Acute cholecystitis	–	1	1	2
Pathology of the omentum	–	1	1	2
Gastric perforation	–	–	1	1
Torsion of the spleen	1	–	–	1

[a] Adhesions 21, strangulation 9, duplication cyst 3, lymphangioma 3, Meckel 3, intussusception 1, bezoar 1, mesenteric cyst 1.
[b] Ruptured ovarian cyst 3, splenic rupture 1, liver rupture 1, mesenteric laceration 1.

A major problem in laparoscopy for chronic abdominal pain remains the interpretation of so-called pathological findings, and the question whether the finding is really responsible for the pain should always be asked. The matter of chronic appendicitis should certainly be addressed. Does this exists, and if so, what is the incidence? There are believers and nonbelievers. In a series of 660 children in which an identifiable cause for the chronic abdominal pain was found at laparoscopy, Waldschmidt diagnosed so-called chronic recurrent appendicitis in more than half of them. In contrast, in Utrecht this diagnosis is hardly ever made. There is also the difficult matter of postoperative adhesions. After previous surgery there are always adhesions! The questions is, are these responsible for the pain, and if so, does lysis prevent recurrence of the adhesions and complaints? Mimicking the abdominal pain by laparoscopic traction onto the adhesions under local anesthesia has been proposed to make more certain that these adhesions are causally involved (Sotnikov et al. 1994), but diagnostic laparoscopy, at least in children, should be performed under general anesthesia.

Complete disappearance of the symptoms after treatment of the pathological finding is probably the best indicator of whether the pathology found was really responsible for the complaints, although there may be a significant placebo effect from the laparoscopy itself. Leape reported that 18% were relieved of the pain without any therapeutic action (Leape and Ramenofsky 1977), and Baker and Symonds (1992) found disappearance of the pain in 58 out of 60 women with chronic pelvic pain 6 months after a negative laparoscopy. On the other hand, Goldstein et al. (1979) experienced a recurrence of the complaints in 25% of the laparoscoped adolescent girls after initial treatment.

Except for possible overdiagnosis, laparoscopy may overlook pathology. In the series of 660 diagnostic laparoscopies of Waldschmidt there were two false-negative findings (pancreatitis in one child and more seriously a malignant lymphoma in another).

Technique

One should stick to general principles. As in diagnostic laparoscopy for acute abdominal pain, no cause may be found. One can conclude, however, that the laparoscopy has been negative only when the abdomen has been systematically reviewed (see above).

Personal Experience

Table 2 summarizes laparoscopic findings in children with chronic abdominal pain (n=660, February 1979–July 1997, Department of Pediatric Surgery, University Medical Center Benjamin Franklin, Berlin).

Conclusion

Diagnostic laparoscopy should be used selectively in patients with chronic abdominal pain. If complaints, however, persist for, for example, 6 months, and a firm diagnosis cannot be made otherwise in a noninvasive way, a proper diagnostic laparoscopy should be carried out. There are too many patients who have had abdominal pain for a long time, only to be diagnosed after an exploratory laparotomy or diagnostic laparoscopy (Hallfeldt et al. 1995; Lauder and Moses 1995). Goldstein et al. warned in 1979 about not taking pain complains in young adolescent girls seriously. This warning should be extended to at least all growing individuals. Even when laparoscopy has a significant placebo effect, all that matters is a symptom-free person.

The indication for performing a diagnostic laparoscopy is relatively straightforward. The findings, however, should be interpreted with caution. Whether a normal looking appendix should be removed remains questionable. Removal of such an appendix causes an adhesion and may be the cause of subsequent pain! The argument that often pathological abnormalities are found in a clinically healthy appearing appendix may not justify appendicectomy.

Table 2. Laparoscopic findings in children with chronic abdominal pain (n=660)

Finding	n
Chronic recurrent appendicitis	352
Adhesions after previous surgery	108
Congenital pericecal bands	55
Cecum mobile	38
Pathology of the female adnexa	37
Cholelithiasis	21
Meckel's diverticulum	13
Appendix epiploica	9
Pathology of the omentum	7
Transient intussusception	3
Urachal duct	3
Chlamydia infection	2
Intestinal malrotation	2
Carcinoid	2
Chronic gastric volvulus	1
Internal hernia	1
Coloptosis	1
Stump appendicitis[a]	1
Flexura lienalis syndrome	1
Endometriosis	1
Yersinia infection	1
Oyuriasis	1

[a] After conventional appendicectomy.

Regional Enteritis

The diagnosis of regional enteritis is often difficult. The laparoscopic appearance may clarify the diagnosis: superficial inflammation, edema, rigidity, marked migration of the mesenteric fat onto the bowel wall (Leape and Ramenofsky 1977), and loss of the bowel mesenteric angle (Miller et al. 1996).

Unclear Gastrointestinal Bleeding

In the event of unclear gastrointestinal bleeding, laparotomy is usually the last resort when other diagnostic tools such as esophago-gastroduodenoscopy or colonoscopy, radioisotope studies, and angiography fail to identify the exact localization of the bleeding. Nowadays patients who are hemodynamically stable should have a laparoscopy before formal laparotomy, as a few causative conditions may be diagnosed and even treated that way, for example, a Meckel's diverticulum, a small-bowel tumor and a vascular malformation of the bowel wall (Evoy et al. 1996; Huang and Lin 1993; Madsen 1994; Sackier 1992). When the diagnostic laparoscopy is negative, laparoscopic exteriorization of a loop of small bowel with subsequent enterotomy and introduction of a flexible scope may increase the diagnostic yield (Phillips et al. 1994). Several reports in adults have been published regarding endoluminal upper or lower gastrointestinal tract endoscopy to find the causative bleeder in combination with therapeutic laparoscopy (Ferzli et al. 1994; Stellato 1996).

Nonmalignant Liver and Biliary Tree Pathology

Cholestasis in the Newborn and Young Infant

Indications

When a newborn or young infant presents with conjugated hyperbilirubinemia, a surgically correctable cause may be present, and the diagnosis should be made as soon as possible.

Surgical approachable cholestasis in the newborn or young infant include: biliary atresia, choledochal cyst, and inspissated bile syndrome. In the event of dilated ducts, the diagnosis of extrahepatic biliary obstruction is easy. When the whole biliary tree dilates progressively in a rather equal manner, and sludge is seen in the dilated gallbladder or ducts, the diagnosis of the so-called inspissated bile syndrome should be made. This occurs in patients with abnormal bile composition, for example, cystic fibrosis, hepatocellular damage, hemolysis, parenteral nutrition, ileal resection, and dehydration (Holland and Lilly 1992).

When the intrahepatic ducts are visible or dilated, a type I or II biliary atresia is present. In contrast when neither the intra- nor extrahepatic ducts are dilated, it is difficult to differentiate between type III biliary atresia and nonsurgical causes of cholestasis. In such situation it is imperative to look at the biliary tree, which means either laparotomy or laparoscopy. As early as 1973 Gans and Berci, described laparoscopic cholangiography to differentiate between surgical approachable and medical causes of neonatal hyperbilirubinemia.

Technique

The patient lies on the back on the operating table, which is tilted in a slight reverse Trendelenburg position. Cholangiography must be possible during the laparoscopy without moving the patient. The surgeon stands at the lower end of the table, while the monitor stands to the right of the patients head (Fig. 5). The camera person is at the surgeon's left site, and the scrub nurse at the surgeon's right side. The patient is under general anesthesia and complete muscle relaxation. A cannula for the scope is inserted in an open manner through the inferior

Fig. 5. Position of the patient, equipment, and crew for cholangiography and liver biopsy in the newborn or young infant

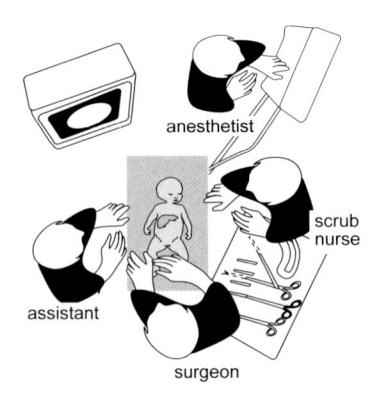

umbilical fold. Next CO_2 is insufflated with a flow of 0.5 l/min. Pressure is limited to 5 mmHg.

The liver is then inspected. The aspect of the liver usually allows differentiation between biliary atresia and other causes of cholestasis. In biliary atresia the liver surface has a dark brownish-green or almost black micronodular aspect with neovascularization in the capsule. The gallbladder is usually hardly visible and retracted within the liver parenchyma. In such an event a cholangiography cannot be made. Under vision a percutaneous biopsy is taken. In Utrecht a fine aspiration needle of 16 or 18 G is used for this purpose (see below). If bleeding at the puncture site occurs, electrocoagulation is applied. Laparoscopy is ended and definitive surgery planned within a few days. Meanwhile the result of the histological examination of the biopsy is available.

When the gallbladder looks normal but collapsed, there may still be biliary atresia. Again, in such circumstances the liver surface looks abnormal in the way as described above. In the absence of biliary atresia the liver surface is usually smooth and shows less neovascularization in the capsule. The gallbladder may be small due to nonuse related to intrahepatic cholestasis but its wall looks normal. In case of the inspissated bile syndrome the gallbladder is packed with sludge.

To carry out cholangiography a grasping forceps is introduced pararectally at umbilical level or somewhat lower, and the gallbladder is grasped and stretched to the right (Fig. 6a). Next the gallbladder is punctured directly (not through the liver substance as has been advocated by Gans) with an intravenous cannula. The needle is directed in such a way that the gallbladder and needle are in line. The needle is then withdrawn, but the cannula left in place (Fig. 6b). The size of the needle depends on the size of the gallbladder. In case of inspissated bile, a large caliber intravenous cannula is used in order to be able to remove the inspissated bile and to flush the gallbladder and biliary tree clean. It is advantageous to use only 2-ml syringes to prevent injection of too much saline or contrast material. Using too much volume may damage the intrahepatic bile ducts. When saline can easily be injected, the cystic and common bile duct must be open. Next radio-opaque contrast material is injected under radioscopic control confirming

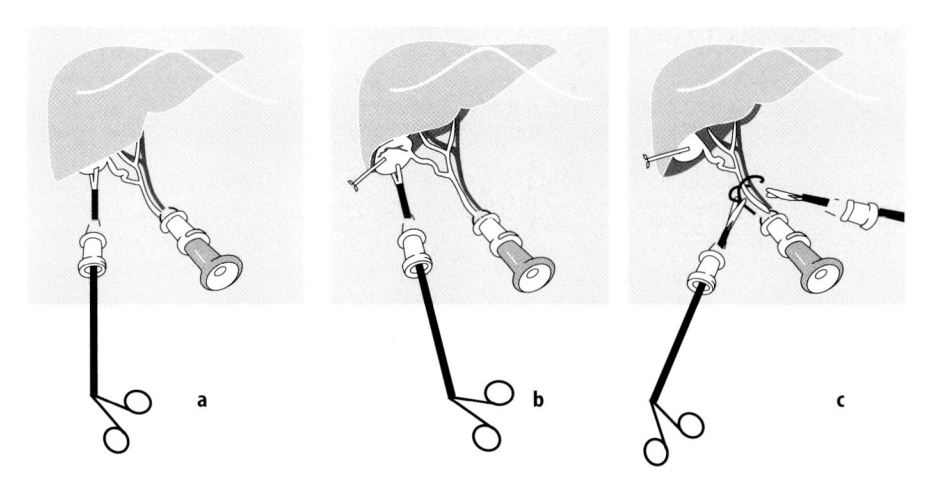

Fig. 6a-c. Cholangiography in the newborn or young infant

distal patency. By using more pressure it is usually possible to obtain some backflow into the liver and to confirm patency of at least the right and left hepatic ducts. If no black flow into the liver can be obtained, a vessel loop is placed around the hepatoduodenal ligament and put on traction, and contrast is injected again (Fig. 6c). No backflow into the liver means hepatic duct obstruction and the need for a formal dissection of the porta hepatis. Otherwise the biliary tree is flushed with saline and the procedure is finished. The small puncture hole in the gallbladder does not need closure. Of course, a liver biopsy is also taken under laparoscopic control. In the event of biliary sludge cleaning of the gallbladder and biliary tree is often therapeutic.

Liver Biopsy

Indications and Technique

A liver biopsy is often needed in the diagnostic workup of liver diseases. When the liver is diffusely involved, a randomly taken biopsy suffices, and a percutaneous technique should be used. Sometimes, however, a specific area must be biopsied. If this area can well be localized by ultrasound, an ultrasound-guided biopsy can be taken. It may be difficult, however, to puncture a small lesion, and in such condition a laparoscopically directed biopsy may offer a solution to the problem. Direct inspection of the liver in case of suspected disease has been considered to be a diagnostic advantage (Crantock et al. 1994; Vargas et al. 1995), and this is also our experience.

A coagulation disturbance is usually considered to be a contraindication for blind puncture or for laparoscopy, and in such a circumstances open biopsy is usually advocated. In Utrecht, however, it is thought that especially when coagulation is disturbed and cannot be improved preoperatively, a laparoscopically

Fig. 7. Needle biopsy of the liver

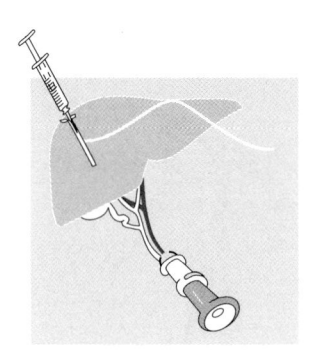

Fig. 8. Wedge biopsies of the liver

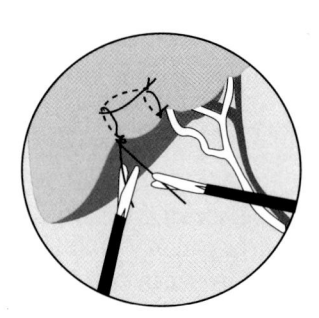

controlled percutaneous puncture of the liver is ideal as in such circumstances bleeding from the puncture place can be controlled endoscopically. In such circumstances an intravenous cannula, appropriate for the needle to be used, is inserted through the abdominal wall at the desired place. The needle is introduced through the cannula. In cases of bleeding the needle in reinserted into the puncture hole and coagulation applied onto the needle. The plastic cannula of the intravenous needle, which is still in place, prevents coagulation of the surrounding abdominal wall (Fig. 7).

In cases of severe coagulopathy it is desirable to have argon gas electrocoagulation available, which is to be used through a 5-mm cannula. As argon gas diathermy uses a rather high gas flow and is not pressure controlled at the time being, another cannula should be opened to allow the gas to escape and to avoid high intra-abdominal pressure. Alternatively, the bleeding puncture hole can be plugged with an hemostatic agent. In cases of coagulopathy apart from the cannula for the scope, at least one other classic working channel should be available for instrumentation. Wedge biopsies of the liver can also be taken as in open surgery, but then two working channels are needed (Fig. 8). Wedge biopsies can also be taken with an endostapler, but this requires the insertion of large caliber cannulae (Lefor and Flowers 1994).

Oncology

Indications for Diagnostic Laparoscopy

While laparoscopy in adults with or without combined laparoscopic ultrasonography is increasingly used for interpretation of resectability of malignant tumors (Babineau et al. 1994; Conlon et al. 1996; van Dijkum et al. 1997; Gouma et al. 1996), its role in pediatric oncology is still limited. At present it is not included in the pediatric oncology protocols, except for the Hodgkin study HD 96 in the German-speaking countries.

Lymphomas. There are several reports on laparoscopic staging in Hogkin's and non-Hodgkin's lymphoma (Childers and Surwit 1992; Coleman et al. 1976; Lefor and Flowers 1994; Nord and Boyd 1996; Zornig et al. 1993). Laparoscopy allows sampling of the lymph nodes, needle and wedge biopsy of the liver (Lefor and Flowers 1994), and ovariopexia. In classic staging the spleen should be removed as well.

Other Malignant Diseases. Laparoscopy is an ideal tool when a biopsy is essential before therapy is started or when residual or recurrent disease is suspected. Holcomb et al. (1995) reported on 60 laparoscopies in children for oncology purposes. Laparoscopy can also be used for cannulation of vessels for regional chemotherapy and for the insertion of thermal or laser probes into tumors and metastases.

Discussion

A few notes of caution should be made. Firstly, as in open surgery, taking a biopsy may change the staging of the tumor, for example, in nephroblastoma, and secondly tumor implants at the laparoscopic cannulae sites have been reported in the sampling of both solid tumors and lymphomas (Aractingi et al. 1993). To prevent metastasis, one should try to take whole lymph nodes if possible. Moreover the specimen should be removed in a recipient bag.

Traumatology

Assessing blunt abdominal injury may be very difficult in children, especially in the event of multitrauma. In such situation the head is often involved as well, and the often resulting decreased consciousness makes interpretation of the clinical picture even more difficult. The decision to open the abdomen is easier to take in the event of penetrating trauma.

To decrease the excessive numbers of negative laparotomies in blunt trauma Root et al. (1965) advocated diagnostic peritoneal lavage. In a number of patients, however, in whom the lavage yields a positive result, at laparotomy the bleeding is insignificant or has stopped. To reduce the number of negative laparotomies, diagnostic laparoscopy for trauma was introduced in the early 1970's (Heselson 1970;

Tostivint et al. 1971) but did not gain popularity. Leape and Ramenofsky in 1977 and Austin and Gans in 1983 wrote about diagnostic laparoscopy in the traumatized child. The rapidly improving new imaging methods such as ultrasonography and computed tomography, in contrast to the cumbersome use of the monocular laparoscope, which had to be held by the surgeon himself, did not contribute to the further development of the latter. With the revival of laparoscopy, due to technical improvements, renewed interest in its use in trauma has emerged.

Indications for Diagnostic Laparoscopy

In Blunt Abdominal Trauma

In cases of multiple injury, decreased consciousness, persisting equivocal abdominal signs after initial survey and assessment, the need for other lengthy neurosurgical or bone operations diagnostic laparoscopy can identify or exclude an unstable abdominal injury such as a bleeding liver injury, mesenteric tear, and splenic laceration. A negative explorative laparotomy under such circumstances unnecessarily adds major morbidity to an already multiple injured patient (Nagy and Sutter 1994). At the present, however, diagnostic laparoscopy in blunt abdominal trauma lacks wide popularity (Leppaniemi and Elliott 1996).

In Penetrating Trauma

There is little doubt that laparoscopy is an excellent tool for looking at possible violation of the peritoneum by both a stab or a gunshot (Ditmars and Bongard 1996).

Stab Wounds. Not every stab wound penetrates the whole thickness of the abdominal wall and not every stab wound that penetrates the whole abdominal wall injures intra-abdominal structures. In the event of an abdominal stab wound, laparoscopy is ideal to see whether the peritoneum has been penetrated (Nagy and Sutter 1994; Poole et al. 1996).

Gunshot Wounds. In the event of a tangential gunshot wound, laparoscopy can be used to see whether the abdominal cavity has been entered (Nagy and Sutter 1994; Poole et al. 1996; Soza et al. 1995).

Technique

Trauma laparoscopy should be carried out under sterile conditions in the operating room under general anesthesia and full muscle relaxation. The general principles of laparoscopy should be followed.

Especially in blunt trauma the abdomen should be taken under view in a systematic manner as in laparoscopy for acute or chronic abdominal pain is important in order not to miss significant pathology. The pancreas should be inspected, and the small bowel should be run from the duodenojejunal flexure to the ileocecal valve. When laparoscopy in penetrating trauma is carried out for more than examining whether the peritoneal cavity has been violated, such a systematic approach is needed as well. Especially hollow viscus perforations are at risk for being missed. A thorough investigation of the abdomen cannot be performed without adequate intra-abdominal equipment and instruments, and one should not hesitate to introduce another cannula. If there is too much blood in the abdomen, or the patient becomes unstable during the procedure, conversion to open surgery should not be delayed.

Discussion

A few notes of caution should be made. There is no place for diagnostic laparoscopy in the unstable patient. The exact role of laparoscopy in blunt abdominal trauma has still to be defined (Leppaniemi and Elliott 1996), but laparoscopy is probably the best diagnostic study for evaluation of diaphragmatic injuries (Poole et al. 1996). Even in penetrating injury one should be careful with diagnostic laparoscopy. The greatest value of diagnostic laparoscopy in penetrating injury is in the evaluation of peritoneal violation, diaphragmatic, and upper abdominal solid organ injuries. It is not ideal for predicting hollow viscus injury (Ortega et al. 1996). One should be careful with laparoscopy in trauma patients with concomitant head injury as the pneumoperitoneum increases intracranial pressure (Este-McDonald et al. 1995; Josephs et al. 1994). Lastly, for success of laparoscopy in trauma one should have a stable patient, good equipment, and an experienced surgeon (Nagy and Sutter 1994).

Ascites

Laparoscopy in cases of ascites in adults may be very helpful. Chu et al. (1994) studied 129 adult patients, of whom 60.5% had carcinomatosis, 20.2% tuberculosis, 5.4%, cirrhosis and 14% no gross abnormality. Ascites in children may as it is in adults be hepatic, renal, cardiac, pancreatic, gastrointestinal, infectious, neoplastic, or gynecological, and it may be of acquired or congenital lymphatic origin. Laparoscopy in children with ascites is rarely indicated. An exception may be lymphatic or chylous ascites. In acquired lymphatic or chylous ascites, laparoscopy may be able to detect or even treat the leak. Intestinal lymphangiectasia can be well diagnosed laparoscopically (Fox and Lucani 1993).

References

Almeida J et al (1995) Acalculous cholecystitis: the use of diagnostic laparoscopy. J Laparoendosc Surg 5:227–231
Aractingi S et al (1993) Subcutaneous localizations of Burkitt lymphoma after coelioscopy. Am J Hematol 42:408
Austin E, Gans SL (1983) Laparoscopy for trauma. In: Gans SL (ed) Pediatric endoscopy. Grune and Stratton, New York, pp 189–194

Babineau TJ et al (1994) Role of staging laparoscopy in the treatment of hepatic malignancy. Am J Surg 167:151-155

Baerlocher C, Engelhart G, Fahrländer H (1973) Die Notfall-Laparoskopie. Leber Magen Darm 3:11-14

Baker PN, Symonds EM (1992) The resolution of chronic pain after normal laparoscopic findings. Am J Obstet Gynecol 166:835-836

Bender JS, Talami MA (1992) Diagnostic laparoscopy in critically ill intensive care unit patients. Surg Endosc 6:302-304

Brandt CP, Priebe PP, Eckhauser ML (1993) Diagnostic laparoscopy in the intensive care patient. Avoiding the nontherapeutic laparotomy. Surg Endosc 7:168-172

Brandt CP, Priebe PP, Jacobs DG (1994) Value of laparoscopy in trauma ICU patients with suspected cholecystitis. Surg Endosc 8:361-364

Burdelski M (1979) Laparoskopie im Kindesalter. Leber Magen Darm 9:259-263

Cadranel S, Rodesch P, Platteborse R (1979) Experience in pediatric laparoscopy. Z Kinderchir Suppl 27:138-141

Childers JM, Surwit EA (1992) Laparoscopic para-aortic lymph node biopsy for the diagnosis of non-Hodgkin's lymphoma. Surg Laparosc Endosc 2:139-142

Chu CM et al (1994) The role of laparoscopy in the evaluation of ascites of unknown origin. Gastrointest Endosc 40:285-289

Coleman M et al (1976) Peritoneoscopy in Hodgkin Disease. JAMA 236:2634-2636

Conlon KC et al (1996) The value of minimal access surgery in the staging of patients with potentially resectable peripancreatic malignancy. Ann Surg 223:134-140

Crantock LR, Dillon JF, Hayes PC (1994) Diagnostic laparoscopy and liver disease: experience of 200 cases. Aust N Z J Med 24:258-262

Ditmars ML, Bongard F (1996) Laparoscopy for triage of penetrating trauma: the decision to explore. J Laparoendosc Surg 6:285-291

Este-McDonald JR et al (1995) Changes intracranial pressure associated with apneumic retractors. Arch Surg 130:362-365

Evoy D et al (1996) Laparoscopic diagnosis and resection of a bleeding Meckel's diverticulum in a thirteen year old female. Ir J Med Sci 165:49

Fahrländer H (1969) Laparoscopy in abdominal emergencies. Germ Med Mon 14:430-432

Ferzli GS et al (1994) Combined use of laparoscopy and endoscopy in diagnosing and treating Dieulafoy's vascular malformations of the stomach. Surg Endosc 8:332-334

Fox U, Lucani G (1993) Disorders of the intestinal mesenteric lymphatic system. Lymphology 26:61-66

Frangenheim H (1974) Die Stellung der Laparoskopie bei gynäkologischen und chirurgischen Problemen im Kindesalter. Padiatr Fortbild K Praxis 39:71-78

Gans SL, Austin E (1983) The technique of laparoscopy. In: Gans SL (ed) Pediatric endoscopy. Grune and Stratton, New York, pp 151-160

Gans SL, Berci G (1971) Advances in endoscopy in infants and children. J Pediatr Surg 6:399-405

Gans SL, Berci G (1973) Peritoneoscopy in infants and children. J Pediatr Surg 8:399-405

Gazzanagia AB, Stanton WW, Bartlett RH (1976) Laparoscopy in the diagnosis of blunt and penetrating injuries to the abdomen. Am J Surg 131:315-318

Gouma DJ et al (1996) Laparoscopic ultrasonography for staging of gastrointestinal malignancy. Scand J Gastroenterol [Suppl] 218:43-49

Goldstein DP et al (1979) New insights into the old problem of chronic pelvic pain. J Pediatr Surg 14:675-680

Hallfeldt KK et al (1995) Laparoscopic adhesiolysis in therapy of chronic abdominal pain. Zentralbl Chir 120:387-391

Heselson J (1970) Peritoneoscopy in abdominal trauma. S Afr J Surg 8:53-60

Holcomb GW III et al (1995) Minimal invasive surgery in children with cancer. Cancer 76:121-128

Holland RM, Lilly JR (1992) Surgical jaundice: other than biliary atresia. Semin Pediatr Surg 1:125–129
Huang CS, Lin LH (1993) Laparoscopic Meckel's diverticulectomy in infants: report of three cases. J Pediatr Surg 28:1486–1489
Josephs LG et al (1994) Diagnostic laparoscopy increases intracranial pressure. J Trauma 36:815–818
Karamehmedovic O et al (1977) Laparoscopy in childhood. J Pediatr Surg 12:75–81
Kelling (1902) Über Oesophagoskopie, Gastroskopie und Koelioskopie. Münch Med Wochenschr 49:21–24
Lauder TD, Moses FM (1995) Recurrent abdominal pain from abdominal adhesions in an endurance triathlete. Med Sci Sports Exer 27:623–625
Leape LL, Ramenofsky ML (1977) Laparoscopy in infants and children. J Pediatr Surg 12:929–938
Leape LL, Ramenofsky ML (1980) Laparoscopy in children. Pediatrics 66:215–220
Lefor AT, Flowers JL (1994) Laparoscopic wedge biopsy of the liver. J Am Coll Surg 178:307–308
Leppaniemi AK, Elliott DC (1996) The role of laparoscopy in blunt abdominal trauma. Ann Med 28:483–489
Madsen MR (1994) Laparoscopy in the diagnosis of bleeding Meckel's diverticulum. Surg Endosc 8:1346–1347
Miller GG, Blair GK, Murphy JJ (1996) Diagnostic laparoscopy in childhood Crohn's disease. J Pediatr Surg 31:846–848
Nagy A, Sutter M (1994) Laparoscopy in abdominal trauma. In: Taterson-Brown S, Garden J (eds) Principles and practice of surgical laparoscopy. Saunders, London, pp 501–514
Nord HJ, Boyd WP (1996) Diagnostic laparoscopy. Endoscopy 28:147–155
Ortega AE et al (1996) Laparoscopic evaluation of penetrating thoracoabdominal traumatic injuries. Surg Endosc 10:19–22
Ozaksit G et al (1995) Chronic pelvic pain in adolescent women: diagnostic laparoscopy and ultrasonography. J Reprod Med 40:500–502
Perry CP (1990) Recognition and treatment of persistent omphalomesenteric ligament. J Reprod Med 35:636–638
Phillips E, Hakim MH, Saxe A (1994) Laparoendoscopy (laparoscopic assisted enteroscopy) and partial resection of the small bowel. Surg Endosc 8:686–688
Poole GV, Thomae KR, Hauser CJ (1996) Laparoscopy in trauma. Surg Clin North Am 76:547–556
Rodgers BM, Vries JK, Talbert JL (1978) Laparoscopy in the diagnosis and treatment of malfunctioning ventriculo-peritoneal shunts in children. J Pediatr Surg 13:247–253
Root HD et al (1965) Diagnostic peritoneal lavage. Surgery 57:633–637
Ruddock JC (1937) Peritoneoscopy in surgery. Surg Gynecol Obstet 65:523–539
Sackier J (1992) Diagnostic laparoscopy in nonmalignant disease. Surg Clin North Am 72:1033–104
Schwöbel MG, Stauffer UG (1980) Der Stellenwert der Laroskopie bei Verdacht auf akute Appendizitis. Z Kinderchir 29:24–29
Selmair H, Wildhirt E (1973) Laparokopie und gezielte Leberpunktion beim Kind. Leber Magen Darm 3:20–22
Sotnikov VN, Erokhin PG, Zakharova IB (1994) Endoscopy in the diagnosis and treatment of abdominal adhesions. Khirurgiia Mosk 6:25–28
Soza JL et al (1995) Laparoscopy in 121 consecutive patients with abdominal gunshot injury. J Trauma 39:501–504
Stauffer UG, Hirsig J (1979) Unsere Erfahrungen mit der Laparoskopie bei Säuglingen und Kindern. Z Kinderchir [Suppl] 27:134–137
Stellato TA (1996) Flexible endoscopy as an adjunct to laparoscopic surgery. Surg Clin North Am 76:595–602
Sugarbaker PH et al (1975) Pre-operative laparoscopy in diagnosis of acute abdominal pain. Lancet I:442–444

Tostivint R et al (1971) Laparoscope dans les traumatismes abdominaux. J Chir (Paris) 102:77–84
van Dijkum EJ et al (1997) The efficacy of laparoscopic staging in patients with upper gastrointestinal tumors. Cancer 79:1315–1319
Vargas C et al (1995) Diagnostic laparoscopy: a 5- year experience in a hepatology training program. Am J Gastroenterol 90:1258–1262
Wildhirt E, Selmair H (1970) Ergebnisse der Laparoskopie im Kindesalter. Endoscopy 2:209–214
Zornig C et al (1993) Staging-Laparoskopie beim Morbus Hodgkin. Dtsch Med Wochenschr 118:1401–1404

**Part III
Abdomen**

Gastrointestinal Tract

CHAPTER 17

Laparoscopic Treatment of Achalasia

G. Mattioli, A. Cagnazzo, P. Buffa, V. Jasonni

Introduction

Achalasia is a functional disorder of the esophagus characterized by abnormal motility of the esophageal body (nonperistaltic waves) and incomplete, delayed, or absent relaxation of the lower sphincter (achalasia) during swallowing [5, 11]. The disease is probably acquired [3, 5, 18]. Its annual incidence in the general population is $4-6/10^6$, and only 5% of patients are aged under 15 years. The patients present with fluid dysphagia ("paroxysmal" dysphagia), retention, and regurgitation of undigested food. Retrosternal pain, sialorrhea, aspiration pneumonia, and failure to thrive are associated symptoms. Contrast barium esophagography, swallowing manometric examination, and endoscopy are the basic tests to confirm the diagnosis [18].

Management of the disease is still symptomatic. Pharmacological agents, for example, Ca blockers, esophageal bougienage, and pneumatic dilations, have been used to treat the disease [2, 15, 16, 20]. The treatment of choice is extramucosal myotomy of the lower esophageal sphincter (LES) to improve esophageal emptying. Heller described a surgical procedure characterized by two parallel anterior and posterior myotomies; Groeneveldt and Zaaijer modified this procedure to a single anterior muscle resection [7–9]. Esophagectomy (Sweet or Lortat Jacob technique) of the lower segment may be necessary if stricture is present [17]. An antireflux procedure can be performed to prevent gastroesophageal reflux and to protect the mucosa from acids. A 360° full-wrap fundoplication (Nissen-Rossetti) is more effective than a 240° (Belsey) or 180° (Dor) partial wrap [6]. The Dor fundoplication is the most effective in reducing the risk of stenosis or recurrence of achalasia and in preventing reflux [19].

The laparoscopic approach is used to reduce operative trauma. The steps of the laparoscopic operation must be similar to the open approach [10].

The need for surgery and its timing are still controversial in the treatment of esophageal achalasia in children. We think that the endoscopic dilations are to be avoided because of the high recurrence rate of symptoms and of the high risk of perforation during the eventual surgical procedure, particularly in small patients. Moreover, surgical treatment offers a better long-term outcome than dilations [1, 4].

Preoperative Workup

All the patients must be studied preoperatively by contrast barium swallowing test, esophageal manometry, and endoscopy to detect the nonrelaxing lower esophageal sphincter and the dilated nonpropulsive esophagus. X-ray esophagography is also used to monitor esophageal distention. Three days before surgery the patients are fed only fluids in order to reduce aliment retention. Enemas are administered both on the day before and early in the morning of surgery to reduce colon distention.

Preoperative Preparation

A nasogastric tube is introduced when the patient is still awake in order to clean the dilated esophagus and stomach and to reduce the risk of aspiration during tracheal intubation. A clean esophagus is mandatory for intraoperative esophagoscopy and minimizes spill of contents in the event of inadvertent perforation. No vesical catheter is needed. Skin preparation with meticulous scrubbing of the umbilicus is needed allowing a good view of the whole abdomen from the pubis to the sternum and laterally to the anterior axillary lines. The patient is supine in the lithotomy position with a reverse Trendelenburg. The surgeon stands between the legs of the patient. The cameraman is on the right and the assistant on the left of the child. The monitor is positioned on the right of the patient at the head of the table (Fig. 1). General anesthesia with tracheal intubation is administered. CO_2 level, heart rate, and blood pressure are constantly and noninvasively monitored [12].

A five-port technique is used (Fig. 2). A Veress needle is inserted through a skin incision 2-cm on the left of the umbilicus. A 12 mmHg CO_2 pneumoperitoneum is created. Similarly as in all laparoscopic hiatal procedures, five cannulas are inserted in a semicircular pattern: (a) left paraumbilical (5-mm) through

Fig. 1. Position of the patient, crew, and monitor

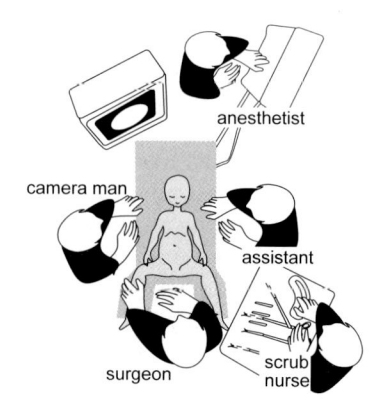

Fig. 2. Position of the trocars. A five-port technique is used. In small patients only 5-mm instruments are used, but in adults a 10-mm telescope and a 10-mm grasper are preferred

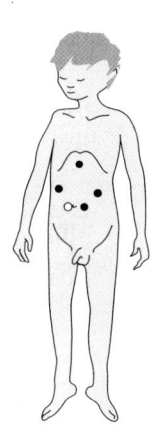

which a Babcock is used for the retraction of the stomach during dissection, (b) right paraumbilical (5-mm) for the telescope, (c) left subcostal (5 mm), and (d) right subcostal (5 mm) as the working ports, and (e) epigastric/subxyphoid (5 mm) for retraction of the liver. We prefer to use the 5-mm ports in children and to use 10-mm ports only in adults [13, 14].

Technique

The liver is retracted through the epigastric port, and the stomach is pulled downward using a Babcock clamp through the left paraumbilical access. The identification of the gastroesophageal junction, using an endoscopic light, is the first operative step to divide the phrenoesophageal ligament; this maneuver allows the anterior esophageal wall to be completely freed from the visceral peritoneal fold. A stationary and dynamic manometric evaluation is performed before and during the dissection of the LES to determine the extension of the myotomy. Only the anterior and lateral walls of the esophagus are dissected, without complete mobilization in order to leave the hiatus intact. The anterior vagus nerve is identified and preserved.

A single anterior myotomy is performed initially with a hook cautery and then using blunt scissors or dissector to spread the musculature. Once the submucosal plane is reached, the mucosa is clearly identified through the myotomy. The distal part of the myotomy is extended over the esophagogastric junction. Care must be taken to avoid the high risk of hemorrhage and mucosal perforation particularly in the patients who have previously been dilated. An intraoperative esophagoscopy aims at reducing the incidence of mucosal perforation. Muscle dissection is stopped when the manometry confirms the reduction in the transitional high pressure zone to values less than 5 mmHg. A strip of the muscle can be resected to promote mucosal herniation and to allow histological examination of the specimen (Fig. 3a).

Fig. 3a,b. Extramucosal myotomy of the lower esophageal sphincter. **a** The transabdominal approach allows a muscle resection to be performed on the abdominal and thoracic esophagus without opening the diaphragmatic hiatus. After opening of the peritoneum and isolation of the anterior wall of the cardia, the circular esophageal muscles are transected using a coagulator hook, and the longitudinal muscles are spread. A strip of muscle is resected to increase the distance between the muscle margins. The myotomy ends when the mucosa completely herniates for a distance of at least 6 cm. **b** Partial fundoplication: an anterior wrap is created using the anterior wall of the stomach. Two sutures are secured on each side of the myotomy. *Numbers,* the sutures between the gastric wall and the esophageal muscle margins

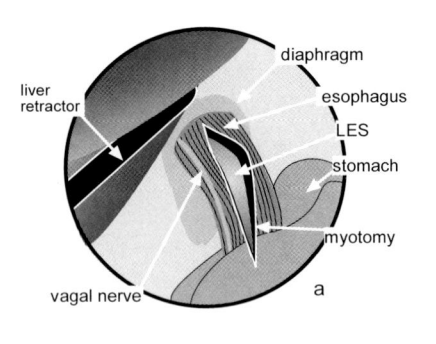

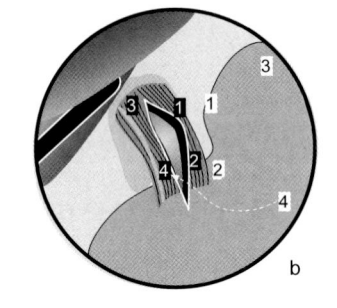

An anterior 180° partial fundoplication is performed in order to prevent gastroesophageal reflux and to protect the herniated mucosa. This is performed by suturing the left and right esophageal muscular edges to the anterior gastric wall and to the right diaphragmatic crura. Four nonabsorbable stitches (two on each side) with intracorporeal knots are used (Fig. 3b). No drains are placed. The parietal holes are closed using an absorbable cuticular suture. A nasogastric tube is inserted and removed the day after surgery. Feeding is allowed when bowel movements start.

Results

We have operated on three children using this approach and on an additional 10 patients younger than 30 years. Mean operative time was 120 min. The patients were discharged 48 h postoperatively. Neither morbidity nor mortality was related to the surgical procedure. We have not experienced mucosal perforation. All the patients were clinically controlled without recurrence of symptoms. A barium meal was administered to detect stasis. No pH analysis was carried out because of absence of symptoms. In all the pediatric cases a manometric postoperative evaluation was performed. Neither recurrence of dysphagia nor gastroesophageal reflux symptoms were evident.

Discussion

Whether the laparoscopic approach is better then the thoracoscopic remains a subject of debate. We prefer the abdominal access as it allows the myotomy to be safely extended to the gastric side (the LES is a subdiaphragmatic anatomical and functional structure), and the fundoplication to be correctly carried out; moreover in young and small patients the one lung ventilation is less easy to perform than tracheal intubation [1].

Controversies exist as to whether a fundoplication should be planned, and which is the best one. The decision to add a fundoplication appears to be a preference of some authors; we think that fundoplication has the main advantages of reducing the risk of gastroesophageal reflux following hiatal and sphincter opening, of protecting the herniated mucosa from the feeding injuries, and of reducing the risk of postoperative perforation [6, 14].

The main disadvantage of the complete wrap (Nissen) is the creation of a high-pressure zone that may become obstructive to the poorly functioning esophagus. The anterior wrap (Dor-Thal) has the advantages of being an easier procedure and of increasing the pressure at the cardia only anteriorly, thus protecting the herniated esophageal mucosa while preventing gastroesophageal reflux. The advantage of the posterior fundoplication (Toupet) is to prevent reflux with minimal risk of obstruction; the disadvantage is the need of a complete esophageal dissection.

We underline that the laparoscopy has modified only the approach while the procedure is the same as for the open classic Heller-Dor extramucosal myotomy that we usually adopt for adults and children with esophageal achalasia. The advantages of the minimally invasive approach are well known and are even more interesting in the cases undergoing functional surgery of the esophagus.

In conclusion, surgery is the most efficient and effective therapy for achalasia, and the minimally invasive approach is the current gold standard in both pediatric and adult populations.

References

1. Ballantine TVN, Fitzgerald JF, Grosfeld JL (1980) Transabdominal esophagomyotomy for achalasia in children. J Pediatr Surg 15:457–461
2. Berger K, McCallum RW (1982) Nifedipine in the treatment of achalasia. Ann Intern Med 96:61–63
3. Berquist WE, Byrne WJ, Ament ME (1983) Achalasia: diagnosis, management and clinical course in 16 children. Pediatrics 71:798–801
4. Caffarena PE et al (1994) Pneumatic dilatations of stenosis of gastro-intestinal tract. Third International Congress for Children Endoscopy-Laparoscopic Surgery, Munster 1–2 February
5. Castell DO (1976) Achalasia and diffuse esophageal spasm. Arch Intern Med 136:571–578
6. Crookes PF, Wilkinson AJ, Johnston GW (1989) Heller's myotomy with partial fundoplication. Br J Surg 76:98–99

7. Ellis FH, Gibb SP, Crozier RE (1980) Esophagomyotomy for achalasia of the esophagus. Ann Surg 192:157–162
8. Ellis FH, Kiser JC, Schlegel JF (1967) Esophagomyotomy for esophageal achalasia: experimental, clinical and manometric aspects. Ann Surg 166:640–645
9. Heller E (1914) Extramukose Cardiaplastik beim chronische Cardiospasm mit Dilatation des Esophagus. Mitt Grenzgeb Med Chir 27:141–145
10. Holcomb III GW, Richards WO, Riedel BD (1996) Laparoscopic esophagomyotomy for achalasia in children. J Ped Surg 31(5):716–718
11. Hurst AF, Rake GW (1930) Achalasia of the cardia. Q J Med 23:491–497
12. Ivani G, Vaira M, Mattioli G (1994) Paediatric laparoscopic surgery: anaesthetic management. Paediatr Anaesth 4:323–325
13. Jasonni V, Mattioli G (1994) Laparoscopic surgery in childhood. J Surg Endosc 8(8):957
14. Jasonni V et al (1994) Nissen fundo-plicatio in children: laparoscopic technique. Third International Congress for Children Endoscopy-Laparoscopic Surgery, Munster, 1–2 Feburary
15. Nakayama DK, Shorter NA, Boyle JT (1987) Pneumatic dilatation and operative treatment of achalasia in children. J Pediatr Surg 22:619–622
16. Okike N, Payne WS, Neufeld DM (1979) Esophagomyotomy versus forceful dilation for achalasia of the esophagus. Ann Thorac Surg 28:119–125
17. Orringer MB, Orringer JS (1982) Esophagectomy: definitive treatment for esophageal neuromotor dysfunction. Ann Thorac Surg 34:237–241
18. Raven RW (1971) Achalasia of the esophagus in children. BMJ 5267:1614–1616
19. Vane DW et al (1988) Late results following esophagomyotomy in children with achalasia. J Pediatr Surg 23:515–519
20. Vantrappen G, Jannssens J (1983) To dilate or to operate? That is the question. Gut 24:1013–1019

CHAPTER 18

Laparoscopic Nissen Fundoplication in Children

A.S. Najmaldin, G.M.E. Humphrey

Introduction

Movement of gastric contents into the oesophagus (gastro-oesophageal reflux (GER) is virtually ubiquitous in neonates [1]. At approximately 2 months of age GER occurs at least twice a day in up to 50% decreasing to less than 1% by 1 year of age [1]. Treatment of GER is only warranted when it is the cause of symptoms or tissue injury. In infants and children the most commonly recognised consequences of GER include recurrent vomiting, oesophagitis, failure to thrive, reactive airway disease and pulmonary aspiration. The majority of children with reflux disease (including those with severe neurological disability) should initially be treated non-surgically, with primary fundoplication being reserved for those with Barrett's oesphagus or reflux induced oesophageal strictures [2, 3].

Common to all of the described methods of performing a fundoplication are the aims to increase the high-pressure zone of the lower oesophagus, to accentuate the angle of His and increase the length of intra-abdominal oesophagus. Although several anti-reflux procedures exist, the Nissen fundoplication first described in 1956 [4] has become the most commonly performed anti-reflux procedure in children with around 80% of children achieving a good result [2, 3, 5].

Laparoscopic Nissen fundoplication was first performed by Dallemagne and associates in 1991 [6]. Since then several large studies have confirmed that the Nissen fundoplication can be safely and at least in the short term effectively performed in both adults and children via the laparoscope with complications rates comparable to those of open surgery [7–9].

Indications and Pre-operative Preparation

The selection criteria for a laparoscopic approach must be the same as those applied to an open operation, i.e. criteria should not be relaxed in the belief that the minimally invasive approach is a lesser procedure than an open one. The indications for surgery are therefore failure to respond to an adequate trial of medical treatment or complications of GER such as Barrett's oesophagus and stricture. The decision for surgery and pre-operative investigations required are greatly influenced by the neurological status of the child and whether a gastrostomy for nutritional support is the primary reason for surgical intervention. Upper gastrointestinal endoscopy with or without biopsy and contrast study to asses the extent and severity of oesophagitis, reflux, presence of a hiatus hernia and adequacy of gastric emptying are indicated. One normally performs 24-h pH monitoring, particularly in those who are neurologically normal. In children who have airway disease and/or recurrent pulmonary aspiration an assessment of the child's respiratory status should be undertaken including chest radiography, blood gas analysis and saturation monitoring.

In our view there is no absolute contra-indication for performing a laparoscopic fundoplication as we have successfully operated on patients who were on heart and lung transplantation programmes at the time of request for fundoplication. However relative contra-indications to a laparoscopic approach are extreme hepatosplenomegaly or portal hypertension, short oesophagus including those with previously repaired oesophageal atresias and scarring from previous upper abdominal surgery when a laparoscopic approach may impose a technical challenge.

The decision to proceed with a laparoscopic approach must be made with full consent from the parents. This should include a discussion of the need to convert to a conventional open procedure should the laparoscopic approach prove difficult and of the complications of surgery. The neurologically impaired child with marked kyphoscoliosis and contractures of the limbs poses specific problems namely positioning on the operating table and access to the operating field. In this group of patients, our experience suggests that a laparoscopic approach is relatively easier than the open route providing the patients are positioned properly and their abdomen and costal margins are examined in order to map out the exact locations for access cannulae.

Equipment/Instruments

In addition to the basic equipment (camera, screen, light source and cables, insufflator, diathermy generator and suction irrigation devices) and a set of laparotomy instruments for emergency or conversion to open surgery if required as in all laparoscopic procedures, the following instruments are required:
- Cannula/trocar ×5 (3.5–12 mm)
- 5 or 10 mm preferably 30° angled telescope
- Atraumatic curved or angled double jaw action grasping forceps without ratchet (3.5–5 mm)
- One soft Babcock, soft bowel clamp or soft atraumatic grasping forceps with ratchet (3.5–10 mm)
- One toothed grasping forceps with ratchet (3.5–5 mm)
- One double jaw action curved scissors with a diathermy point (3.5–5 mm) ensuring that the insulation sleeve extends to the blades
- Unipolar hook diathermy probe. In addition, a bipolar forceps is an advantage.

18 Laparoscopic Nissen Fundoplication in Children

- One needle holder (3.5–5 mm)
- One retractor (3.5–5 mm)
- Suction irrigation probe (3.5–5 mm)
- Non-absorbable suture on needle:-2-0 or 3-0 silk or Ethibond on a curved, ski or straightened out needle (the size and shape of the needle are determined by the internal diameter of access cannulae)
- A piece of nylon or soft rubber tube to use as a sling
- Clips and clip applicator or ultrasound harmonic shear, if short gastric vessels are to be divided

The diameter and length of instruments/cannulae are dependent on the size and shape of the patient as well as the surgeon's preference. It is advisable to use light weight and short working (secondary) cannulae in infants and young children as their surface area for access is small, their abdominal wall thin and peritoneal cavity small.

Technique

The patient is anaesthetised with endotracheal intubation and full muscle relaxation. Theatre layout and positioning of the patient and surgeon are demonstrated in (Fig. 1). A large bore naso-gastric tube in inserted. In all cases the abdomen is palpated to determine presence of enlarged or displaced viscera which might prevent necessary access or predispose to injury during cannula placement. For

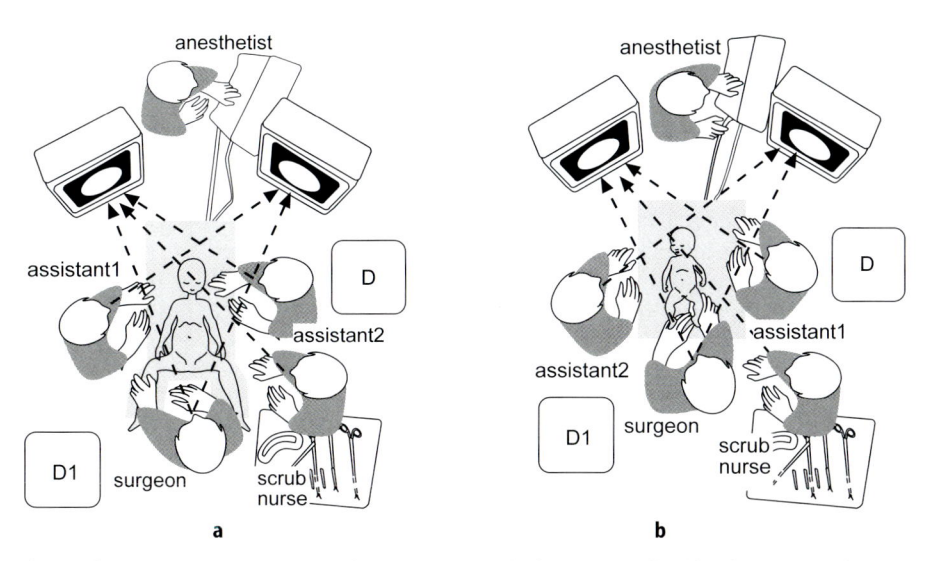

Fig. 1. a-b. Theatre layout and position of large patient **a** and infants and small children **b**. D or D_1, Diathermy generator

example, the extent of the liver and spleen below the costal margin in the infant, the bladder in all ages and a deformed costal margin and spine in the neurologically impaired. If a gastrostomy is to be placed at the time of fundoplication the position of the stoma must be marked before the pneumoperitoneum is created to ensure optimal placement once the operation is complete.

A primary supra-umbilical (peri-umbilical) cannula (5–12 mm for the telescope) is inserted using an open technique [10] and a pneumoperitoneum created using carbon dioxide with a flow rate of 0.2–0.5 l/min and an intra-abdominal pressure of 8–10 mmHg. Following a brief exploration of the upper abdominal cavity, the sites and sizes of four working (secondary) cannulae are selected depending on the patient's size and shape, the presence of hepato-splenomegaly and/or musculo-skeletal abnormalities and whether a concomitant gastrostomy is required (Fig. 2). While a 0° telescope may be adequate and is easier to use, a 30° angled telescope provides a much better view during mobilisation of the oesophagus, particularly when the primary cannula placement fails to give an adequate view because of low position or musculo-skeletal abnormalities. Slight reverse Trendelenberg tilt allows the stomach and other organs to fall away from the oesophageal hiatus and for drainage of peritoneal fluid and blood from the surgical field.

The principles of dissection and suturing are identical to that of the open procedure. In our experience, ligation of the short gastric vessels is not necessary to allow fashioning of a loose complete wrap. A large oesophageal tube or bougie is helpful but not essential during mobilisation of the oesophagus, closure of the hiatus and fundoplication. The liver is gently retracted upwards and the upper part of the stomach is pulled down with an atraumatic grasping forceps (Babcock or soft bowel clamp). During retraction to the stomach care must be taken not to tear the stomach wall. A peritoneal incision a few centimetres long is made at the gastro-oesophageal junction using scissors, diathermy or both. The incision is then extended to the gastro-hepatic omentum superior to the hepatic branches of the vagus nerve. Sometimes the hepatic fibres of the vagus may require sacrificing to allow adequate access to the right side of the oesophagus and the oesophageal hiatus. During this dissection care must be taken to carefully coagulate all small vessels before dividing them, to identify and preserve the vagi and to avoid damage to the oesophagus itself. In most cases the oesophagus can easily be identified and cleared of its attachments on the right and anterior aspects.

The left peri-oesophageal connections are cleared by pulling the stomach downwards and to the right and at this stage the upper border of the gastric fundus is if necessary cleared from the diaphragm (Fig. 3). The oesophagus can then

Fig. 2. Nissen fundoplication, position of cannulae. *A*, Primary cannula for insufflation and telescope; *B1, B2*, secondary "working" cannulae; *C* or *C₁*, retractor; *D*, grasper to retract stomach and hold sling

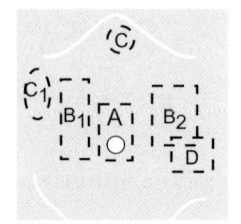

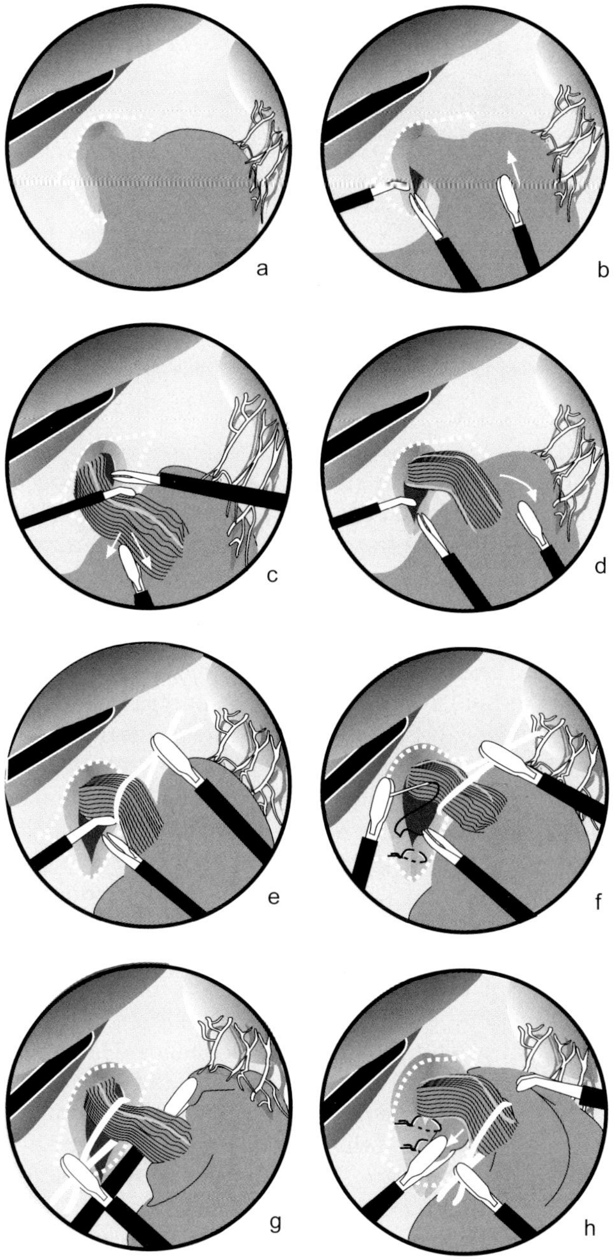

18 Laparoscopic Nissen Fundoplication in Children 167

Fig. 3a–j. Mobilisation of the oesophagus, repair of hiatal defect and fundoplication. *Arrows*, direction of traction/retraction. **a** Incision at cardia. **b** Anterior and right side mobilisation of oesophagus. **c** Mobilisation of the left side of the oesophagus. **d** Creation of a window behind the oesophagus. **e** Sling in place and completion of oesophageal mobilisation. **f** Hiatal repair. **g** Start of wrap. **h** Fundus behind and to the right of oesophagus.

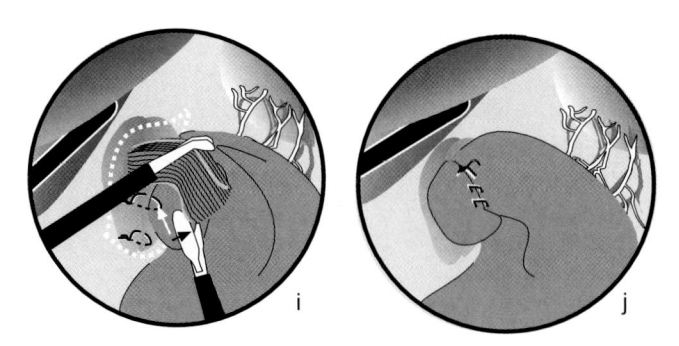

Fig. 3a–j. (continued) Mobilisation of the oesophagus, repair of hiatal defect and fundoplication. *Arrows*, direction of traction/retraction. **i** Fundus to the right and in front of oesophagus; **j** Suturing fundoplication in place

be swept upwards and to the left by using the side of the working grasper/scissors while the stomach is pulled upwards and to the left. A window is created behind the oesophagus from the right. At this stage there is a tendency for the dissection to go deep into the posterior mediastinum and above the left crus. During manipulation behind the oesophagus care must be taken to avoid damage to the oesophagus, posterior vagus, left pleural membrane and spleen. Once the window is created the atraumatic grasper retracting the stomach is replaced by a toothed grasper with ratchet to hold a 10- to 12-cm long sling passed behind the oesophagus. The retro-oesophageal space is now sufficiently cleared to expose both crura and to allow a loose wrap. The posterior vagus is often seen and preserved. The crura are approximated behind the oesophagus using nonabsorbable 2-0 silk or 3-0/4-0 Ethibond sutures. Whilst suturing the crura care must be taken not to damage the liver in front and to the right, spleen behind and aorta underneath the needle especially in small patients as the needles currently available are too long.

Using an atraumatic grasper in the surgeons right hand (left side of patient) the fundus at the greater curve is grasped and the oesophagus lifted using the sling allowing the passage of a second atraumatic grasper this time in the left hand of the surgeon (right side of patient) behind the oesophagus. The fundus is then passed from right hand grasper into the jaws of the left hand grasper and pulled through behind the oesophagus to the right of the patient (Fig. 3). At this point the traction on the sling is released and the toothed grasper replaced by a soft atraumatic grasper with ratchet (Babcock or soft bowel clamp) to hold the wrapped fundus in an optimal position for suturing. The looseness of the wrap is checked and two or three, one or two layers of interrupted 2-0 black silk or 3-0/4-0 Ethibond sutures inserted through stomach-oesophagus-wrapped fundus of stomach preferably using intracorporeal tied knots (alternatively extracorporeal knotting may be utilised). It is advisable, for ease of handling, that sutures are cut to 10–12 cm long before being placed within the abdominal cavity. However, with experience a full length suture may be utilised for insertion of several interrupted stitches. During intracorporeal knotting care must be taken not to inadvertently damage the liver, spleen, diaphragm or pericardium with the needle especially when the surgical space is small as in the infant and small child. It is therefore not unreasonable to remove the needle prior to knot tying. When using extracorporeal knotting techniques care must be taken not to damage tissues by the serration effect of suture traction.

Having completed the fundoplication adjunctive insertion of a gastrostomy if required can be inserted laparoscopically using one or two purse string with or without hitching sutures [11]. Alternatively a percutaneous endoscopic approach may be utilised with the laparoscope confirming optimal placement of the tube on the wall of the stomach and prevention of visceral injury [12].

At the end of the procedure the large bore naso-gastric tube/bougie is replaced by a smaller tube. The pneumoperitoneum is evacuated and fascial incisions greater than 4-mm closed with 3-0 absorbable sutures. Skin closure is achieved using subcuticular absorbable sutures or adhesive strips. Infiltration of local anaesthetic agents into the wounds may be helpful.

Post-operative Care

Post-operative opiate analgesia using an epidural or continuous intravenous infusion may be used in the first 12–24 h particularly in those who require intensive physiotherapy such as the neurologically impaired and those with cystic fibrosis. Other patients may receive adequate pain relief with local wound infiltration of anaesthetic agents.

The children are allowed to take small volumes of clear fluids and drugs on the first post-operative day either orally or via the naso-gastric tube/gastrostomy. Full volume of liquids and nutrition are commenced on the second post-operative day. The naso-gastric tube is removed between 12 and 48 h following operation. Introduction of full feeds in those children who have a gastrostomy and require peritoneal dialysis for chronic renal failure should be delayed for a few days.

Children who are otherwise well may be discharged on the third post-operative day. Discharge of patients with neurological impairment, respiratory or chronic renal failure is generally determined by their underlying condition and need for concomitant therapy. Patients who have had a gastrostomy tube inserted require longer hospitalisation than others because of graded introduction of full volume feeding and the need to educate the child's care givers in the management of the gastrostomy.

Results

Over a 3.5-year period, 52 consecutive patients underwent Nissen fundoplication (38 with gastrostomy) in our institute. Of these, 35 were neurologically impaired,

6 had chronic renal failure and 11 miscellaneous illness (mainly cystic fibrosis). The patients' weights ranged from 3.9 to 42 kg. Two patients were converted to open procedures, one because of an oesophageal tear during mobilisation of the oesophagus and in the second child who had Fallot's tetralogy because of hypercapnia and difficulty retracting an enlarged liver. Both of these children made uneventful post-operative recoveries. There were no other intra-operative complications. The average operating time for fundoplication alone was 2.1 h (range 1.4-3) and for fundoplication with gastrostomy 2.9 h (range 2.3-4.1).

Patients who had fundoplication alone were discharged home on the third or fourth post-operative day. Those who had fundoplication and gastrostomy were discharged at five to seven days post-operatively.

There were no respiratory or wound complications. Gastric bloat was common post-operatively, and diarrhoea developed in four patients. These problems resolved spontaneously within a few months. During follow-up (average 20 months) one neurologically normal child developed dysphagia which settled spontaneously within 4 months of the operation. One neurologically impaired child developed recurrent pain 4 months following laparoscopic fundoplication and required further surgical intervention. At laparotomy the wrap was found to be intact but the hiatus hernia had recurred. Interestingly this patient had no intra-abdominal adhesions below the diaphragm.

Potential Complications

The laparoscopic approach is not immune to the complications of any conventional surgical procedure – namely complications of anaesthesia, cardiovascular, bleeding, visceral injury, chest and wound infections, and incisional hernia. Complications specific to laparoscopy include those associated with trocar insertion and creation of a CO_2 pneumoperitoneum which may largely be avoided by close attention to operative and anaesthetic techniques.

Experience with laparoscopic Nissen fundoplication in childhood is limited [8, 9, 13, 14]. However, a recent review of 2453 adults undergoing laparoscopic Nissen fundoplication reveals results comparable to conventionally performed procedures [7]. The mortality rate for this series was less than 0.2% (4 patients), two deaths were attributed to complications of missed visceral perforation (one duodenal and one oesophageal), one to development of mesenteric thrombosis and in the remaining one myocardial infarction.

Intraoperative events in this adult patient series include conversion to an open procedure in 5.8%, gastric or oesophageal perforation in 1%, pneumothorax in 2% and splenic injury resulted in splenectomy in 0.1%. Early post-operative complications include re-operation because of post-operative bleeding (0.2%) and missed perforation (0.4%). Re-operation was required in less than 1% because of crural disruption, peri-oesophageal herniation or gastric volvulus.

Dysphagia was documented in 20% of cases during the early post-operative period falling to 5.5% after an undisclosed period of time. Re-operation for dysphagia was required in less than 1%, endoscopy for food bolus obstruction in 0.5% and dilatation in 3.5%. Recurrent reflux was documented in 3.4% with 0.7% requiring re-operation.

Discussion

From our experience we have found that adoption of the standard technique for performing a laparoscopic fundoplication in adults is not always appropriate for children especially infants and those that are neurologically impaired. Children differ in anatomy, size both absolute and relative to instruments and compliance when compared with normal adults. Long instruments with a noncentrally placed pivot (the abdominal wall) are difficult to manipulate and are more likely to result in port displacement. The child's abdominal wall is relatively thin resulting in poor support of cannulae. Where ever possible the use of small, short and light weight cannulae and instruments should be considered.

Optimal positioning of cannulae for laparoscopic procedures is vital if the operation is to be performed easily and successfully. When deciding where to site cannulae the size of the child and instruments, the need for gastrostomy, presence of a previous scar, the shape of the subphrenic space, limb and chest deformities and the presence of palpable viscera (liver and spleen) must be carefully considered before each cannula is inserted. Particular attention must be paid to the limitations on instrument mobility posed by fixed flexion limb contractures and kyphoscoliosis in those who are neurologically impaired. In addition, these children may have hepatomegaly or liver displacement as a result of their underlying pathology or musculoskeletal deformities. In larger children, a telescope cannula placed a few centimetres above the umbilicus and/or a 30° telescope gives better visualisation of the surgical field than an umbilical port and 0° telescope. However, performing a concomitant laparoscopic gastrostomy may be compromised by a high telescope cannula.

During dissection, identification of essential landmarks for safe operation may be difficult because of the presence of loose connective tissue and dilated veins which are easily traumatised. Meticulous attention to haemostasis is essential if conversion to an open procedure because vision is lost from bleeding is to be avoided. This is particularly so in the presence of a hiatus hernia when no attempt should be made to excise the hernial sac. However, after an initial learning course, dissection and mobilisation of the gastro-oesophageal junction becomes relatively easy.

Suturing within the confined space of the child's abdomen is not without risk, especially in the infant. Although specialised suturing instruments allowing automatic reloading of purpose designed needles exist they are of limited use in paediatric practise because of the size of the instruments and cannula required for their introduction. The needles currently available with appropriate sized suture material are relatively long increasing the risk of visceral injury during closure of the hiatal opening and securing of the oesophageal wrap which require multiple manipulations of the needle. Extreme vigilance with the needle at all times visible is essential if visceral injury is to be avoided.

Conversion to an open procedure during laparoscopic Nissen fundoplication is required in up to 10% of adult cases because of technical difficulties or visceral injury [7,15]. Our experience suggests that the conversion rate may be similar for children although it may be reduced as experience increases and more appropriate instruments become available.

Visceral perforation, both oesophageal and gastric have been documented following conventional [16] and laparoscopically [7, 8, 17] performed fundoplication procedures and may if unrecognised result in unacceptable morbidity and mortality. Careful manipulation, traction and dissection under vision, meticulous attention to haemostasis and awareness of the risks of diathermy current leakage are essential if this complication is to be avoided.

Recurrent reflux may occur in up to 15% of children treated by open procedures [2, 3, 18]. Experience in adults suggests that a recurrence rate of less than 5% may be attainable using the laparoscopic approach [7], however the results of long-term outcome must be made available before the true recurrence rate can be established. To date, our limited experience of laparoscopic Nissen fundoplication in childhood suggests that the incidence of oesophageal perforation and recurrent reflux is well within the limits of previously reported studies on conventionally performed procedures and laparoscopic procedures in adults.

Dysphagia in the first few weeks following both open [16] and laparoscopic [7] fundoplication is not uncommon. However, persistent dysphagia requiring intervention affects approximately 1% of those undergoing laparoscopic fundoplication [7] and between 1% and 2% of those undergoing conventional open surgery [19, 20].

Conclusion

It appears that Laparoscopic Nissen fundoplication can be performed successfully and safely in infants and children with short-term results comparable with the open technique. Meticulous attention to details, proper technique and instruments are essential. The early recovery and absence of wound and chest complications we have witnessed, particularly in those who are already seriously malnourished and disabled are encouraging.

References

1. Orenstein SJ (1993) Gastroesophageal reflux. In: Wyllie R, Hyams J (eds) Pediatric gastrointestinal disease. Saunders, Philadelphia, pp 337–369
2. Johnson DG (1985) Current thinking on the role of surgery in gastro-oesophageal reflux. Pediatr Clin North Am 32:1165–1179
3. Spitz L et al (1993) Operation for gastro-oesophageal reflux with associated severe mental retardation. Arch Dis Child 68:347–351

4. Nissen R (1956) Eine einfache Operation zur Beeinflussung der Refluxoesophagitis. Schweiz Med Wochenschr 86:590–592
5. Kazerooni N et al (1994) Fundoplication in 160 children under 2 years of age. J Pediatr Surg 29:677–681
6. Dallemagne B et al (1991) Laparoscopic Nissen fundoplication: preliminary report. Surg Laparoscopic Endosc 1:138–142
7. Perdikis G et al (1997) Laparoscopic Nissen fundoplication: where do we stand? Surg Laparosc Endosc 7:17–21
8. Humphrey GME, Najmaldin A (1996) Laparoscopic Nissen fundoplication in handicapped infants and children. J Pediatr Surg 31:596–599
9. Collins JB III et al (1995) Comparison of open and laparoscopic gastrostomy and fundoplication in 120 patients. J Pediatr Surg 30:1063–1070
10. Humphrey GME, Najmaldin AS (1994) Modification of the Hasson technique in paediatric laparoscopy. Br J Surg 81:1319
11. Humphrey G, Najmaldin AS (1997) Laparoscopic gastrostomy in children. Pediatr Surg Int 12:501–504
12. Croaker GDH, Najmaldin AS (1997) Laparoscopically assisted percutaneous endoscopic gastrostomy. Pediatr Surg Int 12:130–131
13. Lobe TE (1993) Laparoscopic fundoplication. Semin Pediatr Surg 2:178–181
14. Longis B et al (1996) Laparoscopic fundoplication in children: our first 30 cases. J Laparoendosc Surg 6:S21–S29
15. Watson DI et al (1996) Laparoscopic surgery for gastro-oesophageal reflux: beyond the learning curve. Br J Surg 83:1284–1287
16. Urschel JD (1993) Complications of anti reflux surgery. Am J Surg 166:68–70
17. Hinder RA et al (1994) Laparoscopic Nissen fundoplication is an effective treatment of gastro-oesophageal reflux disease. Ann Surg 220:472–483
18. Pearl RH et al (1990) Complications of gastro-oesophageal anti-reflux surgery in neurologically impaired versus neurologically normal children. J Pediatr Surg 25:1169–1173
19. DeMeester TR, Bonavina L, Albertucci M (1986) Nissen fundoplication for gastroesophageal reflux disease. Evaluation of primary repair in 100 consecutive patients. Ann Surg 204:9–20
20. Ellis FH, Crozier RE (1984) Reflux control by fundoplication: a clinical and manometric assessment of the Nissen operation. Ann Thorac Surg 38:387–392

CHAPTER 19

Laparoscopic Toupet Fundoplication

P. Montupet, G. Cargill, J.-S. Valla

Introduction

There is no perfect operation for gastroesophageal reflux (GER), as is witnessed by the many procedures that have been described, and that continue to be invented today (Pelissier et al. 1997). The goal of the ideal procedure is to correct the incompetent lower esophageal sphincter, to maintain this result during the entire life, and to avoid side effects. The procedures with only anatomic reconstruction and cardiophrenopexy such as the Allison, Collis, and Lortat-Jacob techniques have been abandoned because of the high rate of recurrence. Today fundoplication is almost the only procedure used in adults and children and is described in this chapter. However, the fundoplication can be total according to Nissen or Nissen Rossetti, or partial with anterior wrap according to Thal, Hill, Boix-Ochoa, or Jaubert de Beaujeu, or partial with posterior wrap according to Toupet (1963).

To minimize side effects occurring after total fundoplication many surgeons have modified the original procedure described by Nissen (De Meester and Stein 1992; Eypasch and Neugebauer 1997; Pelissier et al. 1997). Other authors (Lundell et al. 1991; Mosnier et al. 1995; Patti et al. 1997; Pelissier et al. 1997; Watson et al. 1995) advocate the use of a partial wrap in patients with abnormal esophageal motility, which is usually the case in esophageal atresia or chronic bronchopneumopathy. Partial fundoplication seems less demanding than total fundoplication with regard to lower esophagus motility and offers a more physiological antireflux procedure.

Indication

General indications and contraindications are the same as those described in chapters on Nissen and Thal fundoplication.

Since 1992 our operations for GER have all been undertaken laparoscopically. We did not change our approach in terms of Nissen or Toupet procedures as in our experience both were associated with good results in children and both needed to be evaluated laparoscopically: we operated on 218 patients, of whom 93 had a Nissen's and 125 a Toupet's procedure.

Some indications favor the use of a Nissen procedure with gastrostomy and with or without pyloroplasty as patients with advanced esophagitis, peptic esophageal stricture, Barrett's esophagus, or mental deficiency (24 cases). The latter group is at greater risk for aspiration and would therefore fare less well if they were treated by any method that still allows for vomiting or eructation. Moreover most of these patients need a gastrostomy because of swallowing disorders; such a gastrostomy reduces the consequences of an eventual problem of postoperative dysphagia. On the other hand, the Toupet procedure is preferred in neurologically normal children especially with esophageal dysmotility or with reflux induced respiratory symptoms. Sometimes partial fundoplication is the only feasible procedure because of insufficient gastric fundus to allow a loose total fundoplication (e.g., a small stomach in patients with repaired esophageal atresia).

Preoperative Workup

Routine preoperative assessment includes 24-h pH-metry, manometry, upper gastrointestinal series and fiberoptic examination in most cases. Manometry demonstrates not only anomalies of the lower esophageal sphincter (location, tonus, relaxation), but also dyskinetic anomalies of the esophagus itself. As an upper gastrointestinal series also assesses gastric emptying, other types of dysmotility can be picked up this way.

Patient's preparation includes parental consent regarding the method and the need for prolonged postoperative follow-up in order to check its efficacy. As many of our children have associated respiratory conditions such as bronchitis, asthma or allergy, a preoperative chest X-ray is systematically performed.

Preoperative Preparation

Anesthesia

All the patients receive premedication 1 h before induction of anesthesia with halothane. Intubation and mechanical ventilation are started, a nasogastric tube with a diameter of 10–16 F depending on the size of the child is inserted. General anesthesia is maintained with halothane, while fentanyl is used for intraoperative analgesia and vecuronium is added for muscle relaxation.

Position of the Patient, Crew, and Equipment

The child lies supine; the operating table is tilted head-up (Fig. 1). If the patient is less than 5 years of age, the legs are folded up at the end of the table. If he is older, the legs are stretched out and spread open and the surgeon stands between them. The monitor is placed near the patient's right shoulder. All the cables and tubes are fastened to his right leg. The assistant and instrument table are positioned to the surgeon's right.

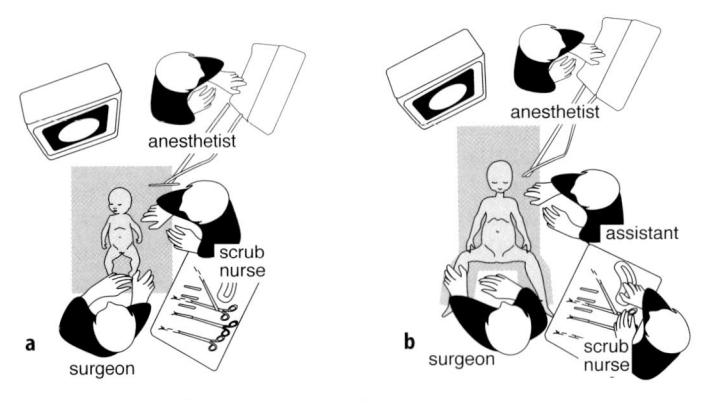

Fig. 1a,b. Position of the patient, crew, and equipment

Positioning of Trocars

Four trocars are used: two for the surgeon's instruments and two for the assistant's instruments (scope and liver or gastric retractor). The position of these trocars varies depending on the size of the child: in children the 0° scope (8 or 10 mm in diameter) is inserted through the umbilicus but in infants the scope (5 or 8 mm) is inserted a few centimeters above the umbilicus, as shown in Fig. 2.

Specific Instrumentation

The trocars are sealed with simple silicone caps in order to facilitate needle passage and also because of the limited of the abdomen. A 0° telescope with panoramic view is used. Sometimes, especially in infants a pediatric Mouret's 2-mm diameter abdominal wall retractor is placed at the xyphoid process. This device enlarges the operative field, it retracts the falciform ligament against the abdominal wall and protects it from injury, it allows for lower abdominal CO_2 pressures, and for suction of blood without causing a collapse of the anterior abdominal wall (Fig. 2a).

The liver retractor can be a palpator, an irrigation-suction cannula, or a "three fingers" retractor. The Johan-type grasping forcepses are broad, have a blunt end and a ratchet device. An additional 3-mm grasper is sometimes inserted directly through the abdominal wall in the left subcostal area. The two needle-holders are light and often used with the safety catch off so as to facilitate grasping, orientation and release of the needle.

For dissection and coagulation we prefer the short and broad hook with a beveled tip, which represents an adequate dissector in children. It is a monopolar instrument but a bipolar hook dissector and a reusable 5-mm clip applier are available in the conventional set of tools.

Fig. 2a,b. Position of the trocars

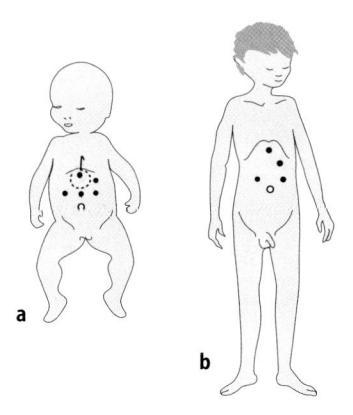

Technique

The pneumoperitoneum is induced with CO_2 via the first cannula, which is inserted in an open way at the umbilicus or a few centimeters above it. Pressure is maintained between 6 and 12 mmHg depending on the age of the child and the presence of an abdominal wall suspensor. The operation involves six steps:

1. The hepatogastric ligament is divided form the lesser curve up to the diaphragm, allowing the right crus and caudate lobe of the liver to come into view. If a sizable pulsatile neurovascular branch heading for the left lobe of the liver is seen, it is left untouched, but this obviously complicates the following steps.
2. The right diaphragmatic crus is bluntly separated from the abdominal esophagus posteriorly all the way to the point where it joins the left crus. For this purpose the retractor is used to compress the caudate lobe, while a grasping forceps is used to pull down the stomach. The esophagus is retracted to the left with a palpator introduced through the left trocar, and the hook introduced through the right trocar *dissects* the right edge of the esophagus, taking care not to damage the esophageal wall, the pleura, or the vagus nerve. The opening in the mediastinal space is cut further down along the right crus, up to the left crus.
3. A window is created behind the abdominal esophagus between the left crus and the gastroesophageal junction.
4. The anterior and left part of the peritoneum and phrenicoesophageal membrane are divided and the left border of the crus is dissected free from the esophagus. The retrocardial opening is widened; only exceptionally short gastric vessels need to be divided.
5. The diaphragmatic hiatus is narrowed with one or two stitches of nonabsorbable 2/0 sutures tied intracorporeally (Fig. 3a). In small children, because of

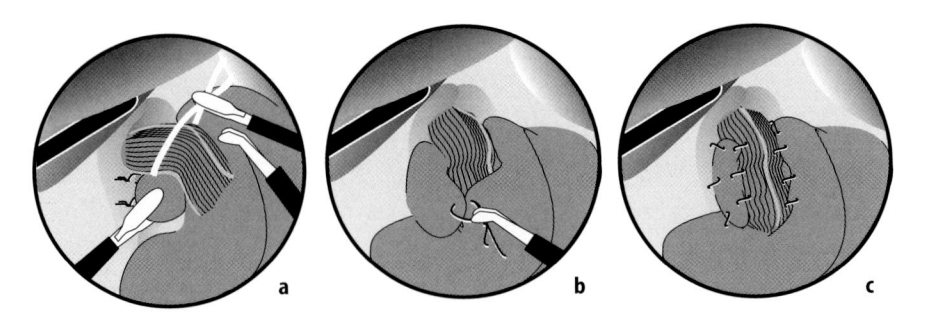

Fig. 3a–c. The actual procedure. **a** The hiatus has been closed behind the esophagus; the fundus is being pulled from the left behind the esophagus to the right. **b** Anterior anchoring stitch to replace the sling. **c** Completed suturing of the wrap to the esophagus and the diaphragm; the anchoring suture has been released

lack of space in the retroesophageal area, extracorporeal knots can sometimes be useful.
6. The gastric fundus is pulled behind the abdominal esophagus and a temporary total fundoplication is made with only one stitch which serves as a tacking stitch and replaces the traction tape (Fig. 3b). A series of three stitches between the right edge of the esophagus and the valve are made one after the other from the bottom to the top. The apical right stitch includes the esophagus, the wrap, and the right crus. Then the valve is loosely attached to the right crus by two more stitches. Three stitches secure the left side of the fundoplication by suturing the greater curvature to the left edge of the esophagus; the apical left stitch here also takes the esophagus, the wrap and the left crus (Fig. 3c).

The tacking stitch is removed allowing the valve to spread out behind the cardia. After complete evacuation of the pneumoperitoneum, the fascia is closed with absorbable thread; adhesive strip is used to close the skin.

Postoperative Care

During the first 24 h, analgesia is obtained with opiates, at the patient's request. In some cases O_2 saturation is monitored. The nasogastric tube is removed on the morning following surgery, and oral feeding is resumed 2 h later, liquid at first followed by a progressively solid diet over 48 h. The amount given depends on each patient's tolerance, and care is taken to avoid hard, dry or irritating foods. In case of nausea or vomiting, metoclopramide is prescribed for 10 days, but medication is discontinued as a rule after the operation.

A postoperative check is scheduled on the 10th postoperative day. After 6 months, another check is performed and includes pH-metry and manometry.

Upper gastrointestinal series is performed at 6 months, 2 years, and 5 years postoperatively.

Results

Between 1992 and 1997, 125 Toupet's procedures were performed. Children were aged 1 month–14 years (mean 5.8 years). In this series there were no neurologically impaired children. No additional procedure such as gastrostomy or pyloroplasty were performed.

Operative Results

None of the patients died, and none of the 125 procedures needed to be converted. The operating time currently ranges from 40 to 90 min.

There were no anesthetic complications, and the intraoperative respiratory changes were of minor importance. Sometimes injury of the liver parenchyma caused by the retractor or the needles complicated the procedure but in all instances the bleeding stopped spontaneously. There was no splenic injury. There were nine (7.2%) intra- and early postoperative complications: three cases of left pneumothorax needing drainage, two of accidental vagus nerve division, and one of ischemia of the upper pole of the spleen after transection of the short gastric vessels without clinical consequences, and three times (2.4%) a reoperation was required. One child underwent a relaparoscopy a few hours after the primary operation for bleeding. Bleeding had perhaps occurred from laceration of one of the short gastric vessels, but no active bleeding was present at the time of the repeat laparoscopy. In another child omentum protruded through the umbilical incision 48 h after surgery which required repair under general anesthesia. In a last child the nasogastric tube, not visible at endoscopy, had been caught in a suture, and the Toupet procedure needed to be repeated. The median hospital stay was 3 days.

During the first 2 weeks, some patients transiently complained of pain, moderate dysphagia, or diarrhea. Acute gastric dilation was never observed, and the dysphagia never persisted. No child got infection or atelectasis, nor wound infection. No patients required esophageal dilatation.

Postoperative Results

Minimal follow-up is 6 months and all patients have had upper gastrointestinal X-rays. Mean follow-up was 16 months with 75 pH studies and 65 manometries.

All patients were clinically improved except for one boy who developed a small but invalidating paraesophageal hernia 3 months after surgery. He was reoperated on first by laparoscopic approach, but conversion was necessary. He is currently free of symptoms. In all cases the upper gastrointestinal series showed that the valve was adequately placed below the diaphragm. In 1.6% mild esophageal reflux was visible.

In 67 of 75 cases (87%) pH returned to normal. Eight (13%) patients had persistent GER documented by pH studies, but in all cases 24 h esophageal pH probe monitoring had improved, and only one child had mild symptoms. These eight cases are being managed nonoperatively.

Esophageal manometry studies showed a restored sphincter with a mean pressure of 12.7±5.3 cmH$_2$O in 59 of 65 (91%); 42% had normal relaxation, 58% had a partial achalasia, and 26% had residual dyskinesia of the lower part of the esophagus.

There were no bowel obstructions, no perforation, no intrathoracically slipped wraps, and no dumping syndrome.

Discussion

About the Laparoscopic Technique in Children

In children a reduced space, fragile liver, protruding caudate lobe, and very little fat are specific features that modify the operative strategy. Dissection most often takes very little time in children, but the risk of perforation, as in open surgery, is greater than of bleeding. We wish to insist that in children instruments should be moved with great caution and quasimillimetric accuracy, especially the coagulation hook. Despite this increased difficulty comparing to adults, laparoscopic fundoplication in children and infants is feasible and effective (Humphrey and Najmaldin 1996; Lobe et al. 1993; Longis et al. 1996; Montupet 1996; Schier and Waldschmidt 1994). In our experience, the operative time has declined from 3 h at first to an average 1 h now.

The Choice of Toupet's Procedure

This discussion is not specific to laparoscopic surgery.

Surgery of GER is "functional" surgery, so the choice for Nissen fundoplication, which is the most widely used procedure in children (Fonkalsrud et al. 1989; Gounot et al. 1989; Lobe et al. 1993; Schier and Waldschmidt 1994) could be discussed, not for its efficacy on reflux but for its high rate of complications such as dysphagia, inability to belch or vomit, gas bloat syndrome, intrathoracic ascension of the valve (Hanimann et al. 1993; Wetscher et al. 1997). In children no comparative studies between Nissen and Toupet have been published; in adult some studies are available in conventional surgery (Segol et al. 1989; Taylor et al. 1994; Thor and Silander 1989) and also in laparoscopic surgery (McKernan 1994; Wetscher et al. 1997) their conclusions are concordant: partial posterior fundoplication is associated with nearly the same efficacy on GER and a lower incidence of postoperative digestive complications such as dysphagia than Nissen.

Although the post-Nissen dysphagia resolves within the 3–4 months after surgery in our experience and in that of Lundell et al. (1991), this side effect may lead to a loss of weight, which is harmful for the growing individual. In his comparative study Wetscher et al. (1997) found a significant reduction in dysphagia following the Toupet fundoplication and a significant improvement of esophageal peristalsis. In our series we noticed a lower incidence of invalidating dysphagia with Toupet's procedure (0/125) in comparison with Nissen (8/93). Concerning the whole complications rate, our results with the Nissen procedure are poorer than with the Toupet procedure (conversion 4 cases, esophagogastric perforation 3 cases, mortality 1 case because of pulmonary complications in a neurologically impaired child, pulmonary infection or atelectasis 3 cases), but we cannot compare our 125 Toupet's procedure and our 93 Nissen's procedure for two reasons: first at the beginning of our laparoscopic experience we favored Nissen's procedure to avoid too much knot tying, second, we reserve now Nissen's procedure with gastrostomy for patients with mental deficiency.

Partial Toupet fundoplication requires a lesser degree of fundus mobilization than total Nissen fundoplication. Division of short gastric vessels was necessary six times in the Nissen procedure but never in the Toupet procedure. The Toupet type valve is adaptable and never very tight; as lesser tension is applied to the valve, the risk of valve dismantling is less. The risk of anterior vagus nerve lesion is also reduced by using a posterior wrap as the wrap is not sutured to the anterior part of the esophagus. As a result the laparoscopic Toupet technique is more and more used by adult surgeons (Mosnier et al. 1995; Patti et al. 1997; Wetscher et al. 1997).

Now, why choose a posterior wrap instead of an anterior wrap? No studies, which compare the two procedures are available but the posterior wrap is more adaptable, and more solid. More adaptable because with an anterior wrap, a more than 180° fundoplication is difficult to do, on the other hand, with a posterior wrap, the surgeon can choose easily between a 180° and an 270° fundoplication. More solid, and perhaps more long-lasting, because the intra-abdominal fixation of the esophagus and wrap is secured to the diaphragm and crura by a greater number of stitches. However, all pediatric laparoscopic data need a longer follow-up in order to consider this last point. Routine radiological surveillance at 6–12 months is not predictive of subsequent failure, which can occur with a median interval of 14 or 28 months. This risk of recurrence is especially high in children with chronic lung disease (McKernan 1994) and in neurologically impaired children.

About the Results

In the absence of pediatric prospective comparative studies, it is difficult to compare the results of open and laparoscopic fundoplication. However, our results tend to be currently better than those obtained with a Toupet procedure performed by open surgery (Montupet et al. 1983). In addition to the reduction in scar, pain, hospital stay, recovery, our results show a nearly total disappearance of parietal complications (1/125), and a total disappearance of postoperative intestinal obstruction due to adhesion that ranges between 2% and 10% after classic open surgery (Bensoussan et al. 1994; Fonkalsrud et al. 1989; Gounot et al.

1989; Hanimann et al. 1993; Montupet et al. 1983). Interestingly, in our case of repeated fundoplication as in others series (Humphrey and Najmaldin 1996) no intra-abdominal adhesions below the diaphragm have been noticed.

Conclusion

Our results of laparoscopic Toupet fundoplication in 125 neurologically intact children, are, except for the initial learning curve, excellent with a mean follow-up of 16 months. Generally speaking we think that the use of laparoscopic techniques in surgical treatment of GER in children is very promising, and that after cholecystectomy it will probably become in the near future the next gold-standard technique.

References

Bensoussan AL, Yazbeck S, Carceller-Blanchard A (1994) Results and complications of Toupet partial posterior wrap: 10 year's experience. J Pediatr Surg 29:1215–1217

De Meester TR, Stein HJ (1992) Minimizing the side effects of antireflux surgery. World J Surg 16:335–336

Eypasch E, Neugebauer E (1997) Laparoscopic antireflux surgery for gastroesophageal reflux disease. Results of a consensus development conference. Surg Endosc 11:413–426

Fonkalsrud ZN et al (1989) Operative treatment for the gastroesophageal reflux syndrome in children. J Pediatr Surg 24:525–529

Gounot E et al (1989) La technique de Jaubert de Beaujen pour le traitement des hernie hiatales du nourrisson et de l'enfant. Résultats à propos de 810 malades opérés de 1960 à 1986. Chir Pediatr 30:203–208

Hanimann B, Sacher P, Stauffer UG (1993) Complications and long-term results of the Nissen fundoplication. Eur J Pediatr Surg 3:12–14

Humphrey GME, Najmaldin AS (1996) Laparoscopic Nissen fundoplication in disabled infants and children. J Pediatr Surg 31:596–599

Lobe TE, Schropp KP, Lunsford K (1993) Laparoscopic Nissen fundoplication in childhood. J Pediatr Surg 28:358–361

Longis B et al (1996) Laparoscopic fundoplication in children: our first 30 cases. J Laparo Endos Surg [Suppl] 6:521–529

Lundell L et al (1991) Lower esophageal sphincter characteristics and esophageal acid exposure following partial and 360° fundoplication: results of a prospective randomized clinical study. World J Surg 15:115–121

McKernan JB (1994) Laparoscopic repair of gastro-esophageal reflux disease. Toupet partial fundoplication versus Nissen fundoplication. Surg Endos 8:851–856

Montupet P (1996) Laparoscopic fundoplication in children. In: Tooli J, Hunter JG (eds) Endosurgery. Churchill Livingston, Edinburgh, pp 935–940

Montupet P, Gauthier F, Valayer J (1983) Traitement chirurgical du reflux gastro-oesophagien par hémivalve tubérositaire postérieure fixée. Chir Pediatr 24:122–127

Mosnier H et al (1995) A 270 degree laparoscopic posterior fundoplasty in the treatment of gastro-esophageal reflux. J Am Coll Surg 181:220–224

Patti MG et al (1997) Partial fundoplication for gastroesophageal reflux. Surg Endosc 11:445–448

Pelissier EP et al (1997) Fundoplication avoiding complicated of Nissen procedure: prospective evaluation. World J Surg 21:611–617

Schier F, Waldschmidt J (1994) Laparoscopic fundoplication in a child. Eur Pediatr Surg 4:338–340

Segol P, Hay JM, Pottier D (1989) Traitement chirurgical du reflux gastro-oesophagien: quelle intervention choisir Nissen, Toupet ou Lortat-Jacob? Etude multicentrique par tirage au sort. Gastroenterol Clin Biol 13:873–879

Taylor LA et al (1994) Chronic lung disease is the leading risk factor correlating with the failure (wrap disruption) of antireflux procedures in children. J Pediatr Surg 29:161–166

Thor KBA, Silander J (1989) A long term randomized prospective trial of the Nissen Procedure versus a modified Toupet Technique. Ann Surg 210:719–724

Toupet A (1963) La technique d'oesophasogastroplastie avec phrenogastropexie appliquée dans la cure radicale des hernies hiatales et comme complément de l'opération de Heller dans les cardiospasmes. Mem Acad Chir 89:394–399

Watson A et al (1995) Laparoscopic "physiological" antireflux procedure: preliminary results of a prospective symptomatic and objective study. Br J Surg 82:651–656

Wetscher GJ et al (1997) Tailored anti reflux surgery for gastroesophageal reflux disease: effectiveness and risk of postoperative dysphagia. World J Surg 21:605–610

CHAPTER 20

Laparoscopic Thal Fundoplication in Infants and Children

D.C. van der Zee, N.M.A. Bax

Introduction

Newborn infants frequently have an incompetent lower esophageal sphincter mechanism (Boix-Ochoa 1976; Ramenofsky 1986; Fonkalsrud and Ament 1996). With growth and development the sphincter mechanism usually becomes competent and symptoms subside. If symptoms of gastroesophageal reflux (GER) persist beyond this period reflux becomes pathological (Boix-Ochoa 1976; Ramenofsky 1986; Fonkalsrud and Ament 1996). Apart from this idiopathic or primary form of pathological GER (PR), secondary pathological GER (SR) is encountered in children with motility disorders of the digestive tract: neurologically impaired children, children after esophageal repair, after gastrostomy placement, but also in bronchopulmonary dysplasia, cystic fibrosis, or cervical transection (Fonkalsrud 1986; Fonkalsrud and Ament 1996; Fonkalsrud et al. 1989; Gauderer 1991; Rice et al. 1991; Stringel et al. 1989; Wheatley et al. 1991).

When medical treatment fails, an antireflux procedure is indicated. The Nissen fundoplication has been the most commonly used technique. The procedure, however, is not without morbidity. The Thal partial wrap procedure, originally described by Alan Thal in 1958, and later advocated by Ashcraft (1986) is said to have the same results, but with fewer complications (Van der Zee et al. 1994). With the advent of laparoscopy the Nissen fundoplication has been repopularized. The dilemma arises whether a technique should be changed because of the laparoscopic feasibility. It is our belief that operations should be performed laparoscopically only when they make sense when carried out by the open route, and not only because they are feasible. As we were accustomed to performing the open Thal fundoplication before, we have remained with the Thal fundoplication technique but changed the approach from open to laparoscopic. This chapter describes the laparoscopic Thal procedure.

Indications and Contraindications

Indications for a (laparoscopic) antireflux procedure are primary (idiopathic) or secondary reflux refractory to conservative treatment. Secondary reflux occurs in mentally retarded children, esophageal atresia or other children with esophageal motility disorders, children with feeding difficulties or failure to thrive. Contraindications are theoretically present in children with a right-to-left shunt, or bleeding disorders. A ventriculo-peritoneal drain is not deemed as a contraindication.

Diagnostic Workup

According to protocol, all patients that are referred for laparoscopic antireflux procedure and/or feeding gastrostomy are subjected to preoperative workup consisting of 24-h pH measurement, upper gastrointestinal series, esophagogastroscopy, and a 3-month postoperative 24-h pH-study. Esophagogastroscopy is repeated in case of preoperative esophagitis.

Technique of Laparoscopic Thal Procedure

The patient is under general anesthesia with full muscle relaxation and is placed in a supine position on the operating table. In younger children the legs are put in a frog position and held by an operation sheet to prevent them from slipping down when the table is in reverse Trendelenburg position (Fig. 1a). In older children the legs are placed in flexion and abduction with the surgeon standing in between (Fig. 1b). In children with flexure contraction of the hips alternative position may be necessary. All children receive an urine catheter for the duration of the operation. The surgeon stands at the lower end of the table with the assistant to his left and the scrub nurse to his right. The monitor is placed at the upper right or left side of the patient (Fig. 1).

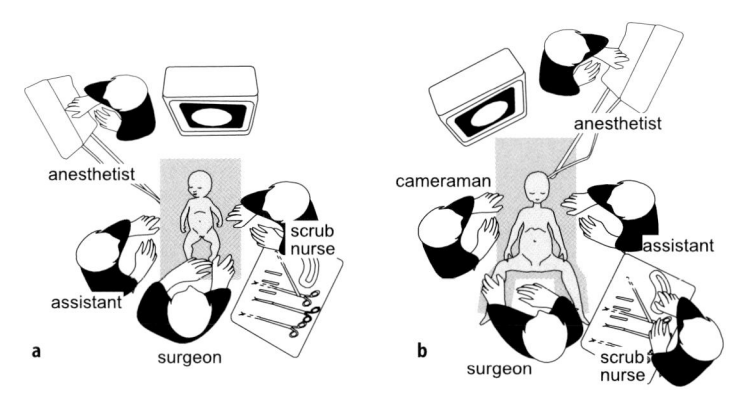

Fig. 1a,b. Position of the patient, crew and monitor. **a** Small patient. **b** Larger patient

Fig. 2a,b. Position of the cannulae. The first cannula is introduced in an open manner through the infraumbilical fold (*1*); the other cannulae are inserted under vision. The scope is then moved to the midepigastrial cannula (*2*). On both sides of the scope working instruments are inserted (*3, 4*). Through the umbilical cannula a Babcock for grasping the stomach is inserted (*1*). A liver retractor can be inserted either through a right subcostal cannula (*5*) **a** or through a subxyphoid cannula (*6*) **b**

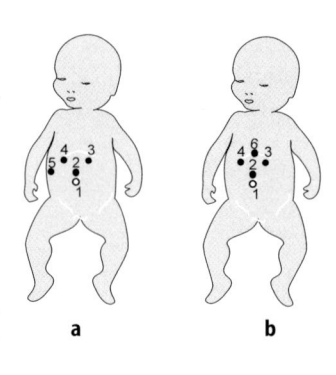

The first trocar is placed at the umbilicus in an "open" way. In younger children a 5-mm trocar is used, in older children a 10-mm trocar can be used (Fig. 2). A 30° optic lens is used. Initial insufflation with CO_2 is 0.5 l/min. with a pressure of 5 mmHg. Maintenance flow is 5 l/min. The following trocars are placed under direct vision: a 5-mm (10-mm) trocar is introduced halfway between xyphoid process and umbilicus. After insertion of all trocars the endoscope is switched to this "epigastric" trocar, and a Babcock stomach retractor is introduced through the umbilical trocar. Laterally from the epigastric port two 5-mm ports are placed for instrumentation.

A liver retractor can be introduced with or without trocar below the right subcostal ridge at the level of the anterior axillary fold or just under the xyphoid, depending on the size of the left liver lobe (Fig. 2a,b). In the case of esophagitis usually a pronounced lymph node is present at the gastroesophageal margin. The peritoneum is incised cranially from the fatpad and the esophagus is freed from the hiatus by blunt and sharp dissection and brought intra-abdominally over a distance of 3–5 cm. The esophagus is kept under traction with an encircled vessel loop (Fig. 3a). Care is taken to avoid injury to the anterior and posterior vagus nerves and its hepatic branches. Depending on the age of the patient a 18- to 22-G esophageal tube is passed through the esophagus into the stomach to determine the supposed hiatal diameter. The posterior crural defect is closed with an Ethibond 3x0 interrupted suture including the dorsal esophageal wall for fixation. If necessary, a second suture can be placed through the crura alone (Fig. 3b).

After closure of the hiatus the tube and vessel loop can be removed. The 180° anterior wrap is performed in two rows with three interrupted Ethibond 3x0 sutures each. The first row of sutures is placed from the fundus of the stomach to halfway the distal part of the esophagus that has been brought down intra-abdominally (Fig. 3c), the second row of sutures runs from the fundus of the stomach to the upper end of the intra-abdominal part of the esophagus and the diaphragmatic ridge (Fig. 3d,e). In the case of gastrostomy placement two 3x0 Vic-

20 Laparoscopic Thal Fundoplication in Infants and Children

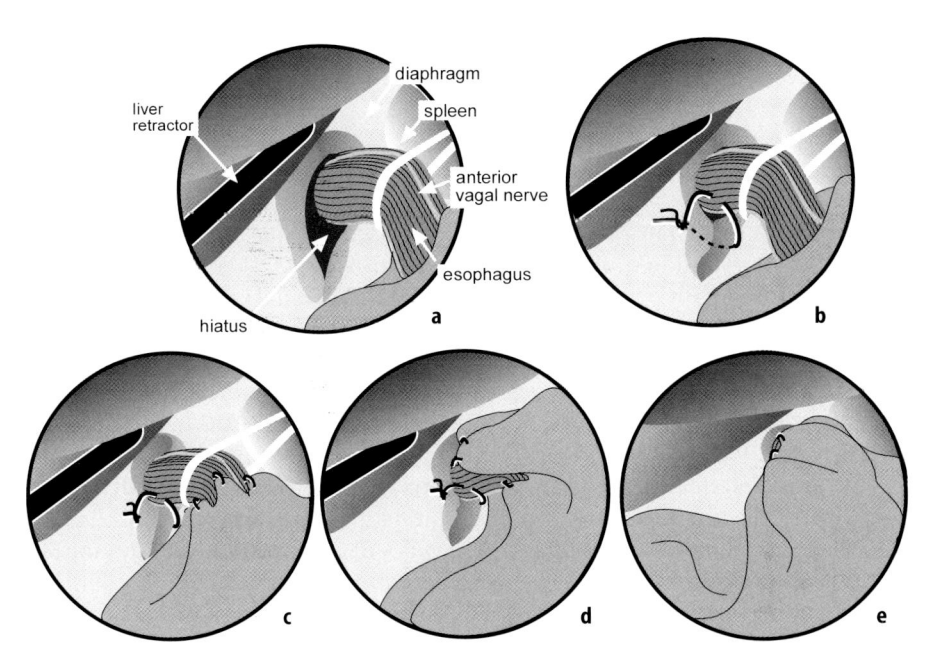

Fig. 3. a The distal intra-abdominal and intrathoracic esophagus, which is encircled with a vessel loop, has been freed from the surrounding hiatus and is brought into the abdomen. **b** The hiatus is closed behind the esophagus, taking a bite of the posterior esophageal wall (to prevent narrowing of the esophagus during this maneuver a large transesophageal probe is present). **c** A first row of three sutures is placed between the anterior wall of the stomach and the mid-intra-abdominal esophagus. **d,e** A second row of three sutures is placed between the anterior stomach and the upper intra-abdominal esophagus including the diaphragm

ryl sutures are introduced through the trocar hole that will be used for the gastrostomy. Either the trocar in the midline or the left-sided trocar is removed. The stomach is hitched with two suture and pulled against the abdominal wall.

The anesthesist insufflates the stomach with air. A 16-F peel-a-way system in introduced into the stomach, and a 14-F gastrostomy catheter can then be inserted into the stomach (in small children a 12-F peel-a-way system can be used for an 10-F button catheter). The balloon is inflated with 3 ml water, retracted against the abdominal wall, and fixed with the external plate. The previously placed sutures are attached to the fascia to fix the anterior stomach wall to the anterior abdominal wall. The gastrostomy catheter can be exchanged for a button after 3 months. All trocars are removed under direct vision and the defects are closed by interrupted Vicryl 4x0 sutures and adhesive strips (Van der Zee and Bax 1996). No nasogastric tube is left behind. In case of a gastrostomy a fluid retaining bag can be attached overnight.

The children receive a continuous morphine infusion 0.25 mg/kg per 24 h over the first 12 h (overnight). The morning after operation the children are allowed feedings to their wish, or they receive half of their gastrostomy feeding over the first 24 h. On the second day the children are put on full enteral feeding and may leave for home or return to the institution by the end of the day.

Personal Experience

Between November 1993 and May 1996 laparoscopic Thal fundoplication was performed in 53 children. In 23 patients a gastrostomy was also placed. There were 18 children with primary reflux and 35 with secondary reflux, of whom 28 suffered from mental retardation. In the second patient laparoscopy was converted into an open procedure because of intractable bleeding that had stopped on exploration. No other intraoperative complications occurred. Feeding was begun on day 1 in 49/53 children and between 2 and 4 days in the other four. Two children with PR had some initial feeding problems that subsided in days. One child was reoperated for a too tight fundoplication. Five children with SR had some initial feeding problems and one child had an inappropriate antidiuretic hormone secretion. Mean hospitalization was 3 days for PR and 5.1 days for SR. Mean hospitalization for mentally retarded children was 5.5 days. In comparison, in our series of open Thal procedure mean hospitalization was 4.5 days for PR and 10 days for MR (Van der Zee et al. 1994).

Follow-up varies from 1–35 months (mean 11 months). Two children with primary reflux had persistent complaints of retrosternal pain or regurgitation. In both instances the results of 24-h pH study were normal. These children showed esophageal motility disorders on manometry. One child with esophageal stenosis displayed persisting vomiting. The 24-h pH study still showed pathological reflux. She was maintained on antireflux medication and required recurrent dilatations. Three mentally handicapped children that underwent a Thal fundoplication and gastrostomy continued to vomit or displayed signs or gagging; the 24-h pH study still showed pathological reflux, although in one child there was a marked improvement.

In total 44/50 children (88%) were ultimately free of symptoms of reflux while 31/41 children (78%) displayed no recurrence of pathological reflux on 24-h pH study.

Discussion

Gastroesophageal reflux is one of the most frequent symptomatic clinical disorders affecting the gastrointestinal tract of infants and children. Gastroesophageal fundoplication is currently one of the three most common major operations performed on infants and children by pediatric surgeons in the United States (Fonkalsrud and Ament 1996). Essential in almost any kind of antireflux procedure is the mobilization of the distal esophagus into the abdomen, repair of the hiatal crura and maintenance of the distal esophagus intra-abdominally by means of some kind of fundoplasty.

In an earlier report we described our favorable results with the open Thal procedure (Van der Zee et al. 1994). In the present series of patients who underwent a laparoscopic Thal fundoplication with or without gastrostomy, 44/50 (88%) were ultimately free of symptoms of GER with a follow-up of 1–35 months (mean 11 months), while 31/41 (76%) displayed no recurrence of pathological reflux on 24-h pH study. Although follow-up over a prolonged period of time is necessary, the majority of complications occur in the first 12 months (Martinez et al. 1992). In the open group 14/18 (78%) was free of symptoms after a mean period of 6.3 years. A 24-h pH study, however, was performed only in a single symptomatic patient. Apparently there appears to be a discrepancy between symptoms and 24-h pH monitoring. In our view 24-h pH monitoring is the only objective evaluation of the postoperative result of the antireflux procedure and should therefore become a standard procedure.

Mentally disabled children in particular seem to benefit from the laparoscopic approach, with hospital stay declining from 10 to 5.5 days. In an earlier report we already described the favorable results in mentally retarded children (Van der Zee and Bax 1996). Also in children with severe scoliosis the laparoscopic approach lends the surgeon the necessary extension of his hands to reach the deep hiatus (Van der Zee and Bax 1995). The results are better than those described by Collins et al. (1995) after laparoscopic Nissen fundoplication: our overall mean hospital stay was 4.4 days versus 6.8 days, while feeding was tolerated 1.2 days postoperative versus 2.3 days.

In conclusion, Thal fundoplication can be performed laparoscopically. The results are comparable to the open procedure and may even supersede those of the Nissen fundoplication in regard to postoperative feeding and hospitalization. In laparoscopy one should therefore remain with the procedure that would otherwise had been performed by the open route. The 24-h pH monitoring should become a standard procedure in postoperative evaluation of the result of the antireflux procedure.

References

Ashcraft KW (1986) Thal fundoplication. In: Ashcraft KW, Holder TM (eds) Pediatric esophageal surgery. Grune and Stratton, London
Boix-Ochoa (1976) Maturation of the lower esophagus. J Pediatr Surg 11:749–756
Collins JB et al (1995) Comparison of open and laparoscopic gastrostomy and fundoplication in 120 patients. J Pediatr Surg 30:1065–1070
Fonkalsrud EW (1986) The role of surgery in the treatment of gastroesophageal reflux and gastric dysmotility disorders in children. In: Ashcraft KW, Holder TM (eds) Pediatric esophageal surgery. Grune and Stratton, London
Fonkalsrud EW, Ament ME (1996) Gastroesophageal reflux in childhood. Curr Probl Surg 33(1):1–70
Fonkalsrud EW et al (1989) Operative treatment for gastroesophageal reflux syndrome in children. J Pediatr Surg 24:525–529
Gauderer MWL (1991) Feeding the neurologically impaired child: evaluation and surgical options. Pediatr Surg Int 6:75

Martinez DA, Ginn-Pease ME, Caniano DA (1992) Sequelae of antireflux surgery in profoundly disabled children. J Pediatr Surg 27:267–273

Ramenofsky ML (1986) Gastroesophageal reflux: clinical manifestations and diagnosis. In: Ashcraft KW, Holder TM (eds) Pediatric esophageal surgery. Grune and Stratton, London

Rice H, Seahorse JH, Touloukian RJ (1991) Evaluation of Nissen fundoplication in neurologically impaired children. J Pediatr Surg 26:697–701

Stringel G et al (1989) Gastrostomy and Nissen fundoplication in neurologically impaired children. J Pediatr Surg 24:1044–1048

Thal A (1968) A unified approach to the surgical problem of the esophagogastric junction. Ann Surg 168:542–550

Van der Zee DC, Bax NMA (1995) Laparoscopic Thal fundoplication in severe scoliotic children. Surg Endoc 9:1197–1198

Van der Zee DC, Bax NMA (1996) Laparoscopic Thal fundoplication in mentally retarded children. Surg Endosc 10:659–661

Van der Zee DC et al (1994) Surgical treatment of reflux esophagitis: Nissen versus Thal procedure. Pediatr Surg Int 9:334–337

Wheatley MJ et al (1991) Redo fundoplication in infants and children with recurrent gastroesophageal reflux. J Pediatr Surg 105:457–761

Laparoscopic Gastrostomy

K.E. Georgeson

Indications

Gastrostomy is commonly employed for children who have swallowing difficulties or failure to thrive (Tunell 1989). Failure to thrive is seen in children with high metabolic demands associated with chronic pulmonary or cardiac disease and children with profound neurological impairment. Other indications for gastrostomy include children with primary aspiration or difficult swallowing due to neurological or esophageal disorders (Tunnell 1989). Any candidate for a gastrostomy should be evaluated for the presence of gastroesophageal reflux. A child with clinically symptomatic gastroesophageal reflux should not have a gastrostomy placed without a concurrent fundoplication. The author prefers laparoscopic gastrostomy to percutaneous endoscopic gastrostomy because the laparoscopic approach is more versatile (Georgeson 1997; Sampson et al. 1996). Laparoscopic gastrostomy can be performed in conjunction with laparoscopic fundoplication. In the instances where fundoplication is not indicated, a laparoscopic gastrostomy can be placed in the lesser curvature which may help deter the development of gastroesophageal reflux after gastrostomy formation (Seekri et al. 1991; Stringel 1991).

Preparation

Patients under the age of 5 years can usually be positioned at the end of the table with the legs folded. Older children can be placed in a similar position with the legs held in stirrups. The patient should be secured to the operating table with tape. The operating surgeon and his assistants stand at the foot of the table. The monitor is usually positioned just to the left of the patient's head.

A nasogastric tube should be passed into the stomach before the procedure. The anesthetist should be prepared with a 60-cc catheter tipped syringe and a clamp to allow for sequential insufflation of the stomach through the nasogastric tube.

Technique

A single 3-mm or 5-mm trocar is used in the umbilicus. In most instances, a 3-mm scope allows adequate visualization for the procedure (Fig. 1). The instruments needed include:
- Scope 0°, 3 mm
- Trocar, 3.5 mm, ×2
- Grasper, 3 mm
- U-stitch
- Needle with guidewire
- Graduated dilators, ×4
- Catheter or MicKey
- Bolsters
- Needle holder (open), ×2

After installation of the pneumoperitoneum to a pressure of 10 cmH$_2$O and placement of the umbilical trocar, a site is selected for the gastrostomy. The gastrostomy site is usually located to the left of the midline and well below the left costal margin. A stab wound is made at the selected site with a number 11 blade pointed in a vertical axis and passed into the peritoneal cavity under laparoscopic surveillance. Care should be taken to keep the site away from the epigastric vessels to avoid bleeding. A 3-mm grasping clamp is passed directly through the stab wound into the peritoneal cavity. The anterior wall of the stomach is grasped at an appropriate site (Fig. 2). For gastrostomy without fundoplication, the stomach should be grasped just to the left of the lesser curvature. A second 3-mm trocar and grasper in the right upper quadrant may be used to retract the liver so that the anterior wall of the stomach can be better visualized. For gastrostomy performed with fundoplication, the gastrostomy may be sited closer to the greater curvature.

Care should be taken to avoid a gastrostomy that is placed close to the pylorus. The stomach is then pulled up adjacent to the anterior abdominal wall.

Fig. 1. One or two trocar sites are used for gastrostomy. The telescope is passed through the umbilical trocar (*1*). The right upper quadrant trocar is optional and is useful for placement of a retractor for the liver to visualize the anterior wall of the stomach (*2*). A 3-mm stab wound is made in the left upper quadrant gastrostomy site

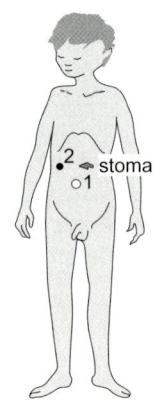

21 Laparoscopic Gastrostomy

Fig. 2. A 3-mm grasping clamp is passed through the stab wound. The anterior wall of the stomach is grasped near the lesser or greater curvature depending upon the preference of the surgeon

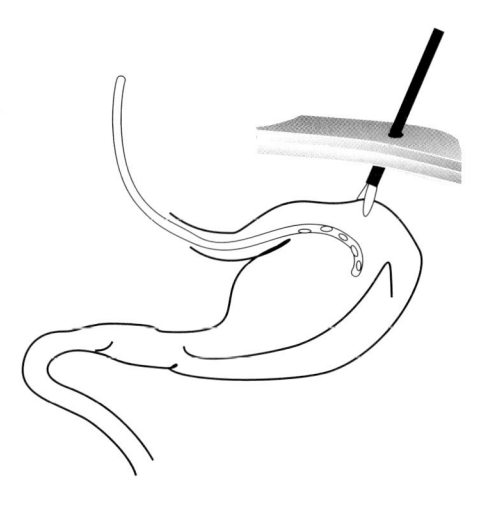

Fig. 3. a Using a large curved needle, two U-stitches are passed through the abdominal wall, through the anterior gastric wall, and back through the abdominal wall in the axis of the telescope. On each side of gastric wall 1 cm is taken. The stomach is then pulled up against the anterior abdominal wall by the U-sutures. A needle is passed through the stab wound into the distended stomach. **b** A guide wire is passed through the needle into the gastric lumen. The needle is withdrawn leaving the guide wire in place. **c** Progressively larger dilators are passed over the guide wire to dilate the gastrostomy tract. **d** A balloon tipped button of appropriate length or a balloon tube is passed over the guide wire into the stomach. The balloon is insufflated. The U-stitches are tied over the wings of the button or over a bolster

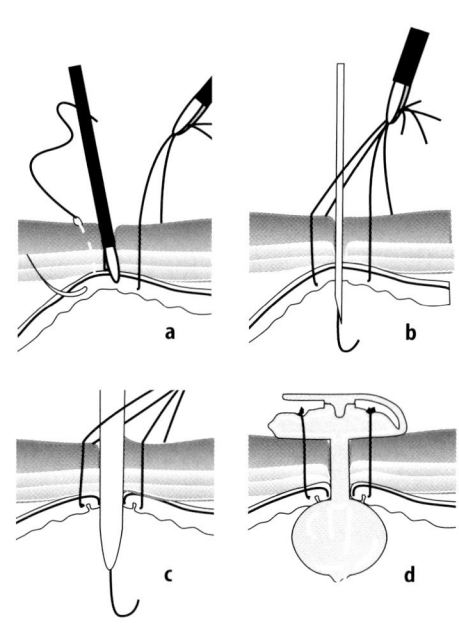

The anesthetist is asked to insufflate the stomach with air using the 60-cc catheter tipped syringe attached to the nasogastric tube. Two U-sutures are passed through the abdominal wall using a large round needle and a monofilament suture. The U-suture should incorporate 1 cm of gastric wall. The suture should be placed through the abdominal wall and stomach parallel to the axis of the telescope (Fig. 3a).

The U-sutures are then secured with a clamp outside the abdominal wall and the 3-mm grasping clamp is removed. The two U-sutures are used to draw the stomach against the abdominal wall. The anesthetist should insufflate the stomach with additional air to induce adequate distention of the stomach at this point. A Seldinger needle is introduced through the abdominal wall through the stab wound and through the gastric wall between the U-stitches. Care should be taken not to introduce the needle too far so that it transverses both the anterior and posterior walls of the stomach. A guide wire is introduced into the stomach through the needle and the needle is withdrawn (Fig. 3b). The stomach should be allowed to fall away from the abdominal wall at this point to make sure the guide wire is in satisfactory position between the sutures. Graduated dilators are then passed over the guide wire using the U-sutures for countertraction of the anterior wall of the stomach until the tract is dilated sufficiently to accept a balloon tube or button (Fig. 3c) Usually the tract should be dilated four French sizes larger than the planned gastrostomy device. A balloon-tipped button or balloon tube is advanced over the guide wire and into the stomach. The appropriate stem length for a button should be premeasured with a dilator. Once the button or tube is seated in place, the U-sutures are tied over the wings of the button or over a bolster (Fig. 3d).

The U-sutures should be tied snugly. Care should be taken not to make them too tight. The umbilical trocar is removed and the trocar site closed. The U-sutures may be removed on the 1st or 2nd postoperative day. Feeding can be commenced within 6–12 h.

Feedings are delivered by bolus, continuous drip, or a combination of the two. The author prefers laparoscopic gastrostomy to percutaneous endoscopic gastrostomy in most cases because of its increased versatility.

Personal Experience

We have performed U-stitch gastrostomy in 60 patients. Complications have been infrequent. Postoperative gastrostomy leakage has occurred in a few patients and is usually prevented by using a small diameter tube (8–10 F) in infants weighing less than 6 kg and in patients with a thin abdominal wall.

References

Georgeson KE (1997) Laparoscopic versus open procedures for long-term enteral access. Nutr Clin Pract [Suppl] 12:S1–S2
Sampson LK, Georgeson KE, Winters DC (1996) Laparoscopic gastrostomy as an adjunctive procedure to laparoscopic fundoplication in children. Surg Endosc 10:1106–1110
SeeKri IK et al (1991) Lesser curvature gastrostomy reduces the incidence of postoperative gastroesophageal reflux. J Pediatr Surg 26:982–985
Stringel G (1991) Gastrostomy with antireflux properties. J Pediatr Surg 25:1019–1021
Tunnell WP (1989) Gastroesophageal reflux in childhood. Pediatr Ann 18:192–196

Laparoscopic Antroplasty

K.E. Georgeson

Introduction

Some children with gastroesophageal reflux and/or failure to thrive also have a delay in gastric emptying (McCallum et al. 1981; Papaila et al. 1989). The formation of a gastrostomy or fundoplication in these children without improving their gastric emptying may lead to bloating, retching, or recurrence of their reflux. The efficiency of gastric emptying is usually tested by a radionuclide scintiscan. Although the practice is controversial, many surgeons perform a gastric outlet enlarging procedure in association with fundoplication and/or gastrostomy in patients with delayed gastric emptying. Fonkalsrud has popularized the antroplasty, which utilizes division of the longitudinal and circular muscles of the pylorus down to the duodenum but leaving the mucosa intact (Fonkalsrud et al. 1992). The seromuscular wall is then closed transversally, enlarging the outlet of the stomach. This chapter describes the technique of laparoscopic antroplasty.

Indications

In patients being considered for gastrostomy and/or fundoplication the preoperative workup includes a gastric scintiscan or evaluation of gastric motility. Patients with delayed emptying are candidates for antroplasty.

Preparation

The instruments needed are:
- Scope, 5 mm
- Trocar, 5 mm
- Trocars, 3–5 mm
- L-hook cautery, 3 mm
- Grasper, 3 mm
- Pyloric spreader, 3 mm
- Needle driver, 3 mm

- Scissors, 3 mm
- Retractor, 3 mm
- 2-0 suture

The patient is positioned with the legs folded and taped at the end of the table. A moderate reverse Trendelenburg position induces the transverse colon to fall away from the pylorus. Patients whose legs cannot be folded under them are placed in stirrups. The monitor is just to the right or left of the patient's head. Trocars positioned for fundoplication can be used.

Technique

A primary antroplasty can be performed using four 3.5-mm trocar sites (Fig. 1). The right anterior axillary trocar site is for retraction of the liver to expose the pylorus. The right and left midclavicular line trocar sites are used by the operator. The telescope is passed through an umbilical trocar site.

A 30° telescope gives an excellent view of the pylorus and keeps the telescope above the working space. The operation is begun by retracting the liver upward.

Fig. 1. Trocar sites for antroplasty are similar to the sites for fundoplication. The pylorus is stabilized and the muscle layers opened with an L-hook electrocautery for a distance of 2.5–3 cm. The muscle is spread with a pyloric spreader. Small circular fibers are elevated from the mucosa and divided with scissors or cautery. The muscular defect is stretched and then closed transversely with interrupted sutures

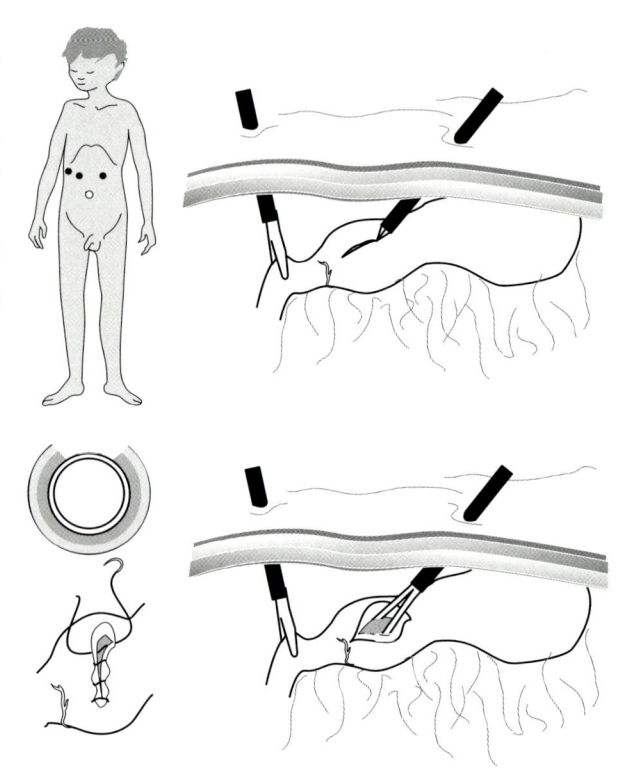

Using a grasper in the left hand, the duodenum is grasped just distal to the pylorus. Cautery is employed to open the longitudinal and circular muscle fibers beginning just proximal to the vein of Mayo. This incision is continued using a cutting electrocautery current for a distance of about 2.5 cm. Great care is taken not to injure the mucosa. A pyloromyotomy spreader is introduced through the left midclavicular trocar site, and the muscle layers are spread gently but forcefully until the muscle has been well separated from the underlying mucosa. The antral muscle fibers are carefully spread distally down to the duodenum. A laparoscopic mosquito clamp can be gently spread under the circular muscle fibers of the distal antrum to separate the muscle fibers from the mucosa. It is important to exercise caution while spreading to avoid making a hole in the duodenal mucosa. The separated muscle fibers are then cut with a L-hook cautery. Once the pyloromyotomy has been completed, 2-0 silk sutures are used to close the defect transversely. Two or three sutures are usually adequate to complete the transverse closure using an intracorporeal knot tying technique.

Feedings are initiated on the day following surgery. Discharge is usually achieved 24–48 h after the procedure.

Personal Experience

We have performed laparoscopic antroplasty on 57 patients. Ten of the 57 patients were randomly selected and were studied postoperatively. All ten showed improvement in gastric emptying 6 months or more after the procedure over their preoperative state. Two patients had transitory dumping which was treated by dividing the bolus feedings into two parts given 15 min apart. There were no mucosal perforations. Antroplasty appears to be a helpful adjunct to fundoplication in children with a preoperative delay in gastric emptying.

References

Fonkalsrud EW, Ament ME, Vargas J (1992) Gastric antroplasty for the treatment of delayed gastric emptying and gastroesophageal reflux in children. Am J Surg 164:327–331

McCallum RW, Berkowitz DM, Lerner E (1981) Gastric emptying in patients with gastroesophageal reflux. Gastroenterology 80:285–291

Papaila JG et al (1989) Increased incidence of delayed gastric emptying in children with gastroesophageal reflux. Arch Surg 124:933–936

CHAPTER 23

Laparoscopic Extramucosal Pyloromyotomy

J.L. Alain, D. Grousseau

Introduction

Laparoscopic extramucosal pyloromytomy is an excellent alternative to the classical management of hypertrophic pyloric stenosis. In May 1990 we performed the first laparoscopic pyloromyotomy (Alain, Grousseau 1991a,b). A careful follow-up of our patients demonstrates the advantages of this approach.

Contraindications

Congenital heart disease and respiratory anomalies must be excluded, and the relative hypovolemia which is often present must be corrected before the operation. Due to the hemodynamic and ventilatory vulnerability of the young infant, utmost care must be provided during anesthesia. Modification of the inspired air concentration has more impact on both alveolar and arterial gas concentrations. Moreover, hypercapnia results not only from the use of CO_2 for the pneumoperitoneum but possibly also from abdominal hyperinsufflation, the Trendelenburg position, or any faulty airway control. An increase in the pulmonary artery pressure secondary to hypercapnia, hypoxia, acidosis, or hypovolemia may lead to a return to fetal circulation as definitive shunt closure takes place only several weeks after birth.

Preoperative Workup

Fluid and pH and electrolyte disturbances should be corrected preoperatively.

Preoperative Preparation

Premedication using an anticholinergic agent precedes the induction of general endotracheal anesthesia with controlled ventilation. Several items need to be monitored during anesthesia:

23 Laparoscopic Extramucosal Pyloromyotomy

- Routine survey in all infants includes arterial blood pressure monitoring, oxyhemoglobin saturation measuring, and ECG monitoring.
- When a pneumoperitonum is created, the following items must be continuously measured as well: the quantity of insufflated gas, the intraperitoneal pressure and the endexpiratory CO_2 by means of capnometry. Capmometry during laparoscopy is very important as it allows for a rapid adjustment of the ventilator settings in order to keep an optimal Pa_{CO_2}. Moreover, capnography allows for early detection of gas embolization or acute hypovolemia.

Instruments

Specific instruments are required. The laparoscope and the ports should have a small caliber (3.5 mm). The laparoscope should have a 0° angle to allow direct vision. Special instruments are used for pyloromyotomy in infants: grasping forceps, scalpel, spatula, and spreading forceps.

Technique

The Infant lies in supine position at the operating table end, either on a mattress or on a table specially warmed for this purpose (Fig. 1). The bladder is evacuated using external pressure (Crede's maneuver). The umbilicus area is carefully disinfected.

For the creation of the pneumoperitoneum a Veress needle is inserted below the left costal margin (Fig. 2). Its intraperitoneal placement is verified by the "syringe test" (Gans and Berci 1971). It is maintained throughout the operation serving to lift up the hepatic border. Alternatively the first trocar may be inserted in an open way. Then CO_2 gas is insufflated slowly and carefully, not exceeding 6–8 cm H_2O in a young child.

The umbilical port is inserted using a blunt trocar through a small incision in its inferior quadrant. The 4-mm direct vision endoscope is now tangentially

Fig. 1. Position of the infant, crew, and monitor

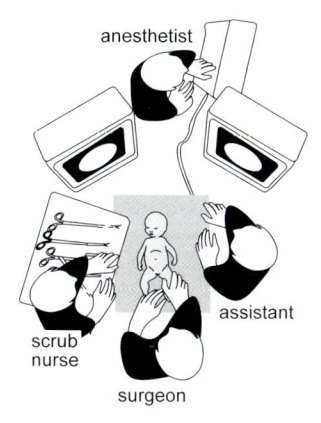

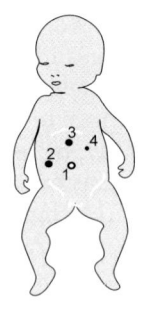

Fig. 2. Position of the Veress needle and trocars. The Veress needle is inserted in the left upper quadrant (*4*). After establishment of the pneumoperitoneum, the 4.5-mm trocar for 0° 4-mm laparoscope is inserted through a small incision in the umbilicus in its inferior quadrant (*1*). Two more 3.5-mm trocars are inserted. A first is inserted 3–4 cm below the hepatic border at the right midclavicular line for the introduction of the atraumatic grasping forceps which grasps the duodenum a few millimeters distal to the pyloric olive (*2*). The duodenum and pylorus now form a single unit and this is preserved until the end of the operation. A second trocar is passed directly above the pyloric olive for the successive insertion of the scalpel, the spatula and the spreading forceps (*3*)

passed through (Fig. 2). To avoid exteriorization of the port during the operation, a suture is passed between its rubber collar and the adjacent skin. The pyloric olive is then visualized through the laparoscope. Its location determines the insertion sites of the remaining ports.

Two 3.5-mm diameter ports are inserted (Fig. 2). The first is inserted 3–4 cm below the hepatic border at the midline on the right side and serves for the application of an atraumatic grasping forceps which is to seize the duodenum a few millimeters away from the pyloric olive. The duodenum and pylorus now form a single unit which is preserved as such until the operation ends.

The second port is passed through the abdominal wall right above the pyloric olive and serves for the successive insertion of the scalpel, the spatula and the spreading forceps.

The scalpel is introduced very carefully through the avascular line where the olive is thicker and only for an optimal distance in order not to injure the gastric mucosa. It is passed depthwise only for making way for the application of the spatula followed by the spreading forceps. A special scalpel is chosen for this purpose with a retractable fixed length blade. The incision is then extended both proximally and distally to cover the whole length of the pyloric olive, paying attention for not injuring the mucosal fold just above the olive (Fig. 3a). Next a blunt spatula is introduced and rotated between the edges of the incision in order to facilitate the application of the spreading forceps (Fig. 3b). The closed tip of the spreading forceps is passed directly through the incision and its arms are spread out towards the two pyloric olive extremities (Fig. 3c). Spreading is carried out slowly and progressively, closing and opening the forceps several times in the same way until complete divulsion of the seromuscular layer. Small spurs are placed on its arms, protecting them from slipping over the muscular edges.

Fig. 3a–c. The actual pyloromyotomy. **a** First the seromuscular layer is incised with a specially designed pyloromyotome. **b** Next a spatula is inserted and turned around its axis to enlarge the incision. **c** Finally the spreader is inserted for spreading of the incised seromuscular layer

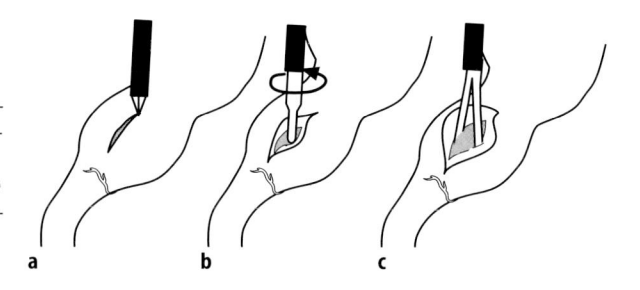

If adhesions still persist, hindering divulsion, it is better to reintroduce the spatula and not the scalpel, to break through the remaining bands. Divulsion is then continued using the forceps, until the gastric mucosa is seen to protrude through the incision bed. Spreading is thus completed. This maneuver causes no bleeding; when bleeding does occur, however, very little coagulation is applied. We have never been faced with this problem.

Intactness of the gastric mucosa must be checked by injection of air through the nasogastric tube. Absence of air bubbles in the incision bed ensures that the gastric mucosa is intact. The slightest suspicion of mucosal injury necessitates immediate conversion to laparotomy to close the mucosal break.

CO_2 is totally exsufflated and the trocars are withdrawn. The insertion sites of the surgical ports are then sutured if necessary.

Postoperative Course

Pain medication is required only during the first few postoperative hours. Pediatric anesthesiologists supervise the smoothness of the postoperative course. The child seems more comfortable and may return to a regular diet on the evening of the same day.

Personal Experience

Since May 1990 we have performed 100 laparoscopic extramucosal pylotomies. There have been no deaths. Two cases of gastric mucosal perforation were not noted by the air injection test. Both patients had a laparotomy the next day. A mucosal perforation was detected at the gastric end of the incision and was closed. As a result of these two patients the scalpel was replaced by another one which possesses a shorter retractable blade. Since this modification no further mucosal perforation has occurred. None of the patients has required a repyloromyotomy.

Discussion

Laparoscopic extramucosal pyloromyotomy has proven its success as a valuable alternative to conventional surgery in infants. Its results compare favorably with those of classical open surgery, "the most consistently successful operation ever described," but with the additional potential benefit of shortened hospital stay and of minimum cosmetic deformity (Greason et al. 1995; Lobe and Schropp 1994; Najmaldin and Tan 1995; Tan 1993). The postoperative course is smoother. With good experience and appropriate surgical instruments the complication rate is small. Prerequisites for a successful laparoscopic intervention include sufficient experience on the part of the surgeon, use of specially adapted instruments and optimal anesthesia. Laparoscopic extramucosal pyloromyotomy should be confined only to surgeons highly reputed in pediatric laparoscopic procedures. Considering the advantages of this new approach for extramucosal pyloromyotomy and its results, its future seems promising.

References

Alain JL, Grousseau D, Terrier G (1991a) Extramucosal pylorotomy by lapararoscopy. J Pediatr Surg 26:1191-1192
Alain JL, Grousseau D, Terrier G (1991b) Extramucosal pylorotomy by lapararoscopy. Surg Endosc 5:174-175
Gans SL, Berci G (1971) Advances in endoscopy of infants and children. J Pediatr Surg 6:199-203
Greason KL et al (1995) Laparoscopic pyloromyotomy for infantile hypertrophic pyloric stenosis: report of 11 cases. J Pediatr Surg 30:1571-1574
Lobe TE, Schropp KP (1994) Pediatric laparoscopy and thoracoscopy. Saunders, Philadelphia
Najmaldin A, Tan HL (1995) Early experience with laparoscopic pyloromyotomy for infantile hypertrophic pyloric stenosis. J Pediatr Surg 30:37-38
Tan HL (1993) Pylorotomy by laparoscopy in children. In: Graber, JN et al (eds) Laparoscopic abdominal surgery. McGraw Hill, New York

Laparoscopic Jejunostomy

K.E. Georgeson

Introduction

Jejunostomy is not commonly performed in children. Most pediatric surgeons prefer to use the more versatile gastrostomy for patients who require long-term enteric feeding (Georgeson 1997). Children can be either bolus or drip fed through a gastrostomy. Nutrients through a jejunostomy tube must be drip fed. Jejunostomy feeding is primarily employed in children requiring tube feeding who cannot tolerate feeding into the stomach (Curet-Scot and Shermeta 1986; Rombeau and Barot 1981; Ryan and Page 1984).

Preoperative Workup

Children with failure to thrive associated with gastroparesis, uncorrected gastroesophageal reflux, and severe chronic retching with intragastric feeds are the primary candidates for laparoscopic jejunostomy. An upper gastrointestinal study and a gastric emptying study are helpful in determining whether a gastrostomy or jejunostomy would be the better procedure for long-term enteric feeding.

Preoperative Preparation

The patient is placed supine on the operating table. The abdomen is prepared from nipples to midthighs. The child is draped widely as for any abdominal operation. The patient should be securely fastened to the table to allow for tilting during the procedure. The surgeon and camera operator are positioned on the patient's left side. The TV monitor is placed on the right side. The scrub nurse is on the patient's right side near the foot of the table.

Procedure

The instruments needed are:
- Scope 0°, 5 mm
- Trocar, 5 mm

- Trocar, 3.5 mm, ×2
- Grasper, 3 mm, ×2
- U-Stitch, ×2
- Needle with guidewire
- Dilator with catheter introducer
- Jejunostomy catheter
- Bolster, ×3

A jejunostomy utilizes the placement of three 5-mm trocars in a line along the anterior axillary border of the abdomen in the left upper quadrant (Fig. 1a) The patient is then tilted to the right and the ligament of Treitz is identified. A loop of jejunum is selected distal to the ligament of Treitz that can be easily brought to the anterior abdominal wall for a distance of at least 10 cm. The jejunum is held at the appropriate point on its antimesenteric surface against the anterior abdominal wall. A U-stitch is passed through the abdominal wall, through the jejunum and back out through the abdominal wall and secured with a clamp or bolster (Fig. 1b,c).

A Seldinger needle is then passed beginning laterally in the midclavicular line of the left upper quadrant. The needle is inserted bevel down. The needle passes deeply through the muscle layers of the abdominal wall to the peritoneum. The needle is carefully advanced extraperitoneally under laparoscopic surveillance (Fig. 3d). After traversing above the peritoneal lining for a distance of 3 cm, the bevel of the needle is rotated 180° and the peritoneum is penetrated just proximal to the jejunum which is held against the abdominal wall by the U-stitch previously placed. The needle is advanced until it penetrates into the jejunal lumen. A guide wire is inserted through the needle and advanced into the jejunum (Fig. 1e). The Seldinger needle is retracted, and the tract is dilated over the guide wire with disposable dilators. The tract is dilated to an appropriate size for the planned jejunal feeding tube.

A catheter introducer and dilator are passed over the guide wire into the jejunum. The dilator is removed; the jejunostomy catheter is passed through the catheter introducer and into the jejunum for a distance of 10 cm (Fig. 1f). The catheter introducer is peeled away, leaving the jejunostomy tube in place. The jejunostomy catheter is secured to the skin. Two more U-stitches are passed through the abdominal wall under laparoscopic surveillance to pass around the subcutaneous tunnel of the jejunostomy tube. The jejunal wall is traversed by the U-stitch which is then brought back through the abdominal wall. A third U-stitch taken several centimeters more proximally on the jejunum completes the jejunostomy. All three U-stitches are tied snugly over a bolster which is left in place for 7–10 days (Fig. 1g,h).

Feedings may be initiated within 6–24 h after placement. No bolus feedings should be administered into the jejunum. Drip feeding is started at a slow rate and advanced as tolerated by the patient. The author has utilized this technique in two patients without complication.

24 Laparoscopic Jejunostomy

Fig. 1. a Port placement for jejunostomy. *Open O*, exit site for the jejunostomy. **b,c** A U-suture is placed through the abdominal wall and jejunum. The sutures can be held by a clamp or tied over a bolster. **d** A Seldinger needle passage is performed under laparoscopic surveillance. The needle is tunneled for a distance of 3 cm just outside the peritoneum. **e** The needle is passed into the jejunum. A guide wire is passed into the jejunal lumen and the needle is removed. **f** An intravenous catheter dilator and peel away introducer is passed over the guide wire into the jejunum. The guide wire and dilator are removed leaving the catheter introducer. A jejunostomy tube is passed through the catheter introducer and into the jejunum. About 10 cm of jejunal catheter should be left in place. **g,h** The introducer is then peeled away. Two more U-sutures are placed through the abdominal wall, through the jejunum and back through the abdominal wall. The jejunostomy tube is secured to the skin. The U-sutures are tied over a bolster

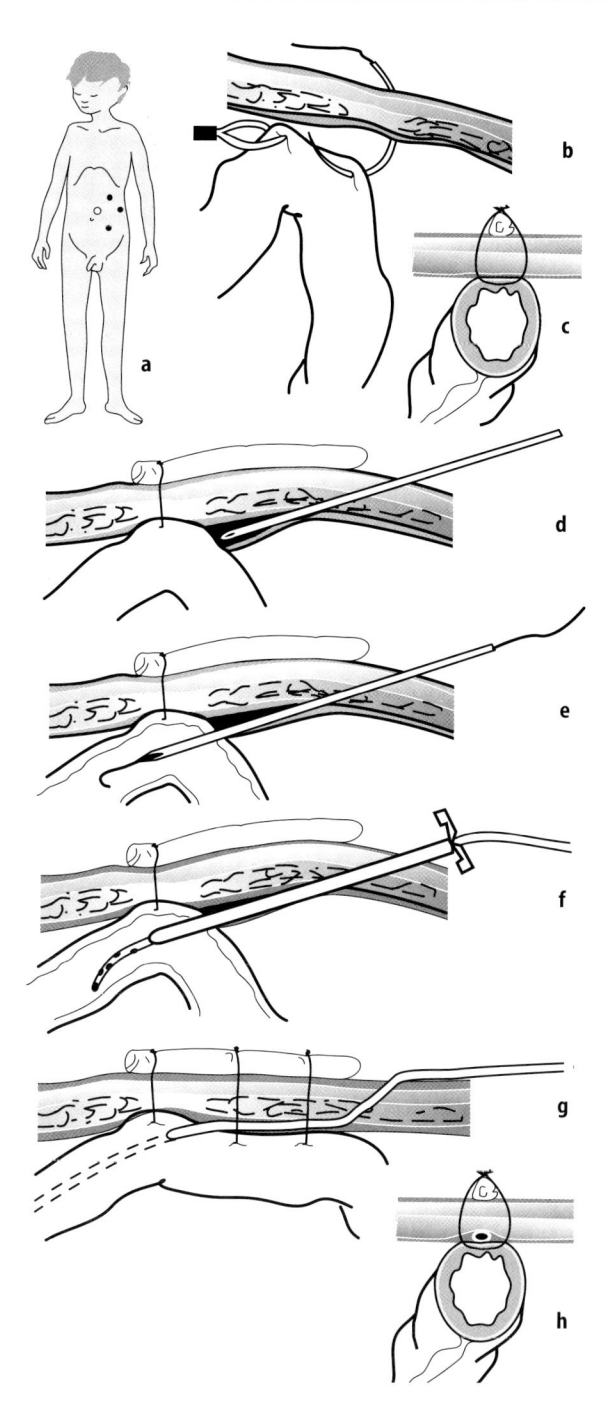

Discussion

This technique is useful in the occasional patient requiring jejunostomy feeding. Because of the difficulty in maintaining the patency of jejunostomy tubes and because bolus feedings cannot be performed through a jejunostomy, this technique is not as useful as a gastrostomy tube. The jejunostomy tube is not as easy to replace as a gastrostomy. Shortening the length of the tunnel results in increased leakage around the jejunostomy tube.

References

Curet-Scot M, Shermeta DW (1986) A comparison of intragastric and intrajejunal feedings in neonatal piglets. J Pediatr Surg 21:552–555
Georgeson KE (1997) Laparoscopic versus open procedures for long-term enteral access. Nutri Clin Pract [Suppl] 12:S1–S2
Rombeau JL, Barot LR (1981) Enteral nutrition therapy. Surg Clin North Am 61:605–620
Ryan JA, Page CP (1984) Feeding: development and current status. JPEN J Parenter Enter Nutr 8:187–98

CHAPTER 25

Laparoscopic Treatment of Anomalies of Intestinal Rotation in Children

N.M.A. Bax, D.C. van der Zee

Introduction

There are many forms of anomalies of intestinal rotation and fixation (Gray and Skandalakis 1972; Grob 1957). The most common form, at least presenting clinical problems, is the form in which the cecum lies to the right of the vertebral column, anterior to the duodenum. The cecum in this form is held in that place by peritoneal adhesions, often called bands of Ladd. There is no fixation of the intestinal mesentery to the posterior abdominal wall, and the mesenterial stalk is narrow which predisposes for volvulus. When volvulus occurs, it always does so in a clockwise direction. It is with this so-called classical form of intestinal malrotation that the authors have accumulated laparoscopic experience, and it is this experience that forms the basis of this chapter.

Indications

Most of the children present in the neonatal period with symptoms of a high gastrointestinal obstruction. Some children, however, may present with intermittent colicky abdominal pain, sometimes in combination with bilious vomiting throughout childhood and even lasting throughout adulthood. It is important to make the diagnosis early, not only to avoid volvulus and necrosis of the whole small bowel but also to avoid a lifetime of misery and misunderstanding.

In symptomatic patients the indication for surgery is obvious, but an anomaly of intestinal rotation is not always clearly symptomatic. According to Kluth and Lambrecht (1994) in about 2% of all barium meals malrotation is found incidentally and the question arises whether all these anomalies of intestinal rotation should be dealt with operatively (Schey et al. 1993). Nowadays many especially mentally retarded children are referred for a feeding gastrostomy. In their preoperative workup, the authors always carry out an upper gastrointestinal tract barium meal in order to identify anatomical abnormalities such as an esophageal stricture, a large hiatal hernia, but also an anomaly of intestinal rotation. Such a rotational abnormality is detected in some of these children, and the question arises as what should be done to this, especially when pathological gastrointestinal reflux is also present. The authors do not think that all these anomalies of intestinal rotation require operative management. Laparoscopic evaluation can be helpful in deciding whether something needs to be done. If there are in fact obstructing bands, they should be divided, but when the mesenterial stalk is wide, the chance for a volvulus is small.

Preoperative Workup

The diagnosis of a rotational abnormality is usually made radiologically by means of an upper GI series. The key to diagnosis during such study is the lack of a normal duodenojejunal junction both in babies and in older children as well as in adults (Berdon 1995). Echo Doppler of the mesenterial vessels can also be diagnostic by showing an inverted position of the superior mesenteric artery and vein, which is a sign of malrotation and not of volvulus (Loyer and Eggli 1989). In nonacute situations it may be wise to washout the large bowel preoperatively, as this increases the laparoscopic working space. It is stressed that this should not be carried out in acute situations.

Technique

Position of the Patient, Team, and Equipment. The child is placed in a supine and slight reverse Trendelenburg position on a short operating table (Fig. 1). The hips are in exorotation and abduction, the knees in flexion, and the feet with the soles against each other. To prevent the patient slipping from the table, the legs are enveloped with the lower end of the sheet covering the table Fig. 2a. As the operation concentrates on the duodenum, a more left lateral decubitus may be advantageous (Fig. 2b). The tower with monitor, camera unit, video, and insufflator stands to the right of the upper end of the table. The surgeon stands at the bottom end of the table with the surgical assistant to his left and the scrub nurse to his right (Fig. 1).

Fig. 1. Position of the patient, team, and equipment

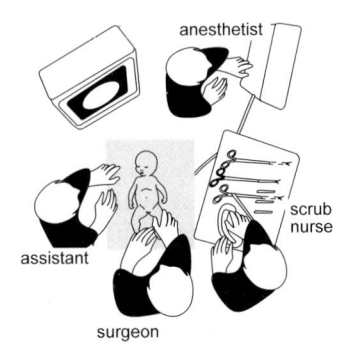

Fig. 2a,b. Position of the patient and of the cannulae. **a** Supine position of the patient, cannula through the umbilicus for the scope, cannulae for the working instruments pararectally on the right and on the left at umbilical level. **b** Alternative slight left decubitus position, cannula for the scope pararectally to the right of the umbilicus, cannulae for the working instruments to the left (umbilicus) and right (anterior axillary line) of the scope

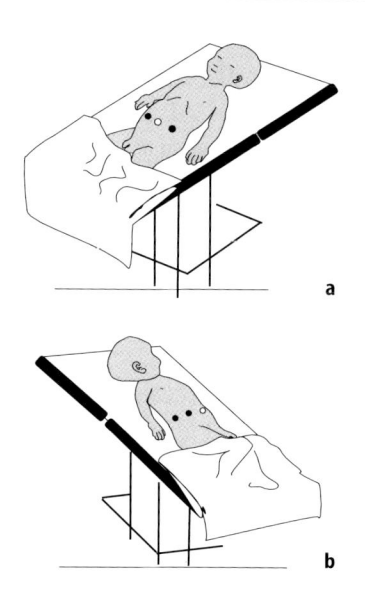

Cannulae. Three 6-mm cannulae are inserted: the first one in an open manner through the inferior umbilical fold for a 5-mm scope, the two others pararectally at the level of the umbilicus, the right one for a forceps (surgeons left hand) and the left one for a pair of scissors (surgeon's right hand) (Fig. 2a). As noted above, it may be better to put the patient somewhat more on the left side and to put two remaining cannulae to the right of the umbilicus and to change the scope from the umbilical cannula to the parectal cannula (Fig. 2b). It may be of assistance if the cannula holding the 5-mm endoscope is lifted by the assistant to allow maximal visibility within the small abdominal space. To prevent pulling out of the cannulae they are fixed to the skin with a 2-0 suture. To prevent pushing in of the cannula a circular tape is put around the base of the cannula, incorporating the suture (Bax and van der Zee 1998a).

Pneumoperitoneum. CO_2 is insufflated at an initial flow of 0.5 l/min and a maintenance flow of 2 l/min. Pressure is limited to 5 mmHg.

Findings

It is not difficult to confirm the diagnosis of intestinal malrotation laparoscopically: cecum and appendix usually are in a high and rather medial position below the liver, to which they are fixed by peritoneal bands (Fig. 3a). The second part of the duodenum looks long and tortuous. In the case of a volvulus, which is always in a clockwise direction, the typical picture is easily identified.

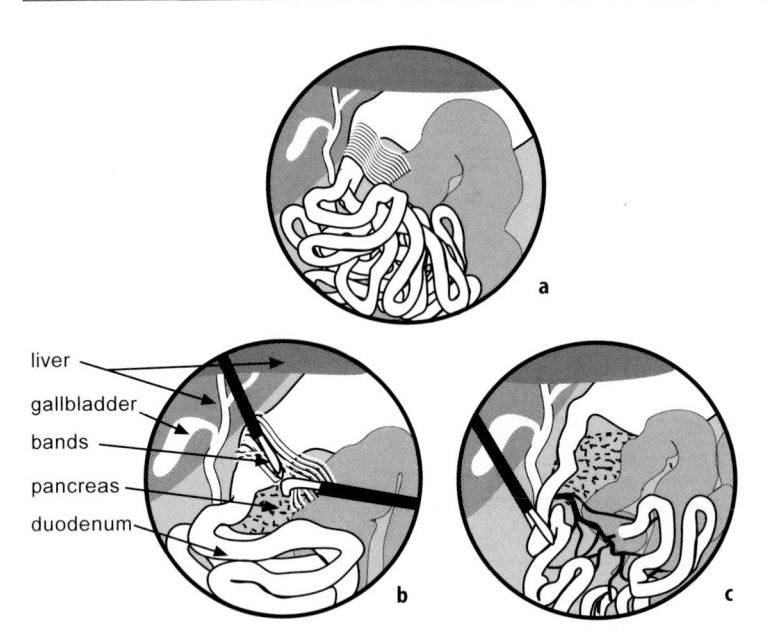

Fig. 3a–c. The actual procedure. **a** Endoscopic view of a classic malrotation before manipulation: small bowel in the right upper quadrant. **b** Transection of the bands of Ladd and moving of the cecum to the left. **c** The duodenum has been kocherized. Further dissection continues in a craniocaudal way first along the duodenum, then along the jejunum and ileum to the terminal ileum

Therapy

As far as therapy is concerned it is very important to concentrate on the stalk of the anomaly and not on the loops of bowel. Even when there is a volvulus but without strangulation, it is far better to leave the volvulus at the time and to concentrate on the second part of the duodenum (van der Zee and Bax 1995; Bax and van der Zee 1998b). First the peritoneal bands fixing the cecum to the duodenum are severed, and the cecum is pushed to the left (Fig. 3b). Next the second part of the duodenum is kocherized. It is very important to stick to the duodenum and to mobilize the distal duodenum further and further while pulling on the more proximal part (Fig. 3c). During this mobilization a peritoneal band in the shape of a ring encircling the duodenum becomes apparent and should be transected anteriorly. This band represents the end of the retroperitoneal part of the duodenum. The proximal jejunum now comes into view. By pulling further and further on the jejunum, the whole jejunum is positioned on the right below the liver. By using this technique an existing volvulus is reduced and the bowel put in a nonrotation position.

The stalk of the anomaly, however, is still narrow and the second part of the duodenum and cecum still lie side by side. By transecting the anterior peritoneal band between the two structures and pushing the cecum to the left, the mesenterial stalk is broadened. The appendix is now grasped and is exteriorized by removing the left cannula. The appendicular vessels are severed, the appendix is ligated at its base and is removed. The right sided cannula is removed as well. After checking the cannula sites for eventual bleeding, the scope is removed and the cannula holes are closed.

Postoperative Care

This care does not differ from that after open surgery.

Results

From November 1994 until July 1997 nine neonates presented with a high gastrointestinal obstruction on a basis of intestinal malrotation. One neonate had obvious necrosis and had an immediate laparotomy. The remaining eight neonates were approached laparoscopically. Four of these eight had volvulus without strangulation, but in one of them there was chylascites and deposits of fibrin, while in another one there had been polyhydramnios and there was more fibrosis as usual indicating that the volvulus has been present for some time. The operation was successfully finished in five of the eight children. In one child the laparoscopic approach was abandoned due to equipment failure. In the remaining two children too little progress was being made, but in these children there was evidence of a longer lasting volvulus.

Four children were referred at the age of 5.5, 11, 18, 28 months for a feeding gastrostomy in the context of feeding problems in relation with mental retardation. During the preoperative workup of these patients which included a pH study, endoscopy of the esophagus, and an upper gastrointestinal tract barium meal, intestinal malrotation was diagnosed. One of these patients proved to have pathological gastroesophageal reflux, and one had associated duodenal stenosis. All had laparoscopic treatment of the malrotation. Two received also a gastrostomy, one a gastrostomy and antireflux procedure according to Thal, and the last had laparoscopic treatment of the malrotation followed by a duodeno-duodenostomy through a minilaparotomy. As the duodenum had been completely mobilized laparoscopically, only a very small laparotomy was needed to do this. No preoperative complications occurred. Postoperatively in one of the two children that also received a gastrostomy the catheter dislodged and acquired an intraperitoneal position. This was recognized before feedings were given, and the catheter was removed. Despite treatment of the malrotation the child continued to vomit, and a repeat pH study demonstrated pathological reflux. A barium meal showed good passage through the duodenum and proximal jejunum. In a second laparoscopic operation the child received a gastrostomy and an antireflux procedure according to Thal. During that laparoscopic operation no adhesions could be noted between the bowel and anterior abdominal. All but one child, who had a pure laparoscopic approach, did well and left the hospital between 4 and 11 days. The child that had antireflux surgery in a second stage had a much longer hospital stay.

Discussion

For laparoscopic procedures in general but particularly in small children optimal muscle relaxation is required to allow as much expansion of the abdomen and thus the greatest possible working space with the least possible CO_2 pressure. If muscle relaxation is optimal experience shows that a pneumoperitoneum pressure of 5 mmHg creates enough room for the laparoscopic treatment of rotational abnormalities of the intestines. By lifting the cannula, holding the scope, even a better view can be obtained.

If a rather incidental rotational abnormality of the bowel has been found during a radiological contrast examination of the gastrointestinal tract, laparoscopy may play an important diagnostic role in those patients, in whom the relationship to the symptoms is not obvious. In such instances laparoscopy is able to identify possible obstructive bands or a small mesenterial stalk, which predisposes to volvulus. If that is the case than laparoscopic treatment should proceed; if not, the anomaly should be left untouched.

The same principles of treatment are followed as in open surgery:
- Transection of the bands of peritoneum, the so-called bands of Ladd, between the cecum and the duodenum as well as between the liver and the duodenum
- Broadening of the stalk of bowel by incising the anterior mesenterial sheet and separating the duodenum and the ileum to prevent volvulus
- Appendectomy to prevent missed appendicitis
- Placement of the bowel in a nonrotation position in the abdomen

Most of these principles were originally described by Ladd (Ladd 1936; Ladd and Gross 1941). In the literature either the bands of Ladd or volvulus are held responsible for the obstruction of the second part of the duodenum. We believe, however, that when obstruction occurs, partial volvulus is always involved in the pathogenesis. By clockwise rotation of the cecum behind the mesenterial stalk obviously the bands fixing the cecum to the duodenum become tightened and obstructive. In the original publications of Ladd, appendectomy was not advocated and broadening of the stalk by incising the anterior mesentery was not clearly described although the latter must have been part of the procedure. Ladd wrote that: If the surgeon attempts to evaluate the findings without delivering all the intestines outside the abdomen, he becomes hopeless confused, wastes valuable time, and seldom find that which he is dealing with (Ladd and Gross 1941). During laparoscopic treatment of malrotation the same happens when the surgeon does not concentrate on the duodenum. Turning around the loops of bowel during the operation does not make the pathological anatomy simpler. Even when a volvulus is present but no strangulation, in the beginning of the procedure it is better to leave the volvulus because access to the proximal duodenum is far better than after derotation. This is at variance with the classical open approach in which a volvulus is immediately reduced. By concentrating on the duodenum and mobilizing the duodenum and later the small bowel further and further, a volvulus is automatically reduced and a nonrotation position obtained. It is advocated that in all cases of malrotation an intrinsic obstruction should be ruled out by passing a tube of adequate size through the duodenum into the jejunum (Kluth and Lambrecht 1995; Smith 1986). We have not adopted this policy as a routine because we think that in the event of a partial obstruction due to a membrane secondary changes, for example, bowel wall thickening, and a difference in caliber is seen laparoscopically. This was obvious in the patient in which we treated the malrotation laparoscopically but who had associated duodenal stenosis. Laparoscopic treatment of the malrotation greatly facilitated the duodeno-duodenostomy as the duodenum had been completely mobilized. As a result only a minilaparotomy was necessary. As in other laparoscopic procedures, when the surgeon is not happy with the procedure, he should convert to an open procedure. We have adopted the policy that when not enough progress has been made within the first laparoscopic hour, conversion is carried out.

The benefit of the laparoscopic approach for the child is obvious: identification of the patients that really need treatment, less postoperative pain, less scarring, and apparently less adhesions.

References

Bax NMA, van der Zee (1998a) Laparoscopic treatment of intestinal malrotation in children. Surg Endosc 12: 1314–1316
Bax NMA, van der Zee (1998b) Trocar fixation during endoscopic surgery in infants and children. Surg Endosc 12:181–182
Berdon WE (1995) The diagnosis of malrotation and volvulus in the older child and adult: a trap for radiologists. Pediatr Radiol 25:101–103
Gray SW, Skandalakis JE (1972) Embryology for surgeons. Saunders, Philadelphia, pp 129–141
Grob M (1957) Lageanomalien des Magendarmtractes. In: Grob M (ed) Lehrbuch der Kinderchirurgie. Thieme, Stuttgart, pp 53–70
Kluth D, Lambrecht W (1994) Disorders of intestinal malrotation. In: Freeman NV, Burge DM, Griffiths DM, Malone PSJ (eds) Surgery of the newborn. Churchill Livingstone, Edinburgh, pp 201–210
Ladd WE (1936) Surgical diseases of the alimentary tract in infants. N Engl J Med 215:705–708
Ladd WE, Gross RE (1941) Abdominal surgery of infancy and childhood. Saunders, Philadelphia
Loyer E, Eggli KD (1989) Sonographic evidence of superior mesenteric vascular relationship in malrotation. Pediatr Radiol 19:173–175

Schey WL, Donaldson JS, Sty JR (1993) Malrotation of the bowel: variable pattern with different surgical considerations. J Pediatr Surg 28:96–101

Smith EI (1986) Malrotation of the intestine. In: Welch KJ, Randoph JG, Ravitch MM, O'Neill JA Jr, Rowe MI (eds) Pediatric surgery. Year Book Medical Publishers, Chicago, pp 882–895

van der Zee DC, Bax NMA (1995) Laparoscopic repair of acute volvulus in a neonate with malrotation. Surg Endosc 9:1123–1124

CHAPTER 26

Laparoscopic Approach to Intestinal Obstruction in Children

D.C. van der Zee, N.M.A. Bax

Introduction

The cause of abdominal symptoms in infants and younger children is usually congenital abnormality. Examples include intestinal malrotation, intestinal atresia, meconium ileus, intestinal aganglionosis, omphaloenteric remnants, and intestinal duplication anomalies. Acquired causes of intestinal obstruction include incarcerated inguinal hernia, intussusception, and inflammatory strictures from necrotizing enterocolitis (Holcomb 1997).

The most important cause of bowel obstruction, however, as in adults, is adhesions after former laparotomy. Festen (1982) observed 2.2% adhesive obstructions after 1476 laparotomies in children. Of the obstructions in this series 70% were due to a single adhesion.

Indications and Contraindications for Laparoscopic Approach

If a child presents with symptoms of obstruction, usually a fairly precise diagnosis as to the level and cause of obstruction can be made by history, clinical presentation, plain abdominal X-ray, and sometimes contrast studies from above or from below. Occasionally, however, especially when the symptoms occur beyond the neonatal period and in absence of previous abdominal surgery, this may be more difficult, and diagnostic laparoscopy may be of value.

Obstructive symptoms in the event of previous abdominal surgery makes adhesive obstruction likely. Again, the level of obstruction is usually easy to define. The question arises how conservative or aggressive one should be in the management of intestinal obstruction. Obviously, in the event of peritoneal signs or signs of overt bowel necrosis, operative exploration should not be postponed. In all children initial treatment should be gastrointestinal decompression and replacement of fluid losses. However, how to proceed further? Some advocate a nonoperative approach, but is it justifiable to wait and see in absence of peritoneal signs? The longer one waits, the more bowel distention, the more pain, and the more difficult a laparoscopic approach. In a review Akgür et al. (1991) managed 149 of 230 adhesive small-bowel obstructions in 181 children conservatively, although 39 needed surgical intervention at a later stage. Ultimately 60% overall required operation. Therefore, why not directly a laparoscopic approach?

Until recently, traditional laparotomy has been the treatment of choice. Although laparoscopic management of acute small-bowel obstruction has been addressed by a number of authors in adult patients (Ibrahim et al. 1996; Francois et al. 1994; Franklin et al. 1994; Keating et al. 1992; Silva and Cogbill 1991; Levard et al. 1993; Federmann et al. 1995), its role in pediatric surgery is still not established. It is our view that if a laparoscopic approach can avoid a formal laparotomy; then early diagnostic laparoscopy has the preference over conservative wait-and-see policy.

Absolute contraindications in laparoscopy in general are bleeding disorders and inability to administer general anesthesia (Reissman and Wexner 1995). Relative contraindications may be severe abdominal distention with massive dilated small bowel; peritoneal signs with compromised or perforated bowel; and unsafe conditions, such as dense adhesions and fused bowel loops.

This chapter deals mainly with the laparoscopic approach of adhesive obstruction in children only. Management of intestinal malrotation, intestinal aganglionosis, and intussusception are dealt with in other chapters.

Preoperative Workup

All potentially obstructed patients should have gastrointestinal decompression and fluid assessment and therapy, including an urinary catheter, before surgery.

Operation

The patient is placed in a supine position on the operating table. Muscle relaxation allows for maximal exposure. Depending on the suspected localization of the obstruction and of the abdominal scars the localization of the first cannula is determined. Ultrasound may be used to determine adhesion of bowel against the abdominal wall.

The first cannula is always inserted using an open technique, preferably in the umbilicus or at another site away from prior incisions if the umbilicus is involved. Working cannulae of 6 mm are placed under direct vision after the abdomen is insufflated to 5–10 mmHg. Tilting the operating table in various positions enables distended bowel to fall away from the laparoscopic line of vision.

A 360° squint gives an overview to determine the area involved. Eventual bands with the ventral abdominal wall can be lyzed with scissors or by diathermy. In the case of small-bowel obstruction the bowel can be run in a retrograde fashion starting at the cecum by grasping the bowel with two atraumatic graspers and using a "hand-to-hand" technique. Care should be taken not to traumatize the obstructed bowel as it is distended, edematous and therefore very fragile. Dilated bowel is prone to perforation from small blunt instruments. The use of 2-mm instruments should be restricted to noninflamed tissues.

Sometimes grasping the mesentery in order to manipulate the bowel decreases the risk of direct trauma. At times it is also indicated, in addition to tilting the table, to change the scope cannula to get a better view. Adhesions can be incised by direct cutting or using diathermy. In a virgin abdomen, however, a band running to a Meckel's diverticulum can be found. If a clear band is seen it is not necessary to perform an extensive adhesiolysis, since it is known that adhesions reformation occurs in 97.1% (Operative Laparoscopy Study Group 1991).

Sometimes adhesions are too extensive or too malignantly adherent to allow laparoscopic dissection. On the other hand, in a number of instances the dissection can be prepared in part laparoscopically, such as the mobilization of the lateral gutter, which allows a restricted laparotomy to complete the release of the obstruction or to perform a limited resection and primary anastomosis.

Laparoscopic resections should be restricted to experienced hands and preferably after meticulous bowel preparation. Care should be taken to obtain meticulous hemostasis and rinse the abdomen clean of blood clots to deter recurrence of adhesion formation. After finishing the procedure cannulae are removed under direct vision, initially leaving the instrument inside to be able to reintroduce the cannula in case of port site bleeding. Muscle relaxation should be continued until the last cannula has been removed to avoid protrusion of omentum through the wound at the time of cannula removal. Fascia closure of 6-mm cannula sites is not necessary except for in the midline and umbilicus, and in infants. Subcutis may be approximated, and the skin is closed with adhesive strips.

Personal Experience

Between December 1993 and May 1997, 35 children presented with an intestinal obstruction syndrome (Table 1). In 16 children a diagnostic laparoscopy was performed. In three instances a laparoscopic assisted minilaparotomy was carried through for segmental bowel resection and anastomosis for jejunal and ileal stenosis, and Meckel's diverticulum, respectively. In one patient extensive malignant adhesions after prior malrotation operation warranted conversion to laparotomy. The single complication occurred in a child with an obstruction of the colon at the hepatic flexure after an antireflux procedure, with massive distension and edema. During the procedure of localizing the adhesion the ascend-

Table 1. Adhesive obstruction in children

	Virgin abdomen	Previous surgery
Open ($n=19$)	–	19
Laparoscopy ($n=16$)	8	8
No conversion ($n=11$)	5	6
Conversion ($n=5$)	3	2
Total ($n=35$)	8	27

ing colon was perforated by a small blunt grasping forceps that was pushing the dilated colon sideways. The procedure was converted, and the patient was given a temporary ileostomy. After a stormy recovery the child is doing well and the ileostomy has been closed.

Eleven children were managed laparoscopically. Six of them had undergone prior laparotomy. In five adhesiolysis was completed laparoscopically. The sixth patient had a history of necrotizing enterocolitis with clinical and radiological signs of obstruction of the descending colon. On laparoscopy no obstruction was found. Intraoperative rectal air insufflation demonstrated no colonic constriction. This patient was spared an unnecessary laparotomy. Two further patients presented with obstructive symptoms where no anatomical cause could be found on laparoscopy. Other causes were a persisting incarcerated hernia after supposed reposition with continued vomiting and abdominal distention, internal small-bowel herniation, and adhesive bands without a prior history in two children.

During the same period 19 children underwent primary laparotomy for obstruction. The majority of these children had a history of laparotomy for necrotizing enterocolitis, and a laparoscopic approach was deemed inappropriate. Five children with a variety of other prior diseases had an obstructing band and might have benefited from a laparoscopic approach.

Discussion

Adhesions are abnormal attachments between peritoneal surfaces; most adhesions are inflammatory in origin and follow either a surgical operation or peritonitis (Macbeth 1977). Surgeons should adjust their major practices by becoming aware of the potential adhesive complications of a procedure; minimizing the invasiveness of surgery; minimizing surgical trauma, ischemia, exposure to intestinal contents, introduction of foreign material into the body, and the use of talc- or starch-containing gloves (Holmdahl et al. 1997; Tulandi 1996).

There are several reports that laparoscopy has less adhesion formation (Bulletti et al. 1996; Tulandi 1996; Pados and Devroey 1992; Moore et al. 1995). Jorgensen et al. (1995) has demonstrated in an experimental model that laparoscopic procedures induce less adhesion formation. Ellis (1997), however, claims that laparoscopy does not seem to eliminate the risk of adhesions and adhesive obstruction. In our own experience we have encountered a reduced incidence of postoperative adhesions after laparoscopic surgery, although the incidence is not zero, as demonstrated by the single complication encountered during adhesiolysis after a laparoscopic antireflux procedure.

A study by the Operative Laparoscopy Study Group (1991) reported adhesion reformation occurred in 97.1%. On the other hand, only 12% de novo adhesions was found by the laparoscopic procedures, in contrast to 51% after open surgery as mentioned by this group. This not only enhances the beneficial effect of laparoscopic surgery, but also justifies the initial laparoscopic approach in adhesive obstruction.

Laparoscopic adhesiolysis has been performed over recent years. Levard et al. (1993) reported fewer than 50% of successful procedures in 25 patients. Federmann et al. (1995) achieved 62% success in resolving small-bowel ileus laparoscopically in 26 patients. Franklin et al. (1994) operated successfully on 20 out of 23 patients by laparoscope. Keating et al. (1992) reported on 5 successfully treated cases in the same fashion with early discharge. Ibrahim et al. (1996) accomplished a 72% success rate in 25 adult patients. However, its role in pediatric surgery has not yet been established. In our own experience laparoscopy is started principally as a diagnostic procedure under antibiotic prophylaxis. In 11 out of 16 cases (70%) adhesiolysis were completed laparoscopically. In three patients segmental resections and anastomoses were performed by minilaparotomy while in two children conversion was carried out.

If massive adhesions are to be expected, such as after extensive necrotizing enterocolitis and other inflammatory diseases, a laparoscopic approach is often inappropriate. On the other hand after (semi)elective (laparoscopic) surgery for congenital abnormalities, such as intestinal malrotation, small intestinal atresia, meconium ileus, intestinal aganglionosis, and intestinal duplication anomalies, diagnostic laparoscopy as a first-stage procedure in postoperative intestinal obstruction syndrome might have avoided a laparotomy in five children.

Ibrahim et al. (1996) describe a number of lessons to be learned that we have mentioned before as well: always open trocar insertion technique, good positioning with tilting of the table, edematous and dilated bowel is prone to perforation, changing of the camera position if necessary, and always look for the cause in a virgin abdomen when difficult or in doubt conversion to laparotomy.

Borzellino et al. (1996) and Caprini et al. (1995) describe the successful use of ultrasound mapping of adhesions as a method of avoiding complications in Veress needle puncture. We have no personal experience with ultrasound mapping, although ultrasound may indicate whether intestinal loops are adherent to the abdominal wall. We agree with Ibrahim et al. (1996) that open initial trocar insertion is mandatory in patients with adhesions, as has also been demonstrated in an experimental study (Elhage et al. 1996).

In conclusion, laparoscopic management of intestinal obstruction in children is feasible and safe in experienced hands. Laparoscopy begins principally as an diagnostic procedure in obstruction after surgery for congenital diseases or acquired diseases without massive general peritonitis. After making an accurate diagnosis the procedure can either be converted to a laparotomy, or partially or totally continued as a laparoscopic procedure.

References

Akgür FM et al (1991) Adhesive small bowel obstruction in children: the place and predictors of success for conservative treatment. J Pediatr Surg 26:37–41

Borzellino G et al (1996) Mappa ecografica delle aderenze peritoneali. Radiol Med Torino 92:390–393

Bulletti C et al (1996) Adhesion formation after laparoscopic myomectomy. J Am Assoc Gynecol Laparosc 3:533–536

Caprini JA, Arcelus JA, Swanson J et al (1995) The ultrasonic localization of abdominal wall adhesions. Surg Endosc 9:283–285

Elhage A et al (1996) Le benefice de la micro-laparotomie ombilicale "open laparoscopy" pour l'abord coelioscopique. Étude experimentale. J Gynecol Obstet Biol Reprod Paris 25:373–377

Ellis H (1997) The clinical significance of adhesions: focus on intestinal obstruction. Eur J Surg [Suppl] 577:5–9

Federmann G et al (1995) Laparoscopic treatment in small-bowel-ileus caused by adhesions. Surg Endosc 9:605

Festen C (1982) Postoperative small bowel obstruction in infants and children. Ann Surg 196:580–582

Francois Y, Mouret P, Vignal J (1994) Occlusion du grêle et viscerolyse coelioscopique. Ann Chir 48:165–168

Franklin Jr ME, Dorman JP, Pharand D (1994) Laparoscopic surgery in acute small bowel obstruction. Surg Laparosc Endosc 4:289–296

Holcomb GW (1997) Clinical principles of abdominal surgery. In: Oldham KT, Colombani PM, Fogera RP (eds) Surgery of infants and children: scientific principles and practice. Lippincott-Raven, Philadelphia, pp 1051–1067

Holmdahl L et al (1997) Adhesions: pathogenesis and prevention-panel discussion and summary. Eur J Surg [Suppl] 577:56–62

Ibrahim IM et al (1996) Laparoscopic management of acute small bowel obstruction. Surg Endosc 10:1012–1015

Jorgensen JO, Lalak NJ, Hunt DR (1995) Is laparoscopy associated with lower rate of postoperative adhesions than laparotomy? A comparative study in the rabbit. Aust NZ J Surg 65:342–344

Keating J et al (1992) Laparoscopy in the diagnosis and treatment of acute small bowel obstruction. J Laparoendosc Surg 2:239–244

Levard H et al (1993) Traitement coelioscopique des occlusions aiguës du grêle. Ann Chir 47:497–501

Macbeth J (1997) Adhesions. In: Sabiston DC Jr (ed) Textbook of surgery, 11th edn. Saunders, Philadelphia, p 894–896

Moore RG et al (1995) Adhesion formation after transperitoneal nefrectomy: laparoscopic versus open approach. J Endourol 9:277–280

Operative Laparoscopy Study Group (1991) Postoperative adhesion development after operative laparoscopy: evaluation at early second look procedures. Fertil Steril 55:700–704

Pados GA, Devroey P (1992) Adhesions. Curr Opin Obstet Gynecol 4:412–418

Reissman P, Wexner SD (1995) Laparoscopic surgery for intestinal obstruction. Surg Endosc 9:865–868

Silva PD, Cogbill TH (1991) Laparoscopic treatment of recurrent small bowel obstruction. Wiss Med J 90:169–170

Tulandi T (1996) Adhesion prevention in laparoscopic surgery. Int J Fertil Menopausal Stud 41:452–45

Laparoscopic Diagnosis and Treatment of Meckel's Diverticulum in Children

J-S. Valla, H. Steyaert

Introduction

As appendix, Meckel's diverticulum seems especially suited for laparoscopic treatment. Meckel's diverticulum is present in approximately 2% of the population but often is a silent lesion. Most symptomatic patients (4%–35% depending on the report) are observed during infancy or early childhood, and the pathology of Meckel's diverticulum has been well known since the description by Meckel in 1808.

The pediatric surgeon can be confronted with this omphalomesenteric remnant in the two following situations:
- It is exposed during an intra-abdominal operation performed for an another purpose: in neonates an abdominal wall or intestinal malformation such as omphalocele, diaphragmatic hernia, intestinal malrotation, atresia, Hirschsprung disease, and Meckel's diverticulum is a part of this more important malformation. Later in childhood Meckel's diverticulum is often an incidental finding during appendectomy.
- Meckel's diverticulum can be the origin of a specific complication such as obstruction, bleeding, and inflammation.

Controversy still exists over systematically searching Meckel's diverticulum in cases of intra-abdominal surgery, making preoperative exploration by echography and scintigraphy in cases of suspicion and removing a pathological Meckel's diverticulum by simple diverticulectomy or by small intestinal resection. Has the introduction of laparoscopic techniques [1, 6, 9–12, 14] affected these controversies?

Indications

We must underline, first of all, that laparoscopic resection cannot concern all the Meckel's diverticulum cases: actually our subject does not include umbilical Meckel's diverticulum cases which appear during the neonatal period and are treated, as before, by classical surgical intervention using an infra-umbilical curvilinear incision.

This study also does not concern either the Meckel's diverticulum cases found during a wide neonatal laparotomy needed by the management of a parietal or intestinal neonatal malformation.

In practice there are two different situations for the laparoscopic pediatric surgeons:
- Meckel's diverticulum is not suspected before laparoscopy and is found incidentally. We think that Meckel's diverticulum must be actively searched during routine appendectomies and other diagnostic or therapeutic procedures on the lower part of the abdomen. Resection of incidental Meckel's diverticulum at the same time is discussed according to the age and the abdominal disease: elective resection is indicated in children under the age of 8 years because of the higher incidence of symptomatic lesions in this group; in older children Meckel resection is more debatable. In cases of very infected peritoneal disease diverticulectomy may add some risk and is performed some weeks later.
- A Meckel's diverticulum is preoperatively suspected because of a classical complication; in the first few months of life, the most common presenting symptoms is intestinal obstruction. Obstruction may be caused by volvulus or strangulation around a fibrous band, ileocolic intussusception with Meckel's diverticulum acting as a lead point, and may be associated with vascular compromise of the bowel. These particular features (abdominal distension, small abdominal cavity, vascular compromise) do not favor of a laparoscopic treatment.

The most common presenting symptom in infants and children is rectal bleeding, painless and without vomiting or hematemesis. The bleeding Meckel is a good indication for laparoscopic removal. The preoperative diagnosis of bleeding Meckel's diverticulum may be made by a ^{99m}Tc-pertechnetate isotope scan, sensitized by a pentagastrin injection [13–15] and after iodine suppression of the thyroid; in some cases, echography is also helpful [10]. However, 5%–15% of results are false negative or false positive. Because laparoscopic exploration is considered a mini-invasive procedure, we must use laparoscopy as a diagnostic method as for intra-abdominal testis and suppress preoperative radiological examinations? Such an attitude does not seem to be justified, as it increases the number of useless laparoscopies.

Inflammation of Meckel's diverticulum is a less common complication and occurs in older children; usually these children are operated on with the preoperative diagnosis of appendicitis and are also a good indication for laparoscopic removal.

Preoperative Preparation

In suspected Meckel's diverticulum the preparation is the same as for all laparoscopic procedures: abdominal and umbilical disinfection, emptying of the bladder by spontaneous miction or Credé maneuver, and emptying of the stomach by a nasogastric tube. In bleeding Meckel's diverticulum preoperative treatment with ranitidine is indicated.

Installation

The patient lies in supine position, the video column is on the right, the surgical team on the left as for appendectomy (Fig. 1) [1]. The position of the surgeon and his assistant could be changed during the procedure, and therefore one must be careful to leave wide mobility of the video column. Apart from the laparoscopic linear stapler there is no need for a specific device for laparoscopic removal of Meckel's diverticulum. The trocar placement is rather the same as for appendectomy (Fig. 2). If a Meckel's diverticulum is suspected, it is useful to put a 12-mm trocar in the umbilicus for the stapler and two 5-mm trocar in the right and left iliac fossa. A 5 mm 0° optic is introduced into the left iliac fossa cannula. If the Meckel's diverticulum is found during an appendectomy, the left sided 5-mm trocar or better the umbilical trocar must be replaced by a 12-mm trocar, for the stapler.

Fig. 1. Position of the patient, crew, and equipment

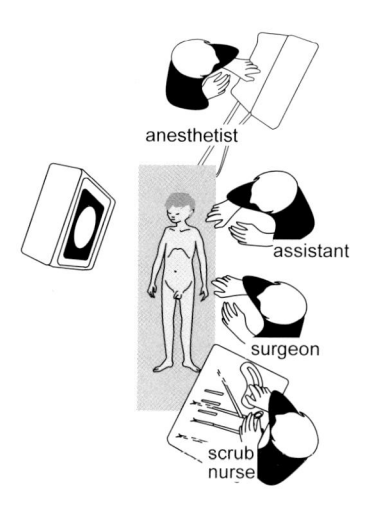

Fig. 2. Position of the trocars. The trocar for the scope is in the left iliac fossa. If the diagnosis of a Meckel's diverticulum is certain preoperatively, a 12-mm trocar should inserted in the umbilicus for use of the linear stapler

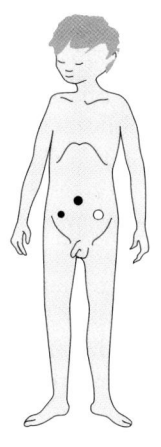

Operative Technique

Search for Meckel's Diverticulum

In a few cases Meckel's diverticulum is found very easily because it is the first visible lesion when introducing the optic in the median line, obliquely towards the small pelvis. Usually one looks for it on the antimesenteric and mesenteric side along the last ileal loops. The quality of this search depends on the surgeon's patience and his technique. He must be helped by the Trendelenburg and the left lateral decubitus to make slide the intestinal mass on his side. Then the intestinal loops are unrolled, beginning at the ileocecal angle, using the superior pelvic strait as a "block." This unrolling and exposing of the intestinal loops is easy done with two grasping forceps in a three-trocar technique. The search for a Meckel's diverticulum during a monotrocar transumbilical appendicectomy with an operating channel optical system is not reliable.

Resection of Meckel's Diverticulum

In symptomatic Meckel's diverticulum managed by classical surgery the most recommended procedure is a 5–10 cm intestinal resection, followed by a primary end-to-end anastomosis. Cuneate resection with transverse closure in order to avoid narrowing of the lumen is another possible procedure, recommended in cases of nonsymptomatic Meckel's diverticulum. The simple diverticulectomy by ligation of the base is advocated by some surgeons [12]. We do not recommend the latter technique because of the risk of leaving ectopic mucosa at the base.

At the beginning of laparoscopic surgery in children, the incidental finding of a Meckel's diverticulum during a laparoscopic procedure was an indication for conversion to an open surgical technique. With more experience it became obvious that Meckel's diverticulum can be safely excised laparoscopically. As for appendicectomy there are two mains steps, hemostasis and bowel resection, and three techniques: (a) a laparoscopically assisted technique, or "out technique," in which the diverticulum and its blood supply are exteriorized through an umbilical incision and treated outside the abdomen, (b) a "mixed technique," in which hemostasis is carried out in the abdomen, diverticulectomy, or small bowel resection out of the abdomen, and (c) a pure laparoscopic technique, or "in technique," in which the two main steps are made in the abdomen. The blood supply of a Meckel's diverticulum usually enters the diverticulum directly from the small bowel mesentery; it must be first separated, then coagulated with bipolar forceps, monopolar hook or laser. Diverticulectomy is made by section following the antimesenteric small bowel border and using an automatic laparoscopic linear stapler. Care must be taken to put the stapler diagonally or perpendicularly to the antimesenteric border to avoid any stenosis of the intestine as it was underlined by Teitelbaum [14] (Fig. 3). The extraction of Meckel's diverticulum through a 12-mm cannula is easy. The

Fig 3a,b. Resection of the diverticulum with the linear stapler. **a** Amputation of the diverticulum in line with the axis of the bowel may result in stenosis. **b** Amputation of the diverticulum in a transverse direction to the axis of the bowel prevents stenosis

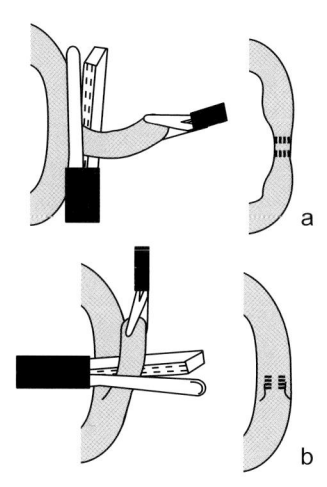

anastomosis is checked by laparoscopy, the umbilical fascia is closed with 2-0 absorbable suture.

Postoperative Care

Antibiotics are discontinued postoperatively after one or two doses. Patients can usually resume oral intake after 24 h. Afebrile children are discharged within 48–72 h and controlled at 10 and 30 days after the operation.

Results

Fifteen children were treated, aged between 6 months and 15 years old (average age: 8.5 years). These included three cases of pathological Meckel's diverticulum (average age: 4 years): an intussusception in a 2-year-old boy, a small bowel obstruction in a 6-month-old boy, and a hemorrhage with pain in a 10-year-old boy (preoperative endoscopy and scintigraphy were negative). In three cases the intestinal loop was exteriorized in the right iliac fossa or through the umbilicus. The affected bowel loop was resected, and an end-to-end anastomosis was performed. In two cases gastric mucosa was found at histology. No complications occurred.

Twelve diverticula were found incidentally during appendectomy (average age: 10 years). Seven diverticula were laparoscopically resected using the laparoscopic linear stapler. Gastric mucosa was found in two of them. No complications occurred. Five diverticula were exteriorized and resected. Gastric mucosa was found in three of them. There was one postoperative complication, namely a perianastomotic abscess after 45 days, requiring a repeat operation. The operation was initiated laparoscopically but was converted later through an incision in the right iliac fossa.

A 4-year-old boy had two recurrent attacks of gastrointestinal hemorrhages associated with pain. In this case the results of preoperative echography, endoscopy from above and below, and scintigraphy were negative. Laparoscopy was also negative.

Discussion

1. *Is the laparoscopic search of the Meckel's diverticulum perfectly reliable?*
   The answer is probably no, as in case of classic surgery, except if the surgeon insists in each case on a careful and meticulous search. The frequency of a Meckel's diverticulum in the population is slightly higher than 2% [2, 3, 8]. This rate has never been reached either in our series or in other important series of appendectomies in the literature [4]. In our experience of 1200 appendectomies using a three-trocar technique, a Meckel's diverticulum was found in 11 cases. Of 300 appendectomies using one-trocar only one Meckel's was found.

2. *Can heterotopic gastric mucosa, the most important element of the Meckel's pathology, be detected by laparoscopy?*
   The answer is no, as in classic surgery, but in classical surgery the surgeon is able to detect by gentle palpation the very rare pancreatic heterotopia (1%–16% depending on the series). Gastric heterotopia, much more frequent (15%–60% in the series), cannot be identified by direct or laparoscopic exterior view. Only histological study can be categorical: it has been shown that the ectopic mucosa can sometimes rather be located at the base of the diverticulum than in the diverticulum itself. So for this reason a small-bowel resection is recommended in cases of pathological diverticulum.

3. *How To Resect a Meckel's Diverticulum?*
   The answer depends on various factors such as symptoms, age, local anatomy, and surgeon's training; in cases of incidental Meckel's diverticulum section with the laparoscopic linear stapler is feasible if the child is old enough, and if the base of the diverticulum is narrow. In case of a symptomatic Meckel's diverticulum in an infant, exteriorization seems to be better because in this age group ectopic mucosa is frequent (40%–75%), the peritoneal cavity is small; it is not simple and safe to manipulate a laparoscopic linear stapler in the small cavity; the umbilical incision needed to introduce a 12-mm trocar is large enough to exteriorize a Meckel's diverticulum and adjacent small bowel in an infant.

   The treatment results of a pure laparoscopic procedure have been very good in all case reports and series, particularly no suture leakage and no wound infection has been reported. In our series the only insufficiency of suture lines was observed after classical resection after exteriorization.

Conclusion

The introduction of laparoscopic techniques has not modified our basic attitude regarding diagnosis and management of Meckel's diverticulum:

- The possibility of a Meckel's diverticulum must be considered in case of a gastrointestinal bleeding or small-bowel obstruction. One must try to make the diagnosis hard preoperatively by echography and scintigraphy, as has been the custom.
- During each submesocolic laparoscopic procedure the pediatric surgeon must systematically look for a Meckel's diverticulum using a technique that follows the same rules as in classical surgery.
- The incidental finding of a Meckel's diverticulum does not require conversion to an open procedure.
- The laparoscopic removal of Meckel's diverticulum follows the same rules as in classical surgery: if the patient is very young and the Meckel's diverticulum complicated, laparoscopically assisted surgery is recommended. Pure laparoscopic removal using the laparoscopic linear stapler is acceptable if the child is old enough, if the Meckel's diverticulum is nonsymptomatic, and if it has a narrow base.

References

1. Attwood S et al (1992) Laparoscopic approach to Meckel's diverticulotomy. Br J Surg 79:211
2. Bemelman WA et al (1995) Meckel's diverticulum in Amsterdam: experience in 136 patients. World J Surg 19:734–737
3. Cullen JJ et al (1994) Surgical management of Meckel's diverticulum. Ann Surg 220:564–737
4. Estour E (1995) Coelio-appendicectomie: revue de 19 séries françaises portant sur 9697 cas opérés entre 1989 et 1994. J Coeliochir13:45–55
5. Grapin C (1990) Diverticule de Meckel et pathologie omphalomésentérique en chirurgie digestive de l'enfant. Helardot P, Bienayme J, Bargy F (eds) Chirurgie digestive de l'enfant. Doin, Paris, pp 449–461
6. Huang CS, Lin LH (1993) Laparoscopic Meckel's diverticulectomy in infants: report of three cases. J Pediatr Surg 28:1488–1489
7. Le Neel JE, Heloury Y (1978) Le diverticule de Meckel. faut-il le rechercher? faut-il l'enlever? A propos de 116 obs. J Chir (Paris) 120:233–237
8. Ludtke FE et al (1989) Incidence and frequency of complications and management of Meckel's diverticulum. Surg Gynécol Obstet 169:537–542
9. Miller K, Hutter J (1993) Videolaparoscopic treatment of Meckel's diverticulum. Endoscopy 25:373
10. Panuel M et al (1994) Ultrasonographic diagnosis and laparoscopic surgical treatment of Meckel's diverticulum. Eur J Pediatr Surg 4:344–345
11. Saw EC, Ramachandra S (1993) Laparoscopically assisted resection of intussuscepted Meckel's diverticulum. Surg Laparosc Endosc 3:149–152
12. Schier F, Hoffmann K, Waldschmidt J (1996) Laparoscopic removal of Meckel's diverticulum in children. Eur J Pediatr Surg 6:38–39

13. St Vil D et al (1991) Meckel's diverticulum in children: a 20 years review. J Pediatr Surg 96:1289–1292
14. Teitelbaum DH, Pollet TZ, Obeid F (1994) Laparoscopic diagnosis and excision of Meckel's diverticulum. J Pediatr Surg 29:495–497
15. Vane DW, West KW, Grosfelp JL (1987) Vitelline duct anomalies: experience with 217 childhood cases. Arch Surg 122:542

CHAPTER 28

Intussusception

A.S. Najmaldin

Introduction

Approximately 80% of intussusceptions are reducible by air or hydrostatic enemas under fluoroscopic or ultrasonographic control [1–3]. Radiological, ultrasonic or clinical evidence of persistence of the intussusception or its complications necessitates laparotomy. During the laparotomy it is not uncommon to see that the intussusception is either already reduced or easily reducible with manipulation [4]. In these situations preliminary laparoscopy may prove effective in avoiding open surgery. Non-operative procedure and/or laparoscopy should be considered inappropriate in the seriously ill child, in those with tense and distended abdomens, or with evidence of perforation.

Pre-operative Preparation

The pre-operative preparation is as in open surgery to include placement of a naso-gastric tube, intravenous fluid and antibiotics. Informed consent is obtained from parents for laparoscopy with permission to undertake laparotomy, bowel resection and/or appendicectomy depending on the laparoscopic findings, or whether the laparoscopy failed in achieving diagnosis or reduction in the intussusception.

Equipment and Instruments

In addition to the camera, screen, light, insufflator, and a laparotomy set of instruments for conversion to open surgery, if and when required, the following instruments are necessary:
- Cannulae × 3 (4–5 mm)
- One 0° or 30° telescope (4–5 mm)
- Atraumatic straight and soft grasping forceps (4–5 mm) × 2

It is important that the jaws of the graspers are broad rather than narrow (Fig. 1). Smaller diameter instruments may cause damage to the delicate dilated bowel.

Fig. 1a,b. Soft, atraumatic grasping forceps. **a** Long and wide jaws appropriate for intussusception. **b** Narrow and/or short jaws may cause bowel injury

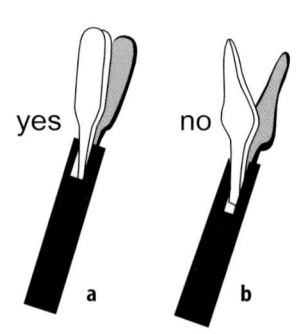

Technique

A general anaesthetic with endotracheal intubation and relaxation is necessary. The patient is placed in a supine position and catheterisation of the bladder is usually unnecessary. Both the surgeon and the assistant (cameraman) stand on the left side of the patient (Fig. 2a). A 4- or 5-mm cannula is placed just below the umbilicus using an open technique, and care must be taken not to damage the dilated intestine often seen directly beneath the peritoneum (Fig. 2b) (see the section on "Open Method" in Najmaldin and Grousseau "Basic Technique," this volume). In spite of mild to moderately dilated loops of bowel, a satisfactory

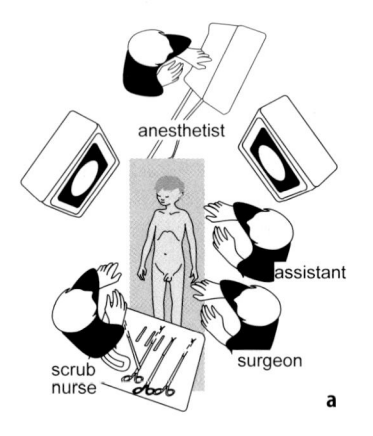

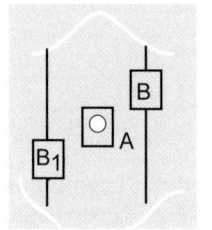

Fig. 2.a. Patient position and theatre layout. **b** Cannulae position for intussusception. *A*, Primary telescope cannula; *B, B1*, two secondary cannulae

pneumoperitoneum is usually achievable at a CO_2 pressure of 6–8 mmHg and a flow of 0.2 l/min.

The initial laparoscopy is carried out using a 4- or 5-mm telescope (0° adequate, 30° preferable). Look around the peritoneal cavity and note the presence, site and status of the intussusception. At this stage of the operation one secondary cannula may be required to gently sweep and retract distended loops of bowel if adequate viewing proved difficult (Fig. 2b). A degree of reverse Trendelenburg and/or lateral tilt may improve exposure. Now one of the three following scenarios may be faced (Fig. 3):

- The intussusception is already completely reduced and no further action is required.
- The intussusception is long and advanced with signs of severe oedema and/or compromised bowel, in which case the laparoscopic procedure should be converted to an open operation unless conditions are right to assess, resect and anastomose bowels via the laparoscope.
- The intussusception is short with a mild/moderate degree of oedema and bruises but no compromised bowel. In this situation, two secondary 'working' 4-mm cannulae are sited in the right iliac fossa and the left upper quadrant enabling atraumatic grasping forceps to be passed for manipulation of the bowel (Fig. 2b). Grasp the proximal bowel gently with an atraumatic grasper and gently and persistently push the neck of the intussusception distally by the side of a second atraumatic grasper over a period of time, which may be more than several minutes. Having confirmed the complete reduc-

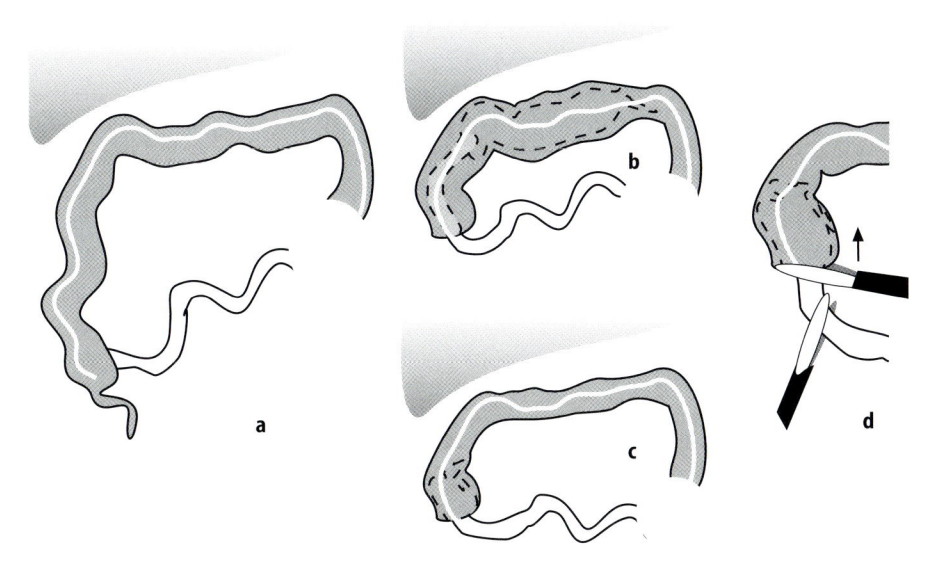

Fig. 3a–d. Laparoscopic view. **a** A completely reduced intussusception. **b** Long-segment intussusception with compromised bowel. **c** Short segment intussusception without sign of compromised bowel. **d** Laparoscopic reduction in short segment intussusception. *Arrow*, Direction of push at the neck of intussusception "distally"

tion, further examination of the bowel is undertaken by the two atraumatic grasping forceps to exclude injury and pathological lead point. At the end of procedure the pneumoperitoneum is evacuated and cannulae removed. The wounds are infiltrated with appropriate local anaesthetic agents and fascial incisions (4–5-mm) are closed carefully using absorbable suture materials.

The laparoscopy is abandoned and the operation continues via an open technique if the intussusception cannot be reduced laparoscopically, or if after reduction there is compromised bowel or a pathological lead point. The laparotomy incision may or may not incorporate one or more of the cannulae sites.

Post-Operative Care

Following a successful laparoscopic reduction in the intussusception, a nasogastric tube is usually not necessary. Appropriate antibiotics and intravenous fluid are continued for 12–24 h. Opiate analgesia is usually not necessary and the patient can resume oral feeds within several hours. The child can go home after 24–48 h and the parents are informed about the usual post-operative complications including recurrent intussusception.

Results

We have applied laparoscopy to six consecutive patients who had one or two failed air enemas for intussusception. A straightforward laparoscopic reduction was achieved in three and the operation time was 15–35 min. In one child the intussusception was already reduced. These patients required no post-operative opiate analgesia, were fed on the first post-operative day and discharged home on the second day. The remaining two laparoscopies were converted to open procedures because of clear signs of long segment intussusception and compromised bowel. These patients made an eventful recovery following appropriate intestinal resection and anastomosis. There were no laparoscopic complications.

Discussion

In spite of a mild to moderate degree of intestinal dilatation, the view that can be obtained with a 4-to 5-mm laparoscope via a periumbilical cannula is usually satisfactory for the purpose of diagnosis and laparoscopic manipulation of the intussusception. It is absolutely critical that an open technique of laparoscopy and not the closed technique laparoscopy (Veress needle and/or blind insertion of primary port) is used in order to avoid injury to the dilated loop of intestine. With the currently available instruments, the key to a successful reduction in the intussusception is in applying gentle and prolonged pressure by the side of an atraumatic instrument against the neck of the intussusception.

Intestinal resection is necessary if the intussusception is advanced and irreducible, or if after reduction there is gangrenous/necrotic bowel or a pathological lead point such as polyp, Meckel's diverticulum or duplication cyst. Sometimes an appendicectomy is required, and small perforations or seromuscular tears in an otherwise healthy bowel may be sutured. All these procedures may be performed via the laparoscope, however, I prefer a suitably placed open incision. This is largely because of concerns about the lack of adequate operative space due to the dilated bowels and the safety of intracorporeal dissection and anastomosis.

At this early stage of experience, I believe that laparoscopy should be considered as a preliminary procedure only if:
- The child is not seriously ill and has no signs of intestinal perforation or tense abdomen.
- The child has had one or more failed air or hydrostatic enemas.

Or as an alternative procedure to open operation if:
- The intussusception is short and contains no compromised bowel.

References

1. Stringer MD, Pablod SM, Brereton RJ (1992) Paediatric Intussusception. Br J Surg 79:867–876
2. Woo SK et al (1992) Childhood intussusception: ultrasound guided hydrostatic reduction. Radiology 182:77–80
3. Beasley SW, Glover J (1992) Intussusception: prediction of outcome of gas enema. J Paediatr Surg 27:474–475
4. Cuckow PM, Slater RD, Najmaldin AS (1996) Intussusception treated laparoscopically after failed enema reduction. Surg Endosc 10:671–672

CHAPTER 29

Laparoscopic Appendicectomy in Children

J-S. Valla, H. Steyaert

Introduction

Appendicectomy is the most common surgical operation in the world: within the context of paediatric abdominal emergencies, appendicitis takes first place because of its frequency and potential gravity. At the beginning of our century, appendicectomy emerged as the most common and most effective abdominal operation. When antibiotics arrived, results improved dramatically: a mortality of around 0.05‰ has now been reached, and 10% of perioperative complications out of only 1% are serious. Accordingly, conventional appendicectomy is often cited as an example of a benign operation, quickly and simply performed, followed by an uneventful recovery, and leaving only a very small scar.

Since the beginning of the 1990's laparoscopic methods have gained widespread use in general surgery. Laparoscopy, commonly used since 1950 as a purely diagnostic tool, has been progressively transformed by gynaecologists, its greatest users, into both a diagnostic and a therapeutic procedure. Therefore it is not surprising that the first laparoscopic appendectomies were carried out at the beginning of the 1980's by a German gynaecologist from Kiel, Kurt Semm [24] and by a French surgeon and gynaecologist from Lyon, Philippe Mouret [21]. Both have been severely criticised and condemned by the surgical community of their respective countries, because this new technique had not been understood. Indeed when only the size of the scar is compared, laparoscopy seems to have few advantages over the MacBurney incision. This view of things, in conjunction with its reputation as a minor operation probably explains why laparoscopic appendicectomy has not met the same success as laparoscopic cholecystectomy, even though the latter was described some years later. Among paediatric surgeons, laparoscopic appendicectomy still gives rise to critical questions: Does it really represent an advance? Does it present its own morbidity?

From our experience with about 1500 cases operated upon between 1989 and 1996, we are going to try to answer these questions, but first of all, we must stress that the introduction of a new technique must not place the child's safety back into doubt, especially in view of the fact that appendectomies are usually performed under emergency conditions and therefore need suitable organisation, specific equipment, and a well-trained team.

Once this is realised, the resistance to change that we initially experienced gradually weakens, and the detractors begin to be converted.

Indications

Regarding abdominal pain syndrome in children, laparoscopy is evidently of some diagnostic interest [13–15, 22]: it is the best and most reliable way to reach the right diagnosis in doubtful cases. However, this diagnostic advantage must not lead to overuse of laparoscopy. The now widespread prevalence of laparoscopic equipment in the operating theatre must not modify the surgical indication in the face of abdominal pain.

At the beginning of our experience [27], with patients under 3 years of age, complicated cases such as generalised peritonitis, localised peritonitis with abscess, and appendicitis with bowel obstruction were considered as counter-indications. What still persists today as a contraindication? Age is no longer a contraindication for a surgical paediatric team which respects all the rules of anaesthesia and intra-abdominal pressure. The uncommon appendicitis complicated by bowel obstruction with abdominal distension (mesoceliac appendicitis) remains for us the only contraindication to the use of laparoscopic techniques. Generalised peritonitis with abdominal contraction represents a good indication for laparoscopy for both diagnostic and therapeutic interests.

There are more controversies about the management of localised peritonitis: at clinical examination there is a palpable painful mass, mobile or fixed, better underlined by examination under general anaesthesia, and the rest of the abdominal wall is supple. After the echography, the surgeon is usually able to distinguish two different situations: either obvious pictures of a purulent collection exist and, in this case, surgical intervention is recommended, or there are no echographic signs of a well-localised abscess: in this case, the paediatric surgeon can choose between immediate intervention or medical treatment with antibiotics followed by daily clinical and echographic control. The latter, very frequently recommended in English-speaking countries but little used in France, allows appendicectomy to be done some weeks later when the conditions are more favourable. On the other hand, when the clinical and echographic situation get worse in spite of medical therapy, prompt appendicectomy is imperative. Anyway, in the face of a right iliac fossa palpable mass, the surgeon must decide, according to his own experience and his settings, whether it is better to perform a conventional or a laparoscopic procedure. Personally we prefer to begin with laparoscopic technique, even if we must convert to open surgery as soon as the dissection becomes dangerous. Here again there is the advantage that laparoscopy can confirm the diagnosis, indicate the exact position of the appendix, and reduce the parietal incision to a minimum.

Fortunately in most of the cases, appendicitis is not complicated; the child is referred to the surgeon, and even hospitalised, because of a right iliac fossa pain. Several situations are possible: sometimes the clinical diagnosis is obvious, an appendicitis can be ruled out or on the other hand asserted. The preoperative assessments such as blood samples, abdominal X-ray, and echography only provide confirmation. The child either returns to his family or is operated upon within 24 h. Most of the time, doubt persists after clinical examination. In that situation there is a two-fold risk: to let a real appendicitis evolve in case of abstention (3% in our series), or on the other hand to perform an unnecessary appendicectomy (12% in our series). For this reason it is necessary to wait 24 h before giving an answer. Antalgic treatment can be given, but no antibiotics. Within this period of time, some blood and urinary tests could be carried out, as well as a pulmonary X-ray. These exams could help to establish a diagnostic score; but these scores are known to be imperfect. A normal abdominal echography cannot negate the diagnosis of appendicitis. Both repetitive clinical examination and complementary examinations help the surgeon to take a good decision. Ultimately, the clinical examination remains the predominant element in any decision. In our experience, half of the children return home without surgery, and the rest take advantage of laparoscopy if right iliac fossa pain persists or increases and no other causes explain these symptoms.

For that matter, laparoscopy has long been proposed to solve diagnostic problems caused by an acute pain located in the right iliac fossa, above all in women where gynaecological diseases can present the same symptoms as appendicitis [22]. In childhood, the use of laparoscopy can be justified in some difficult situations [6–15]: in a child treated with antibiotics, corticoids, or chemotherapy; in a neurologically impaired child; in an obese child, or simply scared by clinical examination; or in girls at puberty.

Sometimes, in spite of the acute abdominal pain syndrome, laparoscopy shows an normal appendix. Must we remove this normal appendix, which could be left in place because of its subsequent usefulness, particularly in a possible urological reconstruction? The answer to this question is not obvious: if another disease which explains the pain syndrome is found and treated, logically the appendix can be left, except in case of Crohn's disease or salpingitis to avoid ulterior confusion between appendicitis and the recurrence of these diseases. On the other hand, if no other anomaly is found, it seems more judicious to remove the appendix in accordance with the following arguments: endo-appendicitis which reaches only the mucosa is rare but possible, and an appendicectomy does away with all forms of psychological anxiety for both the family and its practitioner. Finally, from an economic point of view, if a real appendicitis later occurs, intervention is necessary; it seems better to solve the problem definitively, since laparoscopic appendicectomy has almost never had complications and probably allows for fewer peritoneal sequelae than a traditional appendicectomy.

Finally there is again the problem of chronic abdominal repetitive pain that can occur in both child and adult. Mouret [21] has described caecal and right colonic intra-abdominal adhesion disease: its cause is not obvious and it could explain this chronic pain syndrome. He has gained good results controlling pain with only adhesiolysis without appendix removal. We have encountered this kind of pathology in children 7 years of age and older. Personally we cannot conclude definitively on the efficiency of isolated adhesiolysis, because we always have performed an appendicectomy at the same time. Nevertheless in case of repetitive chronic abdominal syndrome, we must be reluctant to make use of laparoscopic exploration. It could be used as a last resort when all others diagnoses and therapeutic possibilities have been exhausted and if the pain does not allow the child a normal school life.

Preoperative Preparation

In all cases, the child is prepared with a whole abdominal asepsis: a gauze with povidon iodine is left in the umbilicus until the patient enters into the operating theatre. Before this we ask him to urinate; if he cannot manage his bladder, we have emptied it in the operating theatre using the Credé manoeuvre or sondage. In case of peritonitis with septic shock, preoperative resuscitation in the office (intravenous infusion and intravenous antibiotic) is mandatory several hours before surgical intervention. In case of suspected appendicitis, antibioprophylaxy is performed at the beginning of the general anaesthesia.

Installation

Patient is in supine position, both arms along the body, and the asepsis is applied all around the abdomen. The draping includes the xyphoid, pubis and the two iliacs spines. The surgeon is positioned on the left of the patient, the assistant stays on the same side as the surgeon (on his right or on his left side depending upon the technique used), the monitor is on the right and the cables are fixed on the thorax (Fig. 1). The first cannula goes through the umbilicus following the transumbilical open technique. The technique is as follow: The umbilicus is grasped with a Kocher forceps and lifted up strongly; with an eleven blade scal-

Fig. 1. Position of the patient, crew and equipment

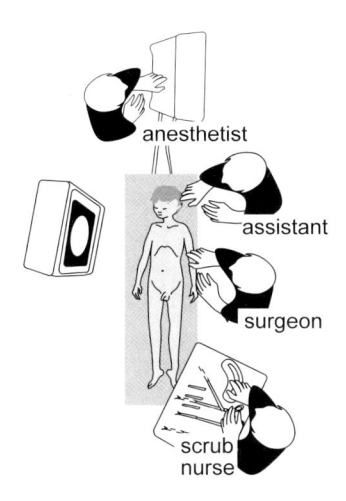

pel, handled horizontally to avoid any intra-abdominal slipping, the umbilical skin is cut longitudinally. The fascia and peritoneum are incised under visual control. The diameter of the hole in the fascia is such that its fits snugly around the cannula for the purpose of air tightness and spontaneous fixation. If the hole is too wide, a purse string suture must be put in place. We use a cannula with a smooth atraumatic trocar, and insufflation is started (8–12 mmHg).

The telescope calibre varies from 5 to 11 mm. Position, number and diameter of the other cannulas are chosen according to the technique used and the appendix pathology. In any case, a cannula is needed for the extraction of the appendix with an internal diameter that is slightly larger than the outer diameter of the telescope.

For the customary three-cannula technique, usually two 5-mm diameter cannulas are necessary, one in the right iliac fossa, and one in the left iliac fossa (Fig. 2). However, others diameters can be chosen: smaller (3 mm or 1.5 mm) or larger (12 mm) if an endoscopic linear stapler must be brought in. These accessory cannulas are put in place under visual control with great care not to injure the iliac vessels, which are very close to the anterior abdominal wall in children. It is more logical to put the left iliac fossa cannula in first and then to choose the position of the right iliac fossa cannula, depending on the localisation of the appendix and the mobility of the caecum.

There is no specific instrumentation for appendicectomy:
- Monopolar hook
- Bipolar coagulation forceps
- Palpator
- Grasping forceps
- Lavage and aspiration cannula

Disposable devices such as endoscopic pretied ligatures and endoscopic staplers are be used only if necessary. The transumbilical "out" technique with only one trocar requires a special telescope with operating channel: personally, we use an 11-mm telescope with 5-mm operating channel. At the beginning of the

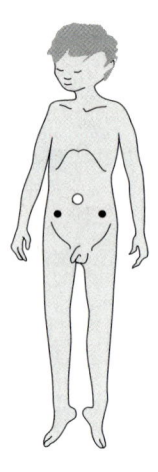

Fig. 2. Position of the trocars in a three-trocar technique

procedure, the operating table is tilted in Trendelenburg position and if required in a left-lateral position necessary in order to isolate the caecal area.

Techniques

There are two steps in appendicectomy: first exploration, then appendicectomy.

The *exploration* allows confirmation of the right diagnosis and choice of technique. It must be well-organised and as complete as possible; we begin with the left internal inguinal ring, bladder, right internal inguinal ring then right iliac fossa, right colon, liver, gall-bladder diaphragm, stomach, spleen, left colon all the way to the beginning point. After the table is put in Trendelenburg position, internal genital organs in girl, cul de sac de Douglas, and ileum are checked. It is possible to take peritoneal liquid samples. In the case of peritonitis a lavage with saline is performed during this exploration before the start of the appendicectomy: this lavage is a time-consuming manoeuvre but must be copious, repeated until the return fluid remains clear.

Often the appendix is immediately visible: the surgeon can assess its pathological condition and also the condition of the caecum and the meso-appendix. Sometimes the appendix is not visible, and the surrounding viscera must be moved away with the help of a palpator or forceps entered into the abdomen through the left iliac cannula. At this time the surgeon is able to choose his operative technique and to put in the accessory cannulas required.

Appendicectomy can then begin: the main steps are the hemostasis of the meso-appendix and the ligature of the appendix base. Depending upon whether these two steps are realised in or out of the abdomen, three different procedures may be described:

- The extra-abdominal or "out" laparoscopic appendicectomy, also called the laparoscopically assisted appendicectomy
- The "mixed" laparoscopic appendicectomy
- The intra-abdominal or "in" laparoscopic appendicectomy

The three techniques are depicted in the Figs. 3–5.
- In the "out" technique (Fig. 3) the appendix is pulled out with the meso-appendix; in order to avoid a too significant traction on the caecum, the pneumoperitoneum must be exsufflated previously or simultaneously, so that extraction can proceed through the umbilicus or a right iliac fossa incision. The transumbilical extraction requires a specific telescope with operating channel, but has the advantage not to require a second incision. The caecal base is held outside of the abdomen with a forceps or a clamp during the time needed to tie, cut and desinfect the appendiceal stump.

This "out" technique is actually our favourite, used in 80% of cases, because it is very simple (only one trocar), quick, safe (no intra-abdominal manipulation and coagulation), cheap and leaves a nearly invisible umbilical scar. The drawbacks of the "out" appendicectomy are the following: it is impossible in

Fig. 3. The "out" technique (laparoscopically assisted appendicectomy) is usually performed with only one trocar. The operating channel telescope is placed through the umbilical port (diameter 11 mm). The appendix is grasped and pulled out with its meso

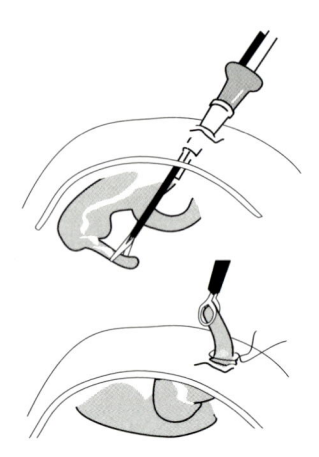

Fig. 4. The "mixed" technique. Three trocars are needed. Hemostasis of the mesentery is performed in the abdomen, while the base of the appendix is ligated outside the abdomen

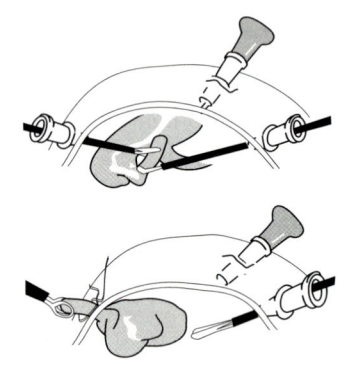

7% of cases because of a retrocaecal position of the appendix, or a very tight caecal adhesion to the posterior wall. This unfavourable anatomical situation requires the placement of one or two additional trocars. The quality of small bowel exploration, the quality of peritoneal lavage is not as good with only one rather than three cannulas: so the single trocar appendicectomy is not a good indication in case of peritonitis. Finally the educational value of the out appendicectomy for surgeons in a learning curve is poor because hemostasis and suture are realised in the same manner as in conventional surgery. Obesity is not a contraindication, because there is no fat in the umbilicus, and thus no risk of leaving an overly long appendiceal stump, but obesity does make the umbilical closure more difficult.
- In the "mixed" technique (Fig. 4), the hemostasis of the meso-appendix is performed in the abdomen while the base of the appendix is ligated outside the abdomen. Three trocars are needed. The forceps introduced in the right iliac fossa (left hand of the surgeon) presents the meso-appendix and puts it under tension; hemostasis is achieved by the device introduced in the left iliac fossa (right hand of the surgeon). We prefer the monopolar hook which al-

lows coagulation and cutting close to the appendix, taking great care not to injure or perforate the appendix; a bipolar forceps or pretied loop can also be used. The monopolar coagulation close to the appendix is a faster and safer technique because the vessels are very small, very easy to coagulate; the diameter of the piece to pull out is reduced at the only appendix without meso: so the extraction through a 5-mm trocar is possible most of the time. The appendix must be grasped exactly at the tip; the jaws of the forceps are positioned along the appendix axis. The pneumoperitoneum is exsufflated in order to facilitate the abdominal wall sinking and the caecal rising. A endo-abdominal visual control is necessary to check that the caecum is in a close touch with the abdominal wall and the appendix completely exteriorised. This checking avoids a appendiceal stump that is too long. The appendix is tied outside of the abdomen as in conventional surgery. The appendicular mucosa is desinfected, coagulated, and the stump goes back into the abdomen, taking great care not to snatch the ligature. Reinsufflation and traction on the caecum makes this return easier.

The mixed technique was the most common at the beginning of our experience because it is educational and cheap. However, it is not advisable in case of obesity (because of the risk of leaving an overly long stump) and in case of fixed or very inflamed caecum (because of the risk of tearing during extraction): this mixed technique exposes one to the accidents of intra-abdominal electrocautery. We now only use it after a failure of the out technique or in case of peritonitis with a good appendicular base.

- The "in" laparoscopic appendicectomy represents the true laparoscopic technique (Fig. 5): all the main steps – liberation, hemostasis, ligature of the stump – are carried out in the abdomen. The ligature can be carried out with a pretied ligature or intracorporeal or extracorporeal tied knot. The stump can be desinfected by direct injection of an antiseptic solution or by application with a small gauze. The mucosa stump coagulation with monopolar hook is not advisable because of the risk of caecal burns and decomposition of the ligature. This "in" technique permits to face all the anatomic and pathological situations. It gives the best training for laparoscopic surgery but it is more complex,

Fig. 5. The "in" technique. Three trocars are needed. All the main steps: liberation, hemostasis, ligature of the stump are realised in the abdomen

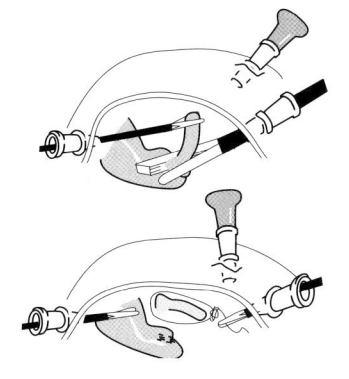

Table 1. Comparative synoptic table of different kinds of laparoscopic appendicectomy

Contraindication	Out transumbilical Peritonitis retrocecal appendicectomy	Mixed Obesity	In None
Efficacy	+	++	+++
Safety	+++	+	+
Speed	+++	++	+
Exploration	+	+++	+++
Aesthetic	+++	+	+
Teaching value	+	++	+++
Cost	+++	++	+

longer and more expensive. In practice we save it for obese children and for peritonitis with caecal inflammation. In such a situation ligature by endoscopic pretied ligature is not reassuring: endoscopic stapler use is indicated and requires a 12-mm cannula, which is useful for the extraction. This 12-mm cannula must be placed in the left iliac fossa, as far as possible from the caecum because endoscopic stapler manipulation in a narrow space is quite difficult; in order to reduce the cicatricial risk, this 12-mm cannula can be placed through the umbilicus and a 5-mm 0° telescope through the left iliac fossa cannula.

All in all, in order to be able to face all situations, the paediatric laparoscopic surgeon must master these three techniques of laparoscopic appendicectomy, the advantages and drawbacks of which are summarised in Table 1. The choice depends upon the anatomic situation, the means at one's disposal and, finally, personal preference.

Some technical points must be clarified:
- First, in case of enormous, preperforative appendix, the manipulation of the appendix is very delicate: appendicular rupture may transform a simple acute appendicitis into a perforated one with peritoneal contamination. The diseased part of the appendix must not be grasped: it is better to grasp, with an atraumatic forceps, the meso-appendix or the appendix base, which usually remains healthy. If the appendix tip is not so diseased, a pretied endoscopic ligature tied at this point can be useful to pull up the appendix, but this technique in not our favourite.
- Burying the stump is possible, as in conventional surgery; a purse string suture can be inserted and tied with two needle-holders. Retrograde appendicectomy is possible with the laparoscopic technique but there is nearly never a need to perform it. Appendicectomy by intracaecal invagination is also possible with the help of a fine device to bury the appendix into the caecum.
- There are three different ways to extract the appendix: the first and the simplest is transparietal extraction without particular protection; the cannula and the appendix are pulled out at the same time. This manoeuvre is possible

with a normal or, occasionally, with an inflamed appendix: in spite of the direct contact between appendix and abdominal wall we have never had parietal infection because the appendix base is cut out of the abdomen, then disinfected, and because the transparietal course is also disinfected after the stump is returned to the abdomen. The second extraction technique consists in putting the appendix into the cannula and extracting it without any parietal contamination. This technique is recommended if the appendix is purulent or after an "in" technique. The third way consists in introducing an extraction bag into the abdomen: endoscopic extraction bag use is advisable in case of perforated appendix with crumbly wall. All the pathological specimens, coprolith, and false membrane are introduced into the bag and pulled out through an enlarged orifice.

- In case of peritonitis the coprolith must be absolutely searched and removed to avoid residual abscess; at the end of the procedure the lavage must be repeated, copious (2–4 l may be sometimes necessary) until the aspirated liquid becomes clear: it is the longest and most tedious part of the operation.
- Localised right iliac abscess or appendicular infiltrate, if operated on, is approached taking great care not to spread pus in the peritoneal cavity and not to injure the bowel. Most of the pus can be aspirated with a large needle directly inserted through the abdominal wall. This puncture is guided by palpation, endoabdominal visual control and if necessary echography. Afterwards, the infiltrate is progressively liberated by gently unsticking adhesions with the help of the aspiration-lavage cannula, which is used as a hydrodissection device, always ready to aspirate each collection as soon it opens. These manoeuvres are made under visual control, unlike in conventional surgery, where these kind of lesions are usually approached in a blind manner with a finger introduced through the right iliac fossa incision. In the face of very inflammatory and bleeding tissues, we do not have to look for hemostasis by electrocoagulation, but to wash and to wait: the situation becomes progressively clear; often the appendix base is healthy and serves as a lead wire to complete the job. If the omentum is too stuck to the appendix it can be removed en bloc; all the pathological tissues are placed into an endoscopic extraction bag and extracted after morcellation.

Whatever the employed technique, whatever the appendix state, a *final check-up* is mandatory. If an out technique has been used this last look needs to reintroduce an umbilical trocar and telescope in order to inspect the stump, mesoappendix, and residual effusions, keeping in mind that table positioning may change declive areas significantly; at the end of the operation putting the table in mild proclive allows an effective final aspiration to be performed in the cul de sac of Douglas.

Each surgeon must determine individually whether to put in a *drain*. Our feeling is that the drainage is necessary in cases of abscess, advanced peritonitis and retroperitoneal space opening. Some anaesthesiologists recommend to leave a xylocaine solution under the diaphragm. Trocars are pulled out under visual control. Exsufflation must be complete. Trocar orifices are cleaned with antiseptic solution. Umbilical fascia is carefully closed with absorbable sutures (a strong thread and a short hemi-circle needle are useful); a dressing with povidon iodine is put on the umbilicus; lateral orifices are closed with sterile skin tapes if small (5 mm) or with absorbable sutures if large (10 or 12 mm) to avoid evisceration. A local anaesthesia around trocar orifices is recommended.

Before sending it to the laboratory, the specimen must be examined from the outside and from the inside to be informed about possible parasite infestation or carcinoid tumour which is managed as usual. We have encountered one case of carcinoid tumour, 1 cm in diameter, located in the middle of the appendix and revealed after appendicectomy. The prognostic factors of appendicular carcinoids are first the size and secondarily the degree of tumourous infiltration of the appendiceal wall and meso-appendix, the position of the tumour along the appendix, and the histological type; in our case, appendicectomy was performed according to the mixed technique, so the meso was coagulated close to the appendiceal wall and it was not possible to know the state of the meso-appendix. A second laparoscopic look was indicated to resect the meso-appendix, which was ultimately not diseased. All in all, carcinoid tumour and laparoscopic appendicectomy are not incompatible: if the tumour is identified during laparoscopy, its removal obeys the usual rule, which is to say, removal of appendix and meso together and in case of a tumour located at the base of the appendix, removal of the lower part of the caecum with endoscopic stapler. If the tumour is identified only on the specimen, the discussion concerns the removal or not of the meso-appendix.

Postoperative Care

Postoperative care depends on whether the appendicitis was complicated. In case of non-complicated appendicitis, the follow-up is only clinical. Analgesic treatment is necessary only during the first 6 h to fight against scapular and umbilical pains. The child is allowed to stand up to drink, but few children wish to go home the same day. They leave 1 or 2 days later; then the practitioner plays a leading part in the follow-up. After a last clinical control between the 6th and 9th postoperative days, the child is allowed to return to all activities.

In case of complicated appendicitis, intravenous antibiotics are continued at least for 3 days and succeeded by oral antibiotics until apyrexia and inflammatory test normalisation; on average the hospital stay is 6.5 days. A clinical and echographic control is programmed between 6 and 10 days after leaving hospital.

Results

We report here two different series.

Lenval Children's Hospital, Nice, 1990–1996

First, we report the results from our own retrospective series of 1500 children operated on over a 6-year period (1990–1996) at the Lenval Children's Hospital in Nice. The results are summarised in Table 2. The distribution according to age is as follows: 0.9% under 3 years old, 2.5% between 3 and 8 years old, 74% between 8 and 18 years old. The distribution according to the pathological state is as follows: 70% acute or gangrenous appendicitis, 16% perforated appendicitis, and 14% macroscopic normal appendix, but in most of these cases histological study showed mucosal and submucosal lesions.

Results vary according to the pathological state: In case of nonperforated appendicitis or normal appendix, conversion rate is 0.08%, mean operative duration is 23 min, mean hospital stay 1.8 days. There is never drainage. Total complications rate is 0.71% and only 0.63% of these complicated cases needed to be reoperated under general anaesthesia.

Table 2. Results of laparoscopic appendicectomy (J.S. Valla, H. Steyaert, A. Grinda, Nice, France)

	Noncomplicated appendicitis ($n=1260$, 84%)	Complicated appendicitis ($n=240$, 16%)	Total ($n=1500$)
Conversion rate	1 (0.08%)	8 (3.3%)	9 (0.6%)
Operation duration (min)	23	55	29
Hospital stay (day)	1.8	6	2.5
Drain	0	72 (30%)	4.8%
Parietal complications			
Abscess	1 (0.08%)	6 (2.5%)	7 (0.46%)
Evisceration	2 (0.16%)	1 (0.4%)	3 (0.13%)
Intra-abdominal complications			
Abscess	2 (0.16%)	14 (6%)	16 (1%)
5th day	1 (0.08%)	0	1 (0.06%)
Bowel obstruction			
Early	1 (0.08%)	3 (1.25%)	4 (0.26%)
Late	1 (0.08%)	5 (2%)	6 (0.4%)
Others	1 (0.08%)	3 (1.25%)	4 (0.26%)
Total complications	9 (0.71%)	32 (13.3%)	41 (2.7%)
Reoperations	8 (0.63%)	14 (6%)	22 (1.4%)

In case of perforated appendicitis, conversion rate rises to 3.3%, mean operative duration 55 min, mean hospital stay 6.5 days, postoperative drainage in 30% of cases, total complications rate 13.3%; 6% of children undergo a second operation by laparoscopy or conventional surgery.

French Group of Paediatric Celiosurgery, 1995–1996

Secondly, a multicentric prospective comparative study was conducted by the French Group of Paediatric Celiosurgery (GECI) for 2 years (1995–1996) on perforated appendicitis in children, open versus laparoscopic surgery. A perforated appendix was defined by operative evidence of a hole in the appendix, the presence of free pus or an abscess cavity noted during surgery, or the growth of enteric organisms from peritoneal cultures. Cases of suppurative or gangrenous appendix that did not meet these criteria and also cases where appendix perforation occurred during the intraoperative manipulation of the appendix were not included in this analysis, even though many such cases were treated by the same protocol.

The results are summarised in Table 3. Of 154 cases, 70 were managed by classical surgery and 84 by laparoscopy, 14 of the latter were converted into open surgery (conversion rate: 16.6%). Conversion was indicated because of advanced localised peritonitis in ten cases and advanced generalised peritonitis in four (no conversion in case of recent peritonitis). The results of these 14 cases were as follows: mean hospital stay 7.7 days and no complications, so these 14 cases were excluded from the statistics, but without risk of miscalculation, since there were no postoperative complications.

Table 3. Results of prospective comparative study: management of appendicular peritonitis in children open versus laparoscopic surgery (GECI 1995–1996)

	Open (n=70)	Laparoscopy (n=70)
Drain	66%	38%*
Hospital stay (days)	9.1	6.5*
Infectious complications		
Wound	4%	3%
Intraperitoneal	4%	10%*
Bowel obstruction	1.7%	0%

154 cases: 70 open surgery, 84 laparoscopic surgery; 14 conversions (conversion rate 16.6%), 0 complications.
*p=0.04.

The two groups: 70 cases operated by laparoscopy and 70 cases by classical surgery were similar concerning median age (9 years) sex ratio (40% boys, 60% girls) pathological lesions (recent peritonitis 50% versus 34%, advanced localised peritonitis 21% versus 32%, advanced generalised peritonitis 29% versus 34%), postoperative antibiotic treatment (combination of two or three antibiotics, given IV for 5 days, and continued per os until the patient was afebrile with normal CRP levels.) The comparison between the two groups was evaluated using the Chi-square test and Student's test. The drainage rate was 66% for open surgery and 38% for laparoscopic surgery ($p=0.04$).

Results are as follows: there are no significant differences between the two groups concerning the rate of total postoperative complications, postoperative bowel obstruction, wound infection rate, reoperation rate under general anaesthesia rate. There are four significant differences. Postoperative intestinal ileus duration (2.2 versus 3.2 days), delay of return to oral diet (2.8 versus 3.9 days) and hospital stay (7.3 versus 9.4 days) are significantly shorter in the laparoscopic group.

The number of postoperative intra-abdominal residual abscesses is higher after laparoscopy (10% versus 4%; $p=0.04$).

Discussion

The discussion should establish a balance between the advantages and drawbacks of laparoscopic and conventional appendicectomy.

1 Advantages of laparoscopy
At first, advantages are of a diagnosis nature.
Because of its global vision, incomparably better than the vision though a short MacBurney incision, laparoscopy provides, a quick and complete solution in the face of abdominal pain in children: in others words, it provides at the same time positive diagnosis, differential diagnosis and topographic diagnosis. Nothing is more frustrating than to have to enlarge a MacBurney incision in order to find an ectopic appendix (22% of appendiceal ectopia in our series). After finding a normal appendix, nothing is more frustrating than having to enlarge a MacBurney incision in order to perform an abdominal exploration, which is in any event restricted to the ileocecal area and the right adnexa. The whole abdominal exploration, which is the initial part of all laparoscopy, allows bringing to the fore an associated lesion which could be left undiagnosed by preoperative echography: mesenteric adenolymphitis (128 cases), rupture of ovarian follicule (18 cases), torsion of embryonic residual appendix of the fallopian tube (20 cases) salpingitis (3 cases), infectious ileitis (10 cases), Crohn's disease (2 cases), Meckel diverticulum (12 cases).

Some associated lesions could be missed by a MacBurney incision: omentum torsion or necrosis (3 cases), torsion of epiploic sigmoid appendix (2 cases) abnormal anterior pericecal adhesions (87 case) patent peritoneo vaginal ductus

(30 cases), disease of the submesocolic area such as cholecystis (1 case). In three cases of peritonitis, operated on with the diagnosis of appendicular peritonitis, laparoscopy allowed to correct the diagnosis. These three cases were primary pneumococcal peritonitis; laparoscopy allowed a normal appendix to be shown, a pus sample to be taken, and the whole peritoneal cavity to be cleaned at the price of very small scars. All in all, the advantage of laparoscopy versus a small right iliac fossa incision seems obvious in the field of diagnosis. If a disease other than appendicitis is brought to view, it could be managed by laparoscopy with the same trocars.

Postoperative Results
The postoperative results analysis allowed one to distinguish between the improvement of recovery and the reduction in complications rate. The assessment criteria for recovery are as follows: postoperative pain and required analgesic doses, oral feeding delay, getting-up delay, hospital stay duration, and convalescence duration until return to unrestricted activities. The study of postoperative complications needs to record all possible complications, both parietal or intra-abdominal complications and early or late complications.

Nonperforated Appendicitis
Regarding nonperforated appendicitis, a better recovery after laparoscopic appendicectomy is not yet proved definitively. Between two groups of children operated by laparoscopic and conventional techniques, the prospective data of Lejus et al. [16] do not show any significant differences concerning postoperative analgesia, oral feeding delay, and getting-up delay. In the laparoscopic group 35% versus only 10% in the conventional group complain about shoulder pain, which are pneumoperitoneum-specific pains. However, this data concerns recovery after a three-trocar appendicectomy during 72 h. It proves that pains generated by pneumoperitoneum and three orifices of trocars are equivalent to pain generated by a MacBurney incision, and we agree with that. However, transumbilical monotrocar appendicectomy may be less painful than three-trocar appendicectomy, and after this delay of 72 h, the parietal pain produced by MacBurney incision may last longer than pain produced by one or more trocars. The inspection of the child's walk during the clinical control 5 or 7 days after the operation is quite instructive about that. It is logical to think that laparoscopy generates, in the early postoperative course, a pain of peritoneal origin but decreases postoperative pain due to wound cicatrisation, which is a pain prolonged for 8–10 days.

From an economical point of view, the argument of a rapid return to work is worthless in children but a cessation of school activity often has great repercussions on a child's life. Moreover, when both parents work, one must stop working to keep the children at home during recovery. Finally, the ability to resume sport activities quickly is an important argument for an athletic teenager.

The difference in mean hospital stay after noncomplicated appendicitis is debatable: in our series the mean hospital stay is 1.8 days; however, after a MacBurney incision, a child is sometimes able to return home the next day. In the comparative study of Gilchrist [7], patients operated by laparoscopy spent significantly fewer days in the hospital and returned to unrestricted activities faster than patients operated by classical surgery. The Varlet's comparative retrospective study [28] brings favourable results for laparoscopic appendicectomy: hospital stay goes from 6 days after conventional surgery to 4 days after laparoscopic surgery. Moreover, the additional hospital stay due to postoperative complications goes from 25 days after laparoscopic surgery to 182 days after conventional surgery.

The decreasing rate of postoperative abdominal wall complications such as abscesses is certainly underscored by all published data on adults [1, 8, 12, 23, 26] or children and adults [4, 17, 19, 20]. Our parietal abscess rate after noncomplicated appendicitis is as low as 0.08%. This very good result can be explained by the lack of contact between appendix and abdominal wall and by the reduced parietal trauma: small incision, no dissection of various layers, no ischaemia due to retractors, and no or little suture material left in place. The frequency of other parietal complications such as hematoma, evisceration, or eventration is probably decreased by the use of laparoscopy but no data have studied this particular point. In our series two eviscerations of omentum through the umbilicus occurred because of stitch rupture.

It is curious that few studies have precisely recorded the occurrence of other complications much more severe than parietal complications, particularly intra-abdominal residual abscesses. In Varlet's data [28], the total complications rate is significantly lower after laparoscopic surgery, including intra-abdominal abscesses. Two cases of intra-abdominal abscess and one case of fifth-day syndrome occurred in our series after nonperforated appendicitis.

Postoperative small bowel obstruction is another classical complication after an ordinary appendicectomy. Appendicectomy is the big supplier of bowel adhesive obstruction in children; 80% of these obstructions occur during the year following operation: a follow-up of 2–3 years could be enough to make up an opinion on that, but we find a lack of prospective studies. Out of 1260 cases of noncomplicated appendicitis we have recorded only one case of bowel obstruction. We side with surgeons who are convinced by the advantages of laparoscopic versus laparotomy regarding the risk of postoperative peritoneal adhesions [2] with its bowel (obstruction) or fallopian tube (sterility) consequences; but no definitive argument has yet been published. Interestingly postconventional appendicectomy small bowel obstruction is one of the best indications for laparoscopic management.

The aesthetic benefit provided by laparoscopic management of nonperforated appendicitis is difficult to quantify. This is often the first argument of laparoscopic users. We consider it the least important of the advantages provided by laparoscopy, except in girls and in cases where an enlargement is necessary (ectopic appendix, obese child).

Perforated Appendicitis
Several points can be discussed concerning the results achieved after management of perforated appendicitis in the GECI prospective comparative study.

Postoperative pain and aesthetic results were not specifically studied; however it is clear that all the children operated on by classical surgery have had a large incision; moreover 20% have had a median laparotomy; so, although the postoperative wound infection rate in the two groups is similar, the reduction in the abdominal wall trauma provided by laparoscopy in case of perforated appendicitis seems obvious, and the aesthetic gain is not negligible, especially in girls (60% of cases).

Results concerning the rate of postoperative bowel obstruction and reoperation under general anaesthesia are similar in the two groups. In the same manner, the risk of septic diffusion because of CO_2 intra-abdominal pressure, a risk that has been demonstrated experimentally [3], is not encountered in clinical data, particularly in the two groups of the GECI data (1 pneumopathy + 1 transient bacteremia in the 70 cases of the laparoscopic group, 1 septic pleural effusion in the 70 cases of the open group).

Three statistically significant results plea in favour of laparoscopic management: postoperative intestinal ileus, delay in resumption of oral diet, and hospital stay are shorter in the laparoscopic group; this last point must be considered to contain cost. These advantages are confirmed by the data of Frazee and Bohannon [5].

On the other hand, the intra-abdominal abscess rate is higher after laparoscopy (10% versus 4%; $p=0.04$). Tang [25] in a study of adults obtained similar results. This disappointing difference seems paradoxical because laparoscopy is renowned for providing a better and more extensive peritoneal lavage than a right flank incision. Tang [25] suggests that laparoscopic appendicectomy in advanced peritonitis may be associated with a significant learning curve: as a matter of fact the residual intra-abdominal abscess rate is lower in our own data (6%; see Fig. 5) than in the multicentric GECI data (10%; see Table 3). In the retrospective Horwitz' data [10], where the residual abscess rate was 41% after laparoscopy, all operations were performed by surgical residents, conversion rate was as high as 26%, and the converted cases – probably the most advanced peritonitis – were posted with the laparoscopic group and not separately studied. For this reason we do not think, in contrast to Horwitz [10], that laparoscopic appendicectomy should be avoided for complicated appendicitis in children. Another explication for this residual abscess rate probably lies in the lack of drainage: during the GECI's study, the quality of laparoscopic peritoneal lavage misled many surgeons into making less use of intraperitoneal drain after laparoscopic operation than after a classical operation (38% versus 66%; $p=0.04$). In Tang's data [25], where 11% of residual abscesses were found after laparoscopy, no drain was used; on the other hand, in Lund's data [18], all children operated on by classical surgery were drained, and the residual abscess rate was 2.9%. So, only a new prospective study comparing the same peritonitis and the same drainage rate could answer this particular question.

These intraperitoneal residual abscesses may be cured by medical management – three cases (antibiotics and anti-inflammatory treatment) – or may need a reoperation (five cases): percutaneous drainage, transrectal drainage, conventional or laparoscopic drainage. Reoperations for abscesses by laparoscopy are feasible by a well-trained surgeon.

2 Disadvantages of laparoscopy

The drawbacks of the laparoscopic technique as opposed to the classical technique are the following. Laparoscopy is a new technique with a completely different set of procedures: it needs a long and specific training. If this learning curve is not respected, accidents can occur such as visceral or vascular injuries [11], which are intolerable in case of benign pathology such as appendicitis.

The need of a pneumoperitoneum could be considered as a drawback because of hemodynamic modifications and postoperative shoulder pains.

Laparoscopic surgery needs expensive, delicate, equipment which requires maintenance demanding great care. A very serious disinfection is mandatory after appendicectomy, which is a septic operation often repeated on the same day.

The operating time is a false problem: the appendix is the best-suited intra-abdominal organ for laparoscopic removal: the operating time varies according to surgeon's training and temperament; some are fast, some are slow. In our experience, the median time for appendicectomy by senior and resident is 23 min if not complicated and 55 min if perforated.

Howewer if the duration of appendicectomy is the same in conventional surgery as in laparoscopic surgery, on the other hand, the duration of cleaning and disinfection of the devices is longer with laparoscopy; which may be a problem when several appendectomies are to be performed successively. The best solution, but the most expensive, is to possess several sets of devices.

The economic evaluation of laparoscopic appendicectomy is quite difficult because there are numerous factors to consider: cost of equipment, depreciation, maintenance, operation duration, cost of disposable material and, in counterbalance, reduction in hospital stay, complications, and recovery.

The cost of disposable material is a real problem for an operation so frequent as appendicectomy: for that reason, the use of disposable devices must be reduced as much as possible. The only exception is when a difficult pathological situation does not allow the use of a more economical technique: in our series of 1500 appendectomies, we have used 180 endoscopic pretied ligatures and 12 endoscopic staplers.

Conclusion

Laparoscopy and conventional surgery are and must remain complementary methods in matters of appendicectomy. To begin with, laparoscopy allows mastering the safety rules of laparoscopy in children, to give the surgeon the chance to gain experience progressively, beginning with the easiest cases, to see and to understand the pathology, and finally to choose the technique according to the intra-abdominal lesions and his own experience and environment.

Thus laparoscopic technique will emerge naturally because of its advantages whatever the pathological status of appendix. Nonperforated appendicitis poses above all a diagnostic problem: in case of wrong diagnosis, laparoscopy gives the possibility of a complete exploration of the abdominal cavity. This advantage could soon pass a major turning point if, under local anaesthesia, in an ambulatory situation, the introduction of a micro-telescope into the abdomen will allow a direct visual exploration of the appendix in a child presenting a right iliac fossa pain. Then the paediatric surgeon may have to conduct a noninvasive examination to solve the daily problem of the right iliac fossa pain syndrome in children.

Perforated appendicitis poses above all a therapeutic problem, always managed in classical surgery with a wide incision: laparoscopy gives here the advantages of mini-invasive surgery with moderate improvement of results. This improvement can only be moderate because conventional appendicectomy had reached a high degree of perfection. And whatever the subject, the final degrees of perfection are the most difficult to attain. The question of residual intraperitoneal abscess after laparoscopic treatment of perforated appendicitis still needs careful prospective evaluation.

Laparoscopy is only one step in the progress in the management of appendicitis. If tomorrow a new technique – safer and less invasive – emerges, patients and surgeons will switch to it. If we look at the example of cholelithiasis management, it does not appear totally utopian to imagine in a near future a coloscope sufficiently thin and powerful to penetrate into the appendix, show lesions, remove obstructive factors and even perform an endoluminal appendicectomy.

For the moment, following the example of conventional surgery, appendicectomy must be considered as a basic procedure in the training of a paediatric surgeon and his team; the restricting aspect, detected at the beginning of practice, will move slowly into the background to leave place for the elegance and efficacy of the videosurgical technique.

References

1. Attwood SEA et al (1992) A prospective randomised trial of laparoscopic versus open appendicectomy. Surgery 112:497–501
2. De Wilde RL (1991) Goodbye to late bowel obstruction after appendicectomy. Lancet 338:1012
3. Evasovich MR, Clark TC, Horattas MC (1996) Does pneumoperitoneum during laparoscopy increase bacterial translocation? Surg Endosc 10:1176–1179
4. Frazee RC et al (1994) A prospective randomised trial comparing open versus laparoscopic appendicectomy. Ann Surg 219:725–731 (and Br J Surg 1993, 80:1192)
5. Frazee RC, Bohannon WT (1996) Laparoscopic appendicectomy for complicated appendicitis. Arch Surg 131:509–512
6. Gans SL, Berci C (1973) Peritoneoscopy in infants and children. J Pediatr Surg 8:399–405
7. Gilchrist BF et al (1992) Is there a role for laparoscopic appendicectomy in pediatric surgery. J Pediatr Surg 27:209–214
8. Hansen JB et al (1996) Laparoscopic versus open appendicectomy: prospective randomized trial. World J Surg 20:17–21
9. Hedebrand D et al (1994) Laparoscopic or conventional appendicectomy? A prospective randomised trial. Chirurg 65:112–120
10. Horwitz JR et al (1197) Should laparoscopic appendicectomy be avoided for complicated appendicitis in children? J Pediatr Surg 32:1601–1603

11. Juricic M et al (1994) Laparoscopic appendicectomy: case reports of vascular injury in two children. Eur J Pediatr Surg –4:327–28
12. Kum CK et al (1993) Randomized controlled trial comparing laparoscopic appendicectomy to open appendicectomy. Br J Surg 80:1599–1600
13. Kum CK et al (1993) Diagnostic laparoscopy – reducing the number of normal appendicectomy. Dis Colon Rectum 36:763–766
14. Leape LL, Ramenoski ML (1980) Laparoscopy for questionable appendicitis. Can it reduce the negative appendicectomy rate? Ann Surg 191:410–13
15. Leape L, Ramenosky ML (1977) Laparoscopy in infants and children. J Pediatr Surg 12:75–81
16. Lejus C et al (1996) Randomized, simple-blinded trial of laparoscopic versus open appendicectomy in children. Anesthesiology 84(4):801–806
17. Lujan JA et al (1995) Acute appendicitis. Assessment of laparoscopic appendicectomy versus open appendicectomy. A prospective trial. Br J Surg 81:133–135
18. Lund DP, Murphy EU (1994) Management of perforated appendicitis in children: a decade of aggressive treatment. J Pediatr Surg 29:1130–1134
19. McAnena OJ et al (1991) Laparoscopic versus open appendicectomy. Lancet 338:693 (and Br J Surg 1992, 79:818)
20. Montupet PH et al (1993/1994) Appendicites aigües et péritonites appendiculaires chez l'enfant, le traitement coelioscopique. Chirurgie 119:433–435
21. Mouret PH, François Y (1993/1994) Plaidoyer pour l'appendicectomie coelioscopique dans l'appendicite aigüe. Chirurgie 119:436–40
22. Olsen JB, Myren CJ, Haahr PE (1993) Randomized study of the value of laparoscopy before appendicectomy. Br J Surg 80:922–923
23. Schroder DM et al (1993) Laparoscopic appendicectomy for acute appendicitis: is there a real benefit? Ann Surg 59:541–548
24. Semm K (1983) Endoscopic appendicectomy. Endoscopy 15:59–64
25. Tang E et al (1996) Intraabdominal abcesses following laparoscopic and open appendectomies. Surg Endosc 10:327–328
26. Tate JJT et al (1993) Laparoscopic versus open appendicectomy: prospective randomised trial. Lancet 342:633–637
27. Valla JS et al (1991) Laparoscopic appendicectomy in children: report of 465 cases. Surg Laparosc Endosc 1:166–72
28. Varlet F et al (1994) Laparoscopie versus open appendicectomy in children. Comparative study of 403 cases. Eur J Pediatr Surg 4:333–337

Laparoscopic Total Colectomy

D.A. Beals, K.E. Georgeson

Introduction

Total colectomy in the pediatric patient is performed for a variety of reasons. The most common pathological entities requiring total colectomy in children are ulcerative colitis, familial polyposis and total colon Hirschsprung's disease.

Total colectomy is frequently combined with a mucous proctectomy and completed by an ileoanal anastomosis, usually after fashioning an ileal reservoir. This reservoir is often protected with a loop ileostomy for several weeks. It is important to emphasize that no compromise in surgical technique is acceptable when utilizing a laparoscopic approach for total colectomy. The surgeon's preferred techniques for open operations should be utilized laparoscopically. The laparoscopic approach for total colectomy adds the potential for decreased postoperative stress and pain, more rapid return of bowel function and better cosmetic appearance.

Laparoscopic Techniques

Laparoscopic total colectomy requires an advanced level of endoscopic surgical skill and should not be attempted until the surgeon is familiar with partial colonic resection, such as laparoscopic endorectal pull-through procedures. Familiarity with the traditional techniques of ileoanal anastomosis and reservoir formation are also helpful. We always inform our patients as to the possible necessity of conversion to an open procedure at any time during the course of the procedure.

As the colon occupies a position in all four quadrants of the abdomen and the pelvis, it is important that proper visualization of the entire abdomen be obtained for this procedure. This visual access is accomplished by two primary techniques: (a) proper trocar placement and (b) proper patient positioning. We prefer to place a trocar at the umbilicus and in each of the four abdominal quadrants (Fig. 1). The umbilical port can be placed with either a closed or open technique depending on the surgeon's preference. This port should be 12 mm in size to accommodate an angled 10-mm telescope and a stapling device. The trocars in each quadrant can be of variable size. In older patients we prefer at least one

30 Laparoscopic Total Colectomy

Fig. 1. Port placement for total colectomy. Port sizes vary from 3.5 to 12 mm depending on the age and size of the patient

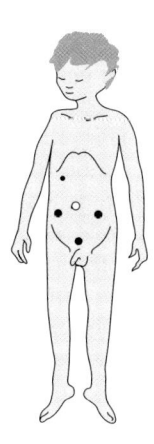

other 12-mm port to accommodate the angled telescope, ultrasonic scalpel and intestinal stapling device. In younger patients and infants 3–5 mm ports are usually adequate as dissection can be readily carried out with a bipolar electrocautery and large vessels controlled with a 5-mm-clip applier. It is advantageous to change the camera and dissecting angle relative to the portion of the colon being dissected. The patient should be secured to the operating table to prevent sliding or rolling during major changes in position. Stirrups are used in children over 3 years of age.

Rectal Dissection

The rectal dissection is initiated in a similar manner to laparoscopic endorectal pull-through for Hirschsprung's disease [1] (see Georgeson, "Endoscopic Endorectal Pull-Through", this volume). The rectosigmoid colon is grasped and held anteriorly.

A window is opened in the rectosigmoid mesentery. In the benign diseases encountered in children, direct mesenteric dissection should be performed as near the rectum as possible to facilitate identification of major blood vessels and avoid injury to other structures in the pelvis. Dissection is carried down toward the pelvis staying just outside the longitudinal muscle of the rectum. The superior and middle rectal arteries can be serially divided with the electrocautery, ultrasonic scalpel or between endosurgical clips. This dissection is usually carried downwards to the level of the prostate in males or the level of the cervix in females. This corresponds to a level approximately 4–8 cm above the dentate line.

Descending Colon and Splenic Flexure

After rectal dissection, the descending colon can be mobilized from the lateral abdominal wall by incising the colonic fusion fascia up to the level of the splenic flexure. When properly performed, this plane is virtually bloodless. Dissection can be facilitated by switching the camera port to the left lower quadrant and operating via the left upper quadrant and umbilical ports. After freeing the descending colon to the splenic flexure the mesentery can be transected utilizing the ultrasonic scalpel or bipolar electrocautery (Fig. 2). Major vessels can be identified and controlled with endosurgical clips, endoscopic suture loops or the vascular endoscopic stapler. The vascular endoscopic stapler should be used sparingly due to the high cost of each staple clip. Once the descending colon has been freed of its mesenteric attachment, the transverse colon can be freed from the overlying omentum. We prefer to leave the omentum attached to the stomach, separating the omentum from the transverse colon with electrocautery or the ultrasonic scalpel. A window is made in the transverse mesocolon and utilizing traction on both the transverse and descending colon, the splenic flexure mesentery is transected.(Figs. 3, 4)

Fig. 2. Dissection should be kept close to the colon for benign diseases. The fusion fascia is incised with sharp and blunt dissection

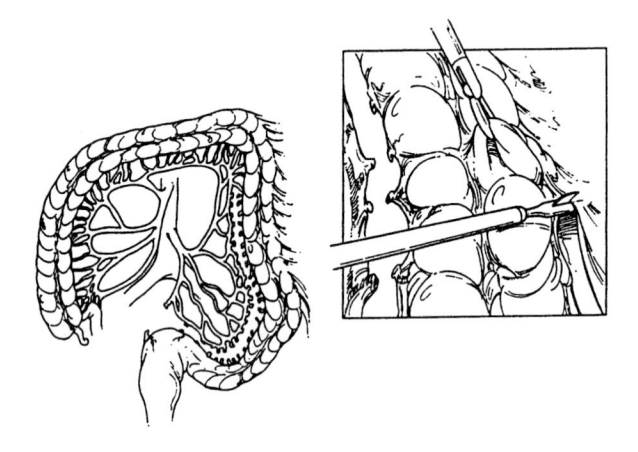

Fig. 3. The splenic flexure should be released from all contiguous attachments. The mesenteric dissection is simplified by stretching the colon between graspers and dividing the vessels with the ultrasonic scalpel or bipolar cautery

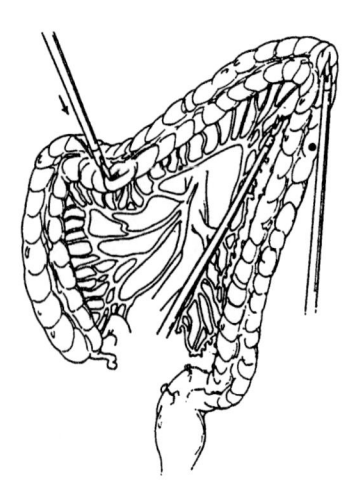

Fig. 4. The mesenteric dissection of the splenic flexure is completed by stretching the transverse mesocolon between graspers and dividing the mesenteric vessels with bipolar cautery or the ultrasonic scalpel

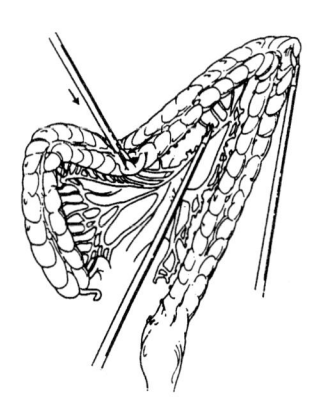

Transverse Colon and Hepatic Flexure

After the distal half of the colon has been completed, dissection is continued along the transverse colon, freeing the omentum from the colon and carefully transecting the mesentery. The middle colic artery should be identified and controlled with endoscopic clips or sutures.

The duodenum is usually in close association with the right transverse colon. The duodenum should be bluntly swept from the colon and mesocolon. In much the same manner as the dissection on the splenic flexure is performed, we prefer to lift an area of the ascending colon from it retroperitoneal position and elevate both the ascending and transverse colon to gain better visualization of the hepatic flexure mesentery. This technique prevents injury to the other right upper quadrant structures and facilitates a rapid mesenteric dissection.

Cecum and Ascending Colon

Dissection of the cecum and ascending colon should be performed carefully to avoid damage to the vascular pedicle of the terminal ileum. The fusion fascia is incised and the ascending colon and its mesentery is carefully dissected. Careful dissection near the colon wall preserves the ileocolic branches providing blood supply to the terminal ileum.

Ileoanal Anastomosis

Minilaparotomy

The surgeon may wish, at this point, to create a small Pfannenstiel incision to facilitate J-pouch formation of the ileum [2]. The stapled anastomosis can be performed in the usual manner for open surgery. This technique is most helpful in children in whom the mesenteric ileal pedicle requires careful dissection to obtain an adequate length for the ileal pouch to reach the anus for anastomosis.

Laparoscopic J-Pouch Formation and Mucosal Dissection with Ileoanal Anastomosis

This technique requires division of the terminal ileum with an endostapling device. The terminal ileum is folded upon itself to make a pouch 10 cm in length and sutures with several alignment sutures. A large traction suture is placed at the apex of the fold and can be left in the abdomen or sutured to the cecum to facilitate passage of the ileum into the pelvis (.Fig. 5).

Anal Mucosal Dissection

The anal mucosal dissection is performed as described elsewhere in this volume (see Georgeson, "Laparoscopic Endorectal Pull-Through"). The entire colon is removed transanally. The ileal pouch is brought down to the anal opening. A small enterotomy is made at the apex of the pouch which is then approximated to the anorectal mucosa with 3.0 absorbable suture in an interrupted fashion. A 10-cm GIA stapler is applied to the J-pouch spur and fired to obliterate the wall between the two limbs of the pouch (Fig. 5). The redundant portion of the J-pouch limb is removed using an angulated endoscopic GIA stapler. A protective loop ileostomy may be performed through an enlarged right lower quadrant trocar site pulling the bowel up to the skin with an endosurgical clamp

Mucosal Dissection and Ileoanal Anastomosis Without Reservoir

If no ileal reservoir is desired, the terminal ileum need not be divided from the colon. In this case, perineal transanal mucosal dissection can be performed in-

Fig. 5. A 10-cm linear stapler is applied transanally to obliterate the septum. The redundant terminal ileum is trimmed with an endoscopic linear stapler

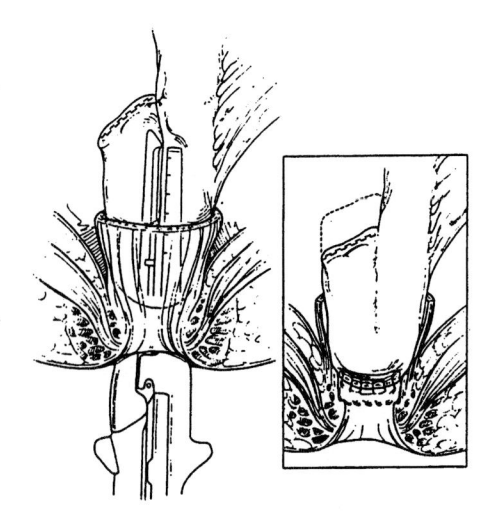

Fig. 6. The J-pouch is formed by laparoscopic placement of tacking sutures in the terminal ileum. Several traction sutures are placed laparoscopically to facilitate pulling the J-pouch to the anus. An incision is made at the apex of the J-pouch and an anastomosis is completed with absorbable sutures

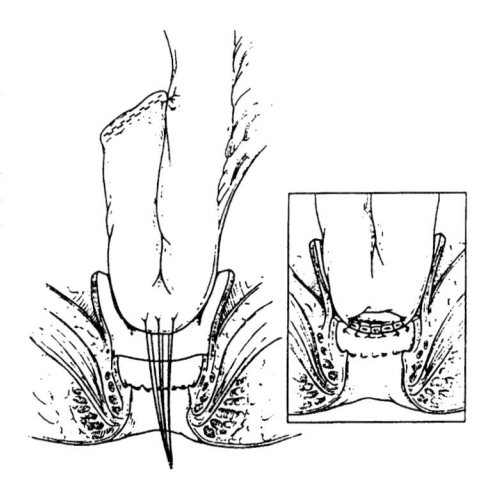

verting the bowel and removing the entire colon transanally. The contiguous ileum is then transected and sutured to the anorectal mucosa with interrupted absorbable sutures as described above. This procedure is primarily useful in patients with total colonic aganglionosis. However, Duhamel's technique is our preferred technique for total colon aganglionosis. The colectomy is performed and the colon is pulled through the anus. The rectal pouch is formed using the terminal ileum for the posterior barrel and is performed in a fashion similar to the technique described by Bax and van der Zee ("Laparoscopic Removal of the Aganglionic Bowel According to Duhamel-Martin," this volume). Protective ileiostomy is performed at the operating surgeon's discretion.

Postoperative Care

Due to the extensive pelvic dissection involved with this procedure, postoperative care often requires bladder decompression. An NG tube is left in place and can usually be removed on the first or second postoperative day. Once bowel function has returned, dietary supplements of fiber increase the consistency of the stool. We also use loperamide to reduce the frequency of bowel movements. Care should be taken to avoid anorectal manipulation for the first 2–3 weeks. Older patients can return to their usual activities within 1–2 weeks after operation.

Personal Experience

Eight patients have had total colectomy performed by the authors. All patients are continent after ileostomy closure. The surgical procedures have taken 3–7 h to perform. A bowel obstruction occurred in one patient at the loop ileostomy site. Two minor wound infections developed in the Pfannenstiel incision.

Conclusion

Laparoscopic total colectomy is an advanced laparoscopic procedure, which can be employed in ulcerative colitis, familial adenomatous polyposis or total colonic aganglionosis [3, 4]. Colonic dissection is similar in each case; however, a variety of methods can be employed to provide anastomosis between the ileum and anus. Decreased postoperative stress and pain and quicker return of bowel function and activity can be expected.

References

1. Georgeson KE, Fuenfer MM, Hardin WD (1995) Primary laparoscopic pull-through for Hirschsprung's disease in infants and children. J Pediat Surg 30(7):1017–2102
2. Bernstein MA et al (1996) Is complete laparoscopic colectomy superior to laparoscopic assisted colectomy? Am Surg 62(6):507–511
3. Thjibault C, Poulin EC (1995) Total laparoscopic proctocolectomy and laparoscopy-assisted proctocolectomy for inflammatory bowel disease: operative technique and preliminary report. Surg Laparosc Endosc 5(6):472–476
4. Wexner DS (1997) Total laparoscopic proctocolectomy and laparoscopic-assisted proctocolectomy for inflammatory bowel disease: operative technique and preliminary report. Surg Laparosc Endosc 7(1):79–80

Laparoscopic Endorectal Pull-Through

K.E. Georgeson

Introduction

The recent trends in surgery for Hirschsprung's disease have been toward early repair and fewer surgical stages (Carcassonne et al. 1982, 1989; Cass 1990; Cilley et al. 1994; So et al. 1980). The laparoscopic technique for colon pull-through continues this trend by combining a primary surgical repair with a laparoscopic technique which can be performed in newborn infants (Georgeson et al. 1995). Patients may be repaired within 1–2 days of diagnosis whether they be neonates or children. Among the procedures currently being performed laparoscopically, the pull-through procedure for Hirschsprung's disease is one of the best validations of the usefulness of minimally invasive surgery in children.

Indications

All patients should have a rectal biopsy to confirm the diagnosis of Hirschsprung's disease prior to laparoscopic pull-through. The absence of ganglion cells and the presence of hypertrophic nerve trunks in combination with high levels of acetylcholinesterase extending up into the mucosal layer confirm the diagnosis of Hirschsprung's disease. A barium enema with a 24-hour follow-up film getting both anterior/posterior and lateral views of the abdomen and pelvis are helpful in planning the operation. In most cases, a definitive transition zone can be identified prior to the planned operation. Contraindications to one-stage laparoscopic pull-through include a diagnosis of total colon Hirschsprung's and an undetermined transition zone. Relative contraindications to laparoscopic pull-through include patients with a long aganglionic segment (the transition zone proximal to the splenic flexure of the colon), a history of severe recurrent enterocolitis, and patients who cannot be adequately decompressed preoperatively.

Preparation

Prior to the pull-through procedure, efforts should be made to decompress the proximal colon and the small bowel. Irrigations with normal saline every 6 h in combination with digital stretching of the anus every 2–3 h usually induce adequate decompression of the colon and small bowel.

Infants and small children are positioned transversely at the end of the operating table. Arm boards placed parallel to the operating table can be used to widen the supporting surfaces for longer infants. The surgeon and his assistants stand over the head of the patient. The torso of the patient is elevated with four or five folded sheets allowing the head to extend backward out of the operating surgeon's way. The camera driver stands to either side of the operating surgeon and the assistant stands at the end of the table to the patient's left side. The monitor is positioned at the foot of the patient. The operation is performed with the patient in a moderate Trendelenburg position to induce the small intestine to slide out of the pelvis. Larger patients are placed on the operating table in a supine orientation. The legs and feet are placed in stirrups with the buttock elevated on towels out at the end of the operating table. Specific instruments utilized include graspers and scissors and a hook cautery. In some patients, a 5-mm clip applier is also useful.

The following is a list of the instruments needed:
- Scope 0°, 5 mm, 1×
- Scope 30°, 5 mm, 1×
- Trocar, 5 mm, 2×
- Trocar, 3.5 mm, 2×
- L-hook cautery, 3 mm, 1×
- Grasper, 3 mm, 1×
- Grasper with ratchet, 3 mm, 1×
- Mosquito, 3 mm, 1×
- Clip applier, 5 mm, 1×
- Open procedure tray, 1×

Technique

The patient is prepared by cleansing all skin surfaces from the buttocks downward. Anteriorly the preparation is extended to the nipples and carried well out laterally so that most of the patient's torso below the nipples is cleansed circumferentially.

One-stage laparoscopic pull-through is begun with the intraperitoneal dissection. Four trocars are placed (Fig. 1). A 5-mm trocar is placed in the right upper quadrant several centimeters to the right of the midline and approximately 2–3 cm below the liver edge. The peritoneal cavity is entered after a pneumoperitoneum is obtained. A 5-mm trocar is also used in the right anterior axillary line about the level of the umbilicus. A 3.5- or 5-mm trocar is placed in the left anterior axillary line above the level of the umbilicus. The fourth trocar (3.5 mm) is placed to the right or left of the midline suprapubically taking care to avoid injury to the bladder during insertion.

Once the peritoneal cavity is entered, the transition zone should be visually identified. If an obvious transition zone is seen, biopsy confirmation is unneces-

31 Laparoscopic Endorectal Pull-Through

Fig. 1. The trocar sites are depicted for laparoscopic pull-through. The telescope is passed through the highest right upper quadrant port

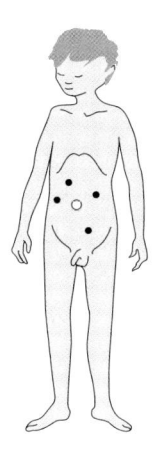

sary. If the transition zone is subtle, biopsies should be taken using a punch biopsy forceps or the endoscopic Metzenbaum scissors to cut through the seromuscular layers. The specimens are sent to the pathologist to aid in identification of the level of ganglionated bowel. The pelvic dissection should not be started until the operating surgeon is certain that the candidate is suitable for a one-stage procedure. If the operating surgeon is in doubt about the level of transition zone, it is much better to perform a leveling loop colostomy than to proceed with a primary pull-through.

The primary pull-through begins with development of a window through the recto-sigmoid mesocolon behind the superior rectal vessels. A 3-mm grasping instrument is passed through the suprapubic trocar and the recto-sigmoid colon is grasped. The colon is then pushed toward the anterior abdominal wall, displaying the rectosigmoid mesocolon. Using scissors or L-hook cautery, a window is developed in the rectosigmoid mesocolon behind the superior rectal artery and vein. The artery and vein are cauterized or clipped and divided. Dissection distally from this point is performed circumferentially close to the rectal wall. Dissection of the mesocolon proximal to this point is performed preserving the integrity of the marginal artery. In this way the colon pedicle retains adequate blood supply.

The pelvic dissection is started by circumferentially clearing the rectum of supporting structures and vessels. The L-hook cautery is very useful for this dissection although endoscopic Metzenbaum scissors can also be used. During the dissection of the rectum, both ureters should be visualized and carefully preserved. The circumferential dissection is stopped just proximal to the prostate or cervix anteriorly. Posteriorly the dissection is continued down to the fourth or fifth sacral vertebra. The middle rectal vessels and supporting tissues are divided with electrocautery to join the anterior and posterior planes.

Once the laparoscopic pelvic dissection is completed, attention is turned to developing an adequate colon pedicle for the pull-through. For a transition zone in the distal sigmoid colon, the fusion fascia of the descending colon can be left

Fig. 2. The laparoscopic dissection begins by making a window through the rectosigmoid mesocolon. The laparoscopic dissection proceeds close to the rectum circumferentially down into the pelvis. Proximally, the dissection is carried inside the marginal artery for appropriate vascularization of the colon pedicle. A transition zone above the midsigmoid colon necessitates division of the lateral fusion fascia

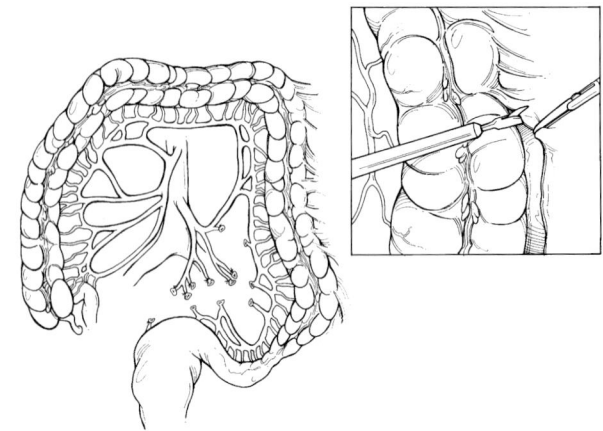

intact. If the transition zone is in the mid or upper sigmoid colon or is in the descending colon, the fusion fascia attaching the colon to the lateral abdominal wall should be divided sharply using Metzenbaum scissors and a grasper. Once the fusion fascia has been divided, attention is turned to the mesocolon. An instrument is passed through the suprapubic trocar site to hold the colon toward the anterior abdominal wall. In this way the mesentery is displayed. Carefully advancing the dissection inside the marginal artery, radially oriented vessels are encountered and either cauterized with the L-hook cautery, coagulated with the ultrasonic scalpel, or clipped with a 5-mm clip applier. This dissection is continued proximally as far as is necessary to bring the ganglionated colon pedicle down for rectal anastomosis without tension (Fig. 2). Once adequate mobilization of the colon and its mesentery is obtained, the pneumoperitoneum is evacuated and the transanal dissection is commenced.

The feet are elevated over the patient's torso exposing the anus. The operating surgeon and assistant move to the other side of the table for this portion of the operation. Six to eight traction sutures are placed through the perianal skin and then through the mucocutaneous junction retracting the anorectum radially in all directions and exposing the rectal mucosa for dissection. Great care should be taken throughout the rectal dissection to not overstretch the anal sphincters. Overstretching of the sphincters during this portion of the operation can lead to fecal incontinence. A site is selected usually about 5–10 mm above the dentate line (Fig. 3). This site is marked using a needle-tipped electrocautery dotting the mucosa circumferentially around the rectum. The cautery is then used to cut through the mucosa but not through the internal sphincter. Fine 4-0 or 5-0 silk sutures are used to secure the cut proximal lip of the mucosa to provide traction for the mucosectomy. Care is taken to stay inside the white circular muscle fibers of the internal sphincter carefully dissecting away the mucosa. Larger blood vessels are cauterized prior to dividing them. Both blunt and sharp dissection is required for this separation to go smoothly. Adequate time should be taken to develop the plane. Once the submucosal plane is established, the dissection goes

Fig. 3. The transanal mucosal dissection begin about 10 mm above the dentate line

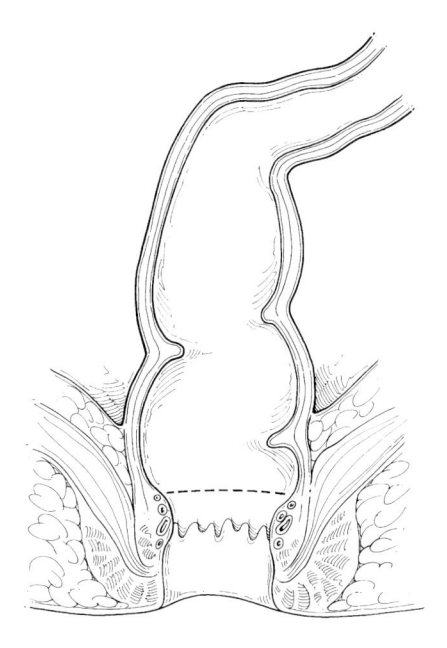

rapidly (Fig. 4). The mucosectomy is continued proximally until the rectal sleeve turns inside out and prolapses through the anus.

A second indication that the dissection is proximal enough is the absence of bleeding during the mucosectomy because the bowel has been previously separated from its blood supply by the laparoscopic dissection. When the rectal sleeve prolapses out through the anus easily the muscular coat is divided posteriorly (Fig. 5). If the intraperitoneal plane is not readily encountered with the first posterior cut through smooth muscle, the mucosectomy is continued up another 2 cm and another attempt to enter the peritoneal cavity is made. Once the dissection plane from above is entered transanally, the muscular cuff is cut circumferentially to free the colon from the surrounding cuff. Redundant portions of the proximal muscular sleeve are also trimmed to leave a sleeve about 5–6 cm in length. The rectal sleeve is then split posteriorly to allow for the development of a neorectal reservoir (Fig. 6). This division of the rectal cuff is optional and may be omitted by surgeons who prefer to leave an intact sleeve of rectal cuff.

The colon is next pulled down through the rectal sleeve until the transition zone is visualized (Fig. 7). The author prefers to pull out an additional 5–10 cm of colon to ensure that the dilated dysmotile segment of the colon is resected. The colon is then transected about half way around its circumference beginning anteriorly. 4-0 absorbable sutures are placed anteriorly and laterally to hold the neorectum in position. The remainder of the colon is then amputated. The specimen is sent to the pathologist for rapid frozen section analysis regarding the presence of ganglion cells in the proximal end of the specimen. The anastomosis is carefully made between the neorectum and the distal mucosal cuff (Fig. 8).

Fig. 4. The circular muscle fibers are dissected away from the mucosa bluntly and sharply. The dissection continues proximally until the laparoscopic dissection is encountered

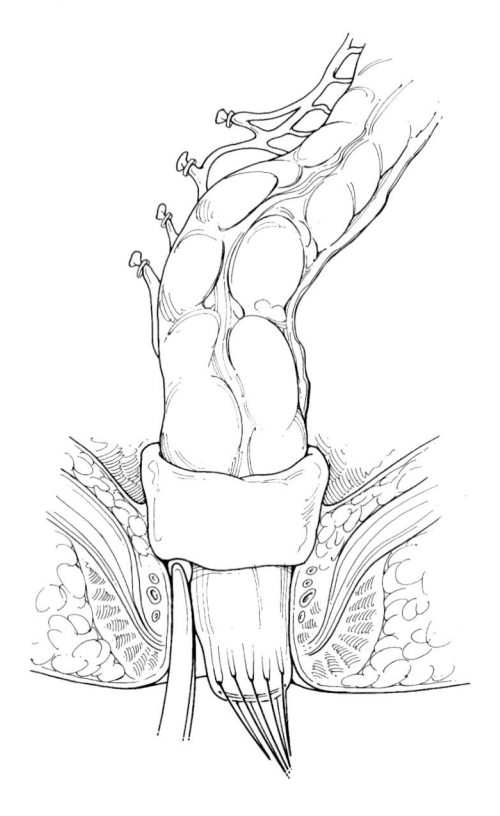

Fig. 5. When the rectum telescopes loosely out through the anus, the muscle layers are transected posteriorly to join the laparoscopic and transanal planes. The rectal muscle layers are divided circumferentially around the rectum

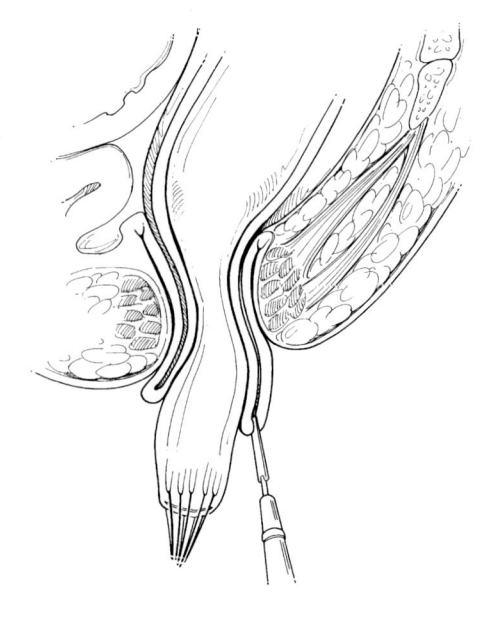

Fig. 6. Excess muscular cuff is trimmed proximally leaving a cuff length of 5–6 cm. Optionally, the cuff should be split posteriorly to allow for development of a rectal reservoir

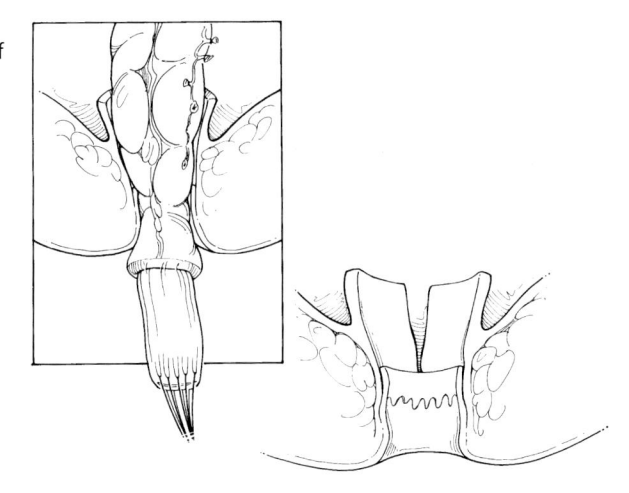

Fig. 7. The mobilized colon is pulled out to a level of 5–10 cm above transition zone. Biopsies are sent to the pathologist for confirmation of the presence of ganglion cells.

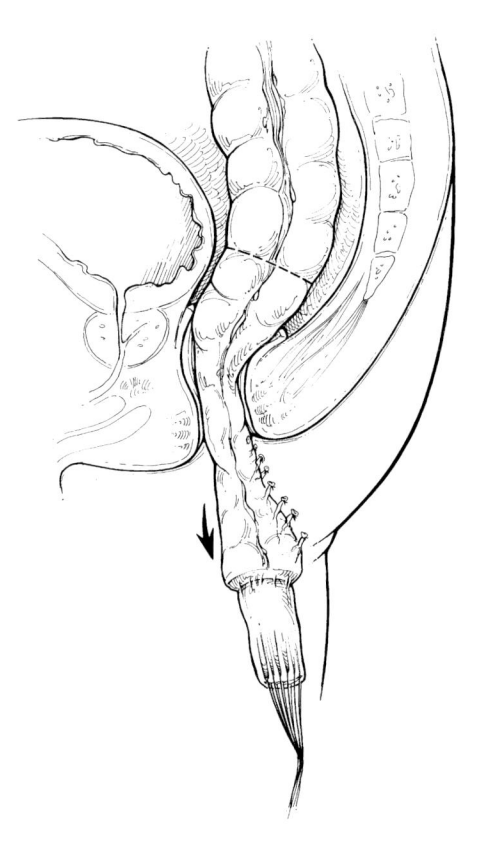

Fig. 8. The careful closure is made with interrupted absorbable suture

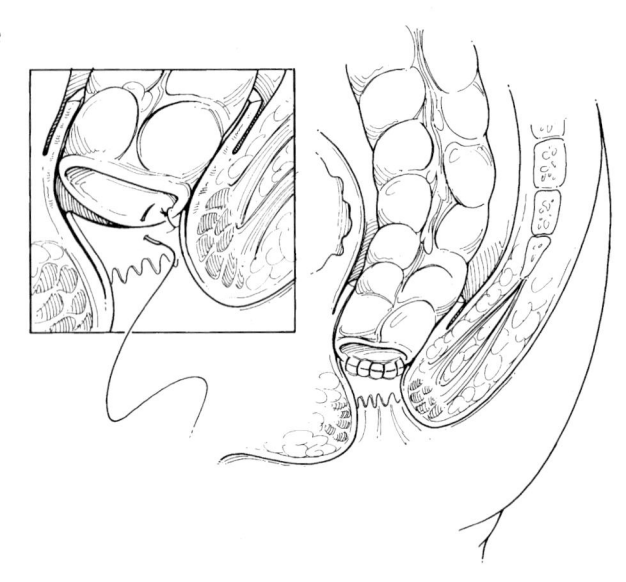

Great care should be taken to avoid any potential anastomotic leaks. The absorbable sutures are left long until the anastomosis has been completed. The long sutures are used to help inspect each portion of the anastomosis to make certain there are no hidden defects in the anastomosis.

Once the anastomosis is completed, the sutures are cut to about 1 cm in length and the anal stay sutures are removed. The anus retracts to a normal position. The little finger, lubricated with saline, is used to evaluate the anastomosis and the neorectum.

The surgeons change their gloves and reinstill the pneumoperitoneum. The colon is observed to make certain it is not twisted as it proceeds into the pelvis (Fig. 9). If there is a potential space behind the mesocolon for herniation of the small bowel, the space is closed using interrupted 3-0 silk sutures. The trocars are then removed and the fascia and the skin are closed in the usual fashion.

Infants and children who are not candidates for a one-stage pull-through should have an initial leveling colostomy. Performance of a leveling loop colostomy is started by taking multiple biopsies as previously described. The transition zone is marked with a suture with the ends left several centimeters long. A 3-cm incision is made at the proposed colostomy site. The marking suture is grasped with a clamp and the colon is pulled up into the wound. A small opening is made through the mesocolon adjacent to the selected loop of colon. The skin is pulled together through the mesenteric defect and approximated with one or two sutures between the proximal and distal portions of the loop. The loop colostomy is opened and matured with absorbable sutures (Fig. 10). Several silk sutures are placed laparoscopically attaching the seromuscular wall of the colon both proximal and distal to the colostomy site to the peritoneum of the anterior abdominal wall. These sutures help to prevent prolapse of the colostomy. They are more easily placed laparoscopically than to place them through the incision.

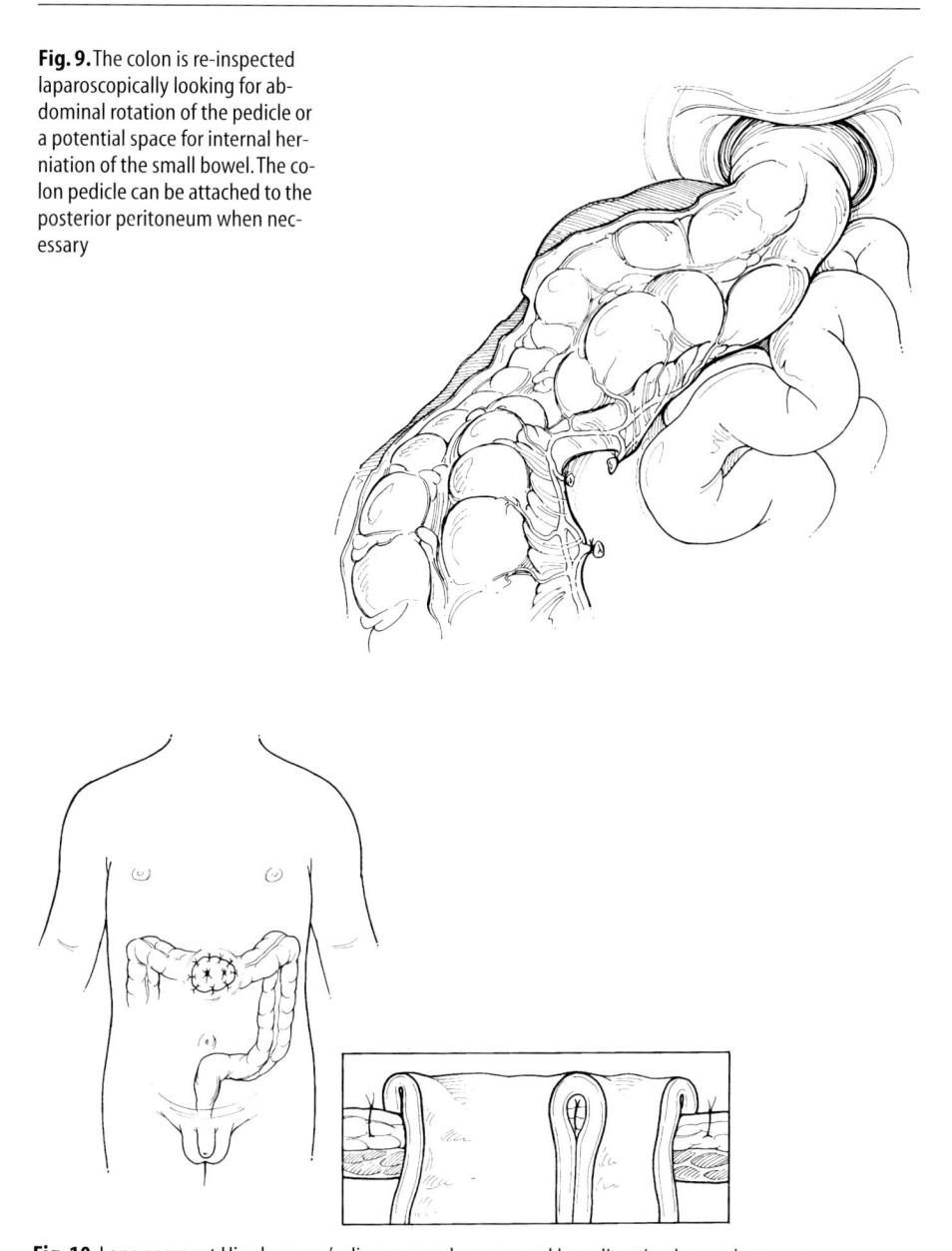

Fig. 9. The colon is re-inspected laparoscopically looking for abdominal rotation of the pedicle or a potential space for internal herniation of the small bowel. The colon pedicle can be attached to the posterior peritoneum when necessary

Fig. 10. Long segment Hirschsprung's disease may be managed by a diverting loop colostomy

Patients who have had a previous loop colostomy are operated secondarily in a fashion similar to a one-stage pull-through operation. The procedure is begun by stapling both the proximal and distal ends of the ostomy closed. Six to eight sutures are then used to approximate the two stapled ends to each other (Fig. 11).

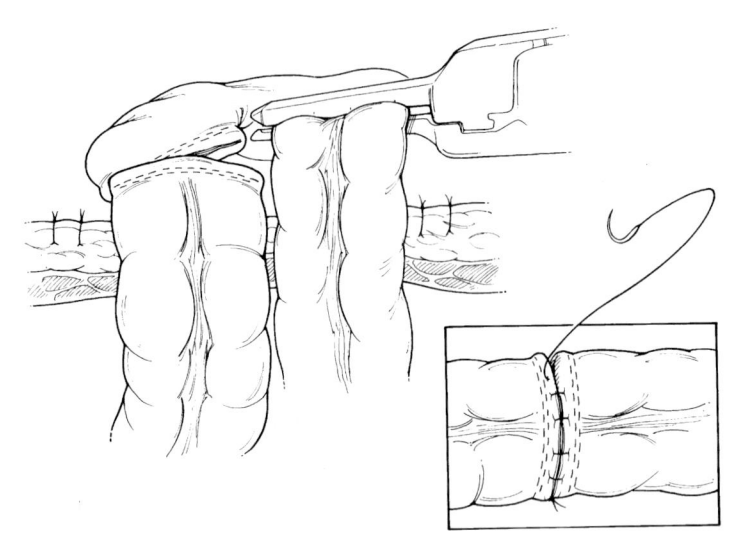

Fig. 11. Second-stage pull-through begins by stapling closed both limbs of the loop colostomy. The ends are approximated with eight to ten sutures. The colon is then dropped inside the peritoneal cavity and the wound closed. The rest of the procedure is performed as with the primary colon pull-through

The stoma is taken down and dropped into the peritoneal cavity. The wound is closed and the procedure is then performed as previously described for the primary pull-through.

Postoperative Care

Postoperatively the patient is not fed overnight. IV fluids are administered at a rate slightly above maintenance. A nasogastric tube can be left in place or may be removed at the end of the operative procedure. Urinary catheterization is usually unnecessary.

The patient is fed on the first postoperative day unless there is no evidence of bowel activity. The diet is advanced as tolerated. Antibiotics are continued for 24–48 h. Patients are discharged on the second to fourth postoperative day depending on their condition. Occasionally a patient requires a longer hospital stay, most commonly in patients with a significantly dilated colon preoperatively.

Personal Experience

Twenty-five patients who had a primary laparoscopic pull-through at our Institution over the last several years have been recently reviewed. Sixteen of the 25 children were under 3 months of age at the time of their pull-through. Average operating time was 183 min. In the patients under 3 months of age, operating time averaged 157 min. Most of the patients were fed by the second postoperative day. Average blood loss was 62 cc. Average time for discharge was 5 days. This time includes our early experience in which the patients were held longer due to our concern about postoperative complications. One of the patients had urinary retention which resolved spontaneously. One patient required an intraoperative blood transfusion due to the transection of the superior hemorrhoidal artery, which retracted and was difficult to control. Two patients developed mild postoperative enterocolitis, which responded to IV hydration and withholding oral feedings. One patient had chronic diarrhea, which responded to loperamide therapy. Two of the older patients experienced fecal soiling which improved with anal dilation and bowel training.

Several of the patients are old enough to evaluate for continence. Those neurologically normal patients over 3 years of age at the time of surgery have all become continent postoperatively. One child with significant mental retardation is not expected to be continent postoperatively. Several patients operated in infancy are now 3 years of age and have achieved fecal continence

Discussion

The laparoscopic endorectal pull-through is an excellent example of the potential advantages of laparoscopy over open surgery in children. The patients appear to recover more quickly and are discharged from the hospital earlier than their counterparts undergoing open procedures. The operation is not difficult to perform and utilizes the same principle of surgery for Hirschsprung's disease that were developed over many years by Drs. Swenson, Soave and others. Adequate preoperative evaluation and preparation are the most essential elements for good results in these patients.

References

Carcassonne M, Morisson-Lacombe G, Letourneau JN (1982) Primary corrective operation without decompression in infants less than three months of age with Hirschsprung's disease. J Pediatr Surg 17:241–243
Carcassonne M et al (1989) Management of Hirschsprung's disease: curative surgery before 3 months of age. J Pediatr Surg 24:1032–1043
Cass DT (1990) Neonatal one-stage repair of Hirschsprung's disease. Pediatr Surg Int 5:341–346
Cilley RE et al (1994) Definitive treatment of Hirschsprung's disease in the newborn with a one-stage procedure. Surgery 115:551–556
Georgeson, KE, Fuenfer MM, Hardin WD (1995) Primary laparoscopic pull-through for Hirschsprung's disease in infants and children. J Pediatr Surg 30:1017–1022
So HB et al (1980) Endorectal "pullthrough" without preliminary colostomy in neonates with Hirschsprung's disease. J Pediatr Surg 15:470–471

Laparoscopic Removal of the Aganglionic Bowel According to Duhamel-Martin

N.M.A. Bax, D.C. van der Zee

Introduction

The treatment of Hirschsprung's disease is usually surgical and consists of removal of all but the most distal part of the aganglionic bowel. The most distal part is conserved for continence purposes. These basic principles have not changed much since its original description by Swenson and Bill (1948). In Utrecht we have adopted the Duhamel-Martin technique (Duhamel 1956; Martin and Caudill 1967). Before the introduction of small stapler apparatuses, infants with Hirschsprung's disease in our centre received a preliminary colostomy and the definitive operation was postponed until the infants were about 6 months of age. Since the introduction of laparoscopic staplers, allowing for earlier definitive operations, we changed our policy and tried to avoid colostomies, bridging the period between diagnosis and definitive treatment with bowel washouts (van der Zee et al. 1993; van der Zee and Bax 1996).

Indications

The indications for a laparoscopic approach regarding Hirschsprung's disease do not differ in essence from the indications for open surgery.

However, there are some general contraindications for a laparoscopic approach as severe cardiorespiratory disease. Till now one child in the authors experience has not been considered to be good candidate for a laparoscopic approach as she had a congenital right left cardiac shunt in the context of trisomy 21. In such a case there is an increased risk for CO_2 embolism. Whether this is the case remains uncertain.

Preoperative Workup

The diagnosis of Hirschsprung's disease is established by means of a rectal suction biopsy. If interpretation of this biopsy is difficult, than a second suction biopsy is taken and rectal manometry is carried out. If the diagnosis is still not clear, a full thickness rectal wall biopsy is carried out. Most of the children have

32 Laparoscopic Removal of the Aganglionic Bowel According to Duhamel-Martin 273

had a contrast enema at one stage. Such a study may give an idea of the extent of the disease but will not influence initial therapy.

We try to avoid colostomies. Instead we try to decompress the bowel by means of colonic washouts. In the newborn this usually requires a short hospitalisation period, but in the older child this often can be carried out on an outpatient basis. The parents are instructed how to keep the bowel decompressed. If the goal of good decompression of the bowel is achieved, than the laparoscopic operation is planned. We have no fixed rules for the timing of this operation although the operation seems easier to perform in the younger patients. Most of the children diagnosed shortly after birth will be operated between 2 and 6 months of age. If decompression of the bowel cannot be achieved in a satisfactory manner, the definitive operation is performed much earlier, even in the neonatal period when needed. The youngest patient in our series was 13 days old.

A colostomy is not a contraindication for laparoscopic surgery.

All patients are admitted the day before the laparoscopic procedure and have both a colonic washout and antegrade bowel washout until the effluent becomes clear.

Technique

The technique has already been described before (Bax and van der Zee 1995) but with time many adjustments have been made.

All patients receive a central venous line and one dosis of antibiotics.

Position of the Patient, Team, and Equipment

The patient is positioned in supine Trendelenburg, half way the table (Figs. 1a, 2a). The anorectum is emptied with a suction catheter.

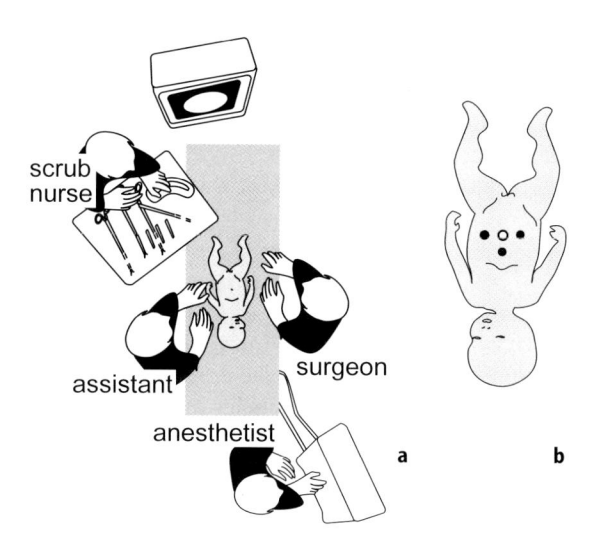

Fig. 1a,b. Small child. **a** Position of the child, crew, equipment. **b** Position of the cannulae. The first cannula in inserted in an open way through the inferior umbilical fold. In small children 5-mm cannulae suffice

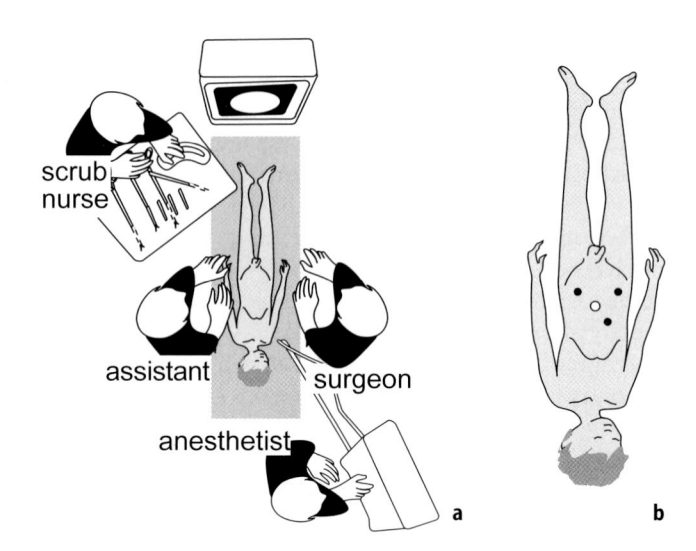

Fig. 2a,b. Bigger child. **a** Position of the child, crew, equipment. **b** Position of the cannulae. The first cannula in inserted in an open way through the inferior umbilical fold. In bigger children a 12-mm cannula should be inserted through the umbilicus to allow for the use of a linear stapler

Skin preparation includes the whole abdomen, lower back and legs. The feet and lower legs are draped in sterile sheets in order to allow for a combined abdominal and transanal approach without the need for repeat skin preparation and draping.

The surgeon stands at the patients right side, the surgical assistant at the left side, and the scrub nurse at the left bottom end of the table.

The tower with monitor, camera-unit, video and insufflator stands at the bottom end of the table. The HF electrosurgical unit, suction apparatus and standard with irrigation fluid stands at the right bottom end of the table.

All cables come from about the same direction, i.e. the right lower end of the table and are positioned in a circle along the patients left site, over the patients thorax, along the patients right side. The cables are joined together with a gauze, which is fixed to the sheet covering the table.

A Foley catheter is now inserted into the bladder which is regularly emptied.

Cannulae

Four cannulae are used (Figs. 1b, 2b). The first 6-mm cannula is inserted in an open way through the inferior umbilical fold and is used for a 5-mm scope. The three remaining 6-mm cannulae are inserted under scopic control after creation of a pneumoperitoneum. In babies one cannula is inserted halfway the xyphoid process and the umbilicus and two other cannulae are inserted pararectally at the level of the umbilicus (Fig. 1b). The epigastrial cannula is used for a forceps, and the right pararectal one for a pair of scissors or for a hook. The left parectal one is used for a forceps to be held by the assistant. In older children, the working instruments must be positioned lower down towards the iliac fossae (Fig. 2b).

In small children the upper rectum can be transected between ligatures, introduced through the 6-mm cannulae. In bigger children, in which the rectum is dilated, transection of the rectum requires a linear stapler introduced through a 12-mm cannula. If this is known preoperatively, than it is better to insert a 12-mm cannula at once through the inferior umbilical fold. Once such a cannula is in place a 10-mm scope can be used.

Pneumoperitoneum

CO_2 is insufflated at an flow of 5 l/min. Pressure is limited to 8 mmHg.

Findings

At initial laparoscopy it is immediately clear that the patient has Hirschsprung's disease as the bowel wall of the involved segment looks thickened. Dilatation of the more proximal bowel is usually absent and proves that the colonic washouts have been successful.

Operation

If the bladder in boys or the uterus in girls is in the way during the dissecting in the small pelvis, both structures can be suspended with a 3 0 suture, brought in directly through the abdominal wall using a curved needle. After taking a bite of bladder or uterus, the needle is pushed back through the abdominal wall at the other site of the midline.

Extramucosal biopsies are than taken in order to define the proximal extension of the aganglionosis, one just above the peritoneal reflection, one at the rectosigmoid junction, one half-way the sigmoid colon, and when needed one ore more biopsies higher up. The harvesting of extramucosal biopsies of the bowel is easy in places of bowel wall thickening. In normal looking areas, however, it is difficult to stay extramucosally, but when the bowel has been well prepared preoperatively a small hole does not lead to spillage of fecal material and is easily closed laparoscopically with one or two 5-0 absorbable sutures.

Rectosigmoid Aganglionosis

Nowadays we start the dissection with the mobilisation of the sigmoid colon by incising the lateral peritoneal fold. This is best carried out with the assistant also standing on the right of the patient while the surgeon uses the right pararectal cannula for a pair of scissors and the epigastrial one for a forceps.

After the assistant has moved back to the left, the rectal dissection is started. The assistant picks up the upper rectum, while the surgeon starts the dissection by opening the border between the bowel and the mesentery on the right (Fig. 3a). The dissection is as close to the bowel wall as possible rather coagulating the bowel wall than the surroundings. After the right leaf of the mesentery has been transected over some distance, the loose, almost avascular areolar tissue between the two leaves is divided. Next the left leaf is transected taking care that the left ureter is not harmed (Fig. 3b). Once a hole is made through the posterior mesentery, then the dissection becomes easier as the left lateral pelvic wall can be observed from the right through this hole. The dissection goes further and further not only posteriorly but also laterally and anteriorly until the pelvic floor is reached. The dissection must go this far because the rectal stump must be evaginated transanally and amputated further in order to leave as little rectal stump behind as possible. The posterior dissection must go right down to the perineum. If the posterior dissection is stopped earlier, it is difficult to find the lowermost dissected area through the posterior rectal incision, which is made later on.

For the dissection we use monopolar dissecting scissors with a short blade and the monopolar hook. During activation of the elcetrosurgical HF apparatus it is important to have the entire noninsulated part of the instrument in view in order to avoid accidental touching of other tissues.

Next the sigmoidal and inferior mesenteric vessels are severed either with diathermy or between 5-mm titanium clips. This usually suffices for a tension free pull through of ganglionic bowel.

The upper rectum is now transected between oo ligatures in a small baby with nondilated upper rectum, or with the linear stapler inserted through the umbilical 12-mm port (Fig. 3c). In the later event a 5-mm scope must be inserted through the epigastrial cannula.

After transection of the upper rectum a 5-mm blunt instrument is inserted through the epigastrial cannula and brought down behind the rectum right

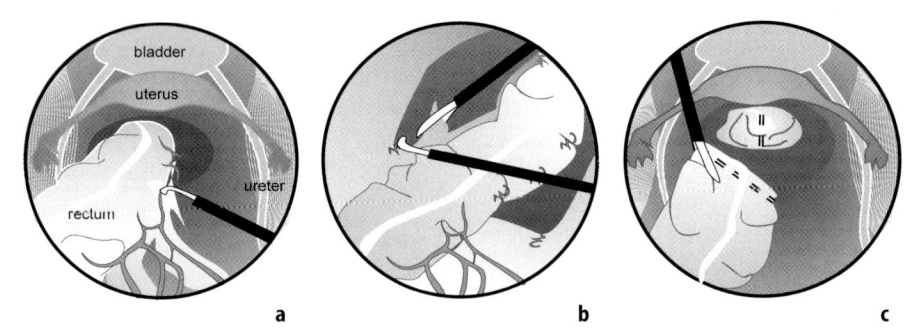

Fig. 3a–c. Mobilisation and transection of the rectum. **a** The dissectum of the rectum is started on the right, close to its wall. First the right mesenteric leaf is opened. Next the middle plane is transected. **b** Finally the left mesenteric leaf is opened. As a hole has now been created through the rectal mesentery, a better overview of the small pelvis is obtained which makes further dissection much easier. **c** After mobilisation of the rectum down to the pelvic floor, the upper rectum is transected, between ligatures in the small child or with the linear stapler in the bigger child

32 Laparoscopic Removal of the Aganglionic Bowel According to Duhamel-Martin

down to the perineum. The assistant exerts some pressure on this instrument in order to keep it in place.

Next the legs of the baby are pulled up, two small Langenbeck retractors are inserted in the anus laterally, and a nearly 180° semicircular incision is made through the posterior rectum 0.5 cm above the dentate line. This incision is deepened till the previously inserted blunt instrument is reached. A grasping instrument is now inserted through the anus into the retrorectal space following the blunt instrument, which is withdrawn. With the grasping forceps the end of the proximal colon is grasped and pulled through till a well-ganglionated bowel area is reached (Fig. 4a). The pull through is scopically controlled in order to avoid torsion. At appropriate level the pulled through bowel is transected and anastomosed to the opening in the lower posterior rectum (Fig. 4b). The side to side anastomosis between the anterior rectum and posterior pulled through bowel is made using the endostapler inserted through the anus (Fig. 4c).

To avoid any blind pouch formation, nowadays, we evert the side to side anastomosis progressively using oo sutures. When the cranial end of the side to side

Fig. 4a–c. Pull-through. **a** The mobilised proximal bowel is pulled through the distal opening in the posterior rectum. **b** The pulled though bowel is amputated in ganglionic area and anstomosed to the hole in the rectum. **c** A side to side anastomosis is made between the remaining rectum and pulled through bowel, using a linear stapler. To avoid pouch formation, the remaining rectal stump is everted, amputated, and closed. Eversion is achieved by putting traction sutures on the stapled side to side anastomosis

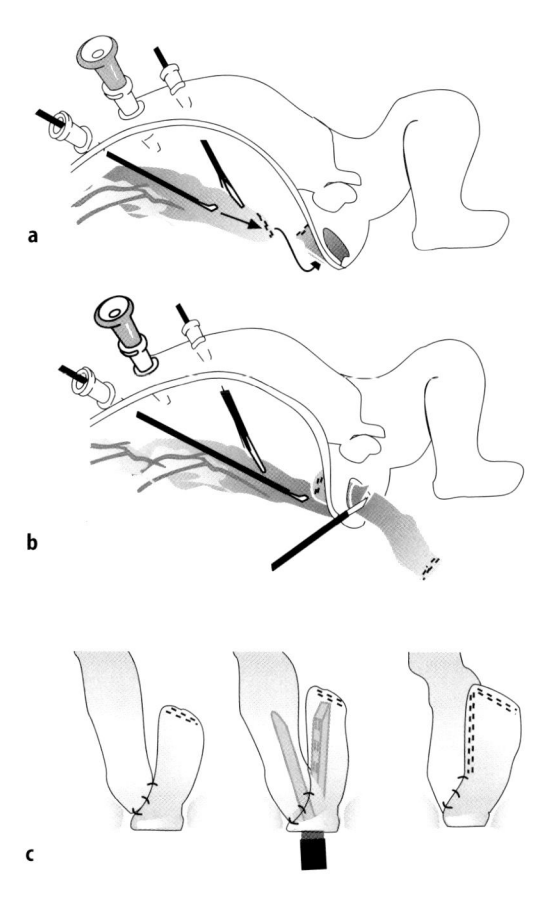

anastomosis is reached, than the posterior rectal wall higher up is pulled down by further oo sutures till the end of the blind rectum is everted. The rectal pouch above the side to side anastomosis is amputated and the remaining hole closed using 3-0 absorbable sutures.

As is standard in our institution at the end of the procedure a F 18 or 24 siliconized cannula is inserted transanally into the pulled through bowel and is fixed with tape. All cannulae are removed under scopic control and the fascial defect at umbilical level is closed with vicryl sutures. If the anterior fascia is easily identifiable at the other cannulae sites, than the holes in the anterior fascia are closed as well. Skin is adapted with adhesive strips.

Extended Aganglionosis

When the aganglionosis extents as far as the middle descending colon, a classical pull through is not possible, and further mobilisation of the colon is necessary. It is possible to dissect the omentum off the transverse colon laparoscopically, to take down the splenic and the hepatic flexures of the colon, to transect the middle and right colic vessels between clips and to turn the right colon down to be anastomosed with the remaining rectum according to Duhamel-Martin method. It must also be possible to bring the terminal ileum down. To do the entire dissection laparoscopically takes substantial time and is not easy. Moreover in such situation at least two screens should be present, one at the left site of the patient and the other one at the right side. These screens should be interconnected with a long cable allowing the screens to be moved cranially or caudally as needed. The scope stays in the umbilicus but, depending on the region to be dissected, the other cannulae are used for different instruments.

Alternatively a tranverse supraumbilical incision can be made to take the omentum down from the transverse colon, to mobilise the transverse colon and both colonic flexures, to transect the middle and right colic vessels between ligatures, and to mobilise the ileocecal region and to turn the right colon down or the bring the ileum down.

Colostomy

A colostomy is not a contraindication for laparoscopic assisted treatment of Hirschsprung's disease. In the rare cases that a colostomy has been unavoidable, this colostomy can be taken down at the definitive operation. The hole were the colostomy was situated can be used for some dissection in the vicinity and can be closed around a large cannula.

Postoperative Care

A nasogastric tube is left in place for the first 24–36 h. Parenteral nutrition is given from day 1 onwards. The transanal cannula is rinced with saline twice a day in order to keep the cannula open until the patient starts to pass stools. As soon as the patient starts to pass stools, the cannula is removed. Postoperative pain medication is given for 48 h and consists of epidural nicomorphine or intravenous morphine. A bladder catheter is left in place for at least 24 h or for as long as epidural morphine is given. Oral feeding is started on day 5 and rapidly augmented. Many patients are discharged the following day.

Personal Experience

So far 19 children with Hirschsprung's disease have had a laparoscopic or laparoscopic assisted approach for removal of the aganglionic bowel. One child was operated by the classic open way as it had a congenital right to left cardiac shunt. In ten of the 19 children the diagnosis was made within the first month of life, in two between 1 and 6 months, in two between 6 and 12 months, and in two after 1 year of age. The timing of the resection of the aganglionic bowel depended on how easily the colon could be kept decompressed by daily washouts. If this was difficult than the resection was planned without much delay, in contrast if this was easy than there was no hurry. The youngest patient was only 13 days old and weighed 2.9 kg. The period between diagnosis and surgery varied from 10 days to 8 months, with a mean of 3.75 months.

Sixteen children had rectosigmoid disease, two whole left colon involvement and one had total colonic aganglionosis. Conversion to an open procedure was only necessary in the second patient as there was doubt about the quality of the side to side anastomosis. Two children had a laparoscopic assisted approach. The first child had whole left colon involvement and had received a right transverse colostomy. In this child the colostomy was taken down, and a large cannula was sutured in place where the stoma had been located. Later on part of the dissection was carried out through the reopened wound. The second child was thought to have near total colonic aganglionosis. In this child a limited upper transverse laparotomy was made for mobilisation of the transverse and ascending colon, and for mobilisation and turning down of the ileocecal region.

No major intraoperative problems occurred but the operation was lengthy, especially in the beginning of the series. As a result many of the patients spent a night in the intensive care. Operative time has come down now to about 3.5 h. Most patients were discharged within 7 days. Follow-up is still relatively short but we have the feeling that the children operated on laparoscopically behave similarly to the children operated on in an open way. Two patients have had an insufficient resection, despite preoperative confirmation of "a normal looking" nervous plexus in the distal bowel end to be pulled through. One patient had rectosigmoidal disease and in the second the pulled through ascending colon appeared aganglionic at the second operation.

Discussion

Whether children that have been operated on laparoscopically are better off than children operated on in an open way, is difficult to prove. Not only are the number of patients with Hirschsprung's disease relatively small, most parents choose for that operation that leaves the least scars. The cosmetic benefit of the laparoscopic approach is beyond doubt and the parents are very pleased with this. Whether postoperative well being is indeed less affected in the laparoscopic group is difficult to say. Not only we but also our nurses have the impression that this is the case; however, critical colleagues may claim that this is due to bias. We do not expect superior long-term results as the operation we are carrying out laparoscopically is basically the same as the operation we do in an open way. In an open Duhamel-Martin we also resect most of the rectum. Some difference, however, is present. In the laparoscopic approach we evert the rectal stump and amputate this stump externally. In the open method, the rectum is amputated deep in the pelvis so there is no stump.

Some persons ask us why we keep performing a Duhamel-Martin laparoscopically as a Swenson is easier to do laparoscopically. We decided not to change our basic technique as we prefer the Duhamel-Martin procedure, which partially transects the internal sphincter. Moreover, by not changing the technique that we are accustomed to, we are able to compare our laparoscopic results with the results of the previous open method. We realise that this is a comparison between historical series, but this is the best we can do.

References

Bax NMA, van der Zee DC (1995) Laparoscopic removal of aganglionic bowel using the Duhamel-Martin method in five consecutive infants. Pediatr Surg Int 10:226–228

Duhamel B (1956) Une nouvelle opération pour le mégacôlon congénitale: l' abaissement rétrorectal et trans-anal du côlon et son application possible au traitement de quelques autres malformations. Presse Med 64:2249–2250

Martin LW, Caudill DR (1967) A method for eliminating of the blind rectal pouch in the Duhamel operation for Hirschsprung's disease. Surgery 62:951–953

Swenson O, Bill AH 1948 Resection of rectum and rectosigmoid with preservation of sphincter for benign spastic lesions producing megacolon. Surgery 24:212–220

van der Zee DC, Bax NMA (1996) Duhamel-Martin procedure for Hirschsprung's disease in neonates and infants: One-stage operation. J Pediatr Surg 31:901–902

van der Zee DC et al (1993) Use of EndoGIA stapling device in Duhamel-Martin procedure for Hirschsprung's disease. Pediatr Surg Int 8:447–448

Treatment of Hirschsprung's Disease by Laparoscopic Dissection of Bowel, Transanal Eversion and Perineal Resection

F. Schier, J. Waldschmidt

Introduction

Prolapsing colon through the anus and performing an extra-anal anastomosis is not new. As early as 1889 abdomino-perineal pull-throughs and extra-anal anastomoses were described by several authors (Hocheneck, Treves, Weir; for literature, see Holschneider [2]). In the late 1940's at the Children's Hospital at Great Ormond Street, London, the colon and rectum were mobilized and – unopenedly – prolapsed through the anus. Denis Browne had suggested the technique. A sigmoidoscope and a long needle were used for the maneuver. The rationale was to avoid intra-abdominal contamination. This is exactly what will be described in this chapter using laparoscopic techniques.

Swenson's contribution was to remove the bulk of diseased colon before pulling the two stumps coaxially through the anus. In 1948 he presented this technique [4]. He already considered primary operation without colostomy in children of good general health. Subsequent technical modifications were designed by Swenson himself and by several other authors. Horizontal anastomosis was replaced by diagonal anastomosis.

Indication

Although historically designed for the treatment of Hirschsprung's disease, the technique described in this chapter can be used for any colon resection. A limiting factor could be the volume of colon to be passed through the anus. In our experience it is only difficult to evert the first few centimeters of colon. Thereafter the process becomes more easy.

We do not know how suitable the procedure is for total colonic aganglionosis. We lack any personal experience with laparoscopic dissection of the right colon and the ileocecal area. Theoretically it should be feasible. The left colonic flexure is not difficult to dissect laparoscopically.

Size and general condition of the child are no factor. Any child considered able to sustain a conventional colon resection would even more be a candidate for laparoscopic colon resection.

We tend to avoid colostomies or ileostomies and prefer early resection as soon as a reliable rectal biopsy reading is available. If there is a colostomy in place it is no major obstacle for laparoscopic colon resection, in contrast, it can may be advantageous by providing a histologically safe level of resection and also serve as an additional point of fixation of the bowel, thus facilitating laparoscopic dissection.

Preoperative Workup

There is no difference in the preoperative workup compared to conventional open surgery. Case history, suction or full thickness biopsy, manometry and radiology remain the procedures to establish the diagnosis.

Preoperative Preparations

The mother is instructed in emptying techniques in order to prevent the distension of the bowel until primary surgery is feasible. If this fails, a stoma is opened and resection delayed.

Prior to surgery the child is admitted for mechanical bowel cleansing, as in open surgery. Older children undergo both antegrade and retrograde irrigation. Newborns are submitted only to retrograde cleaning by enema. Antibiotics are administered prior to surgery in case the bowel is opened inadvertently either during biopsy or during dissection or pull-through. A urinary catheter and a nasogastric tube are placed. The anorectum is dilated digitally and all remaining rectal feces are removed. A rectal tube allows for intraoperative evacuation of feces, liquid and gas still accumulated in the large bowel from previous enemas.

The child is prepped and cleansed in a way that conversion to the open technique is feasible. The skin is disinfected circumferentially from above the umbilicus all the way down to the feet. The feet are wrapped individually so that the legs may be bent in the hip joint for subsequent easy and sterile intraoperative access to the perineum.

A stoma, if present, is closed by tapes. Otherwise, increased intra-abdominal pressure by insufflation might lead to intraoperative spillage of feces.

Operating Room Lay-Out

The procedure may create physical difficulties when performed on a surgical table designed for adults. The instrument grips may clash with the table during horizontal or even upward preparation. A narrow pediatric table seems preferable.

For the positioning of personnel and equipment within the operating room, see Fig. 1. Two surgeons suffice for the intraoperative part of the procedure. For

Fig. 1. Operating room lay-out

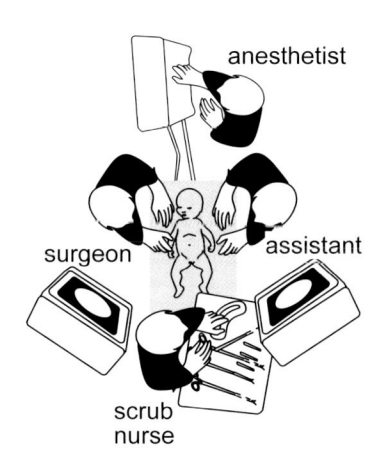

the perineal anastomosis a second assistant would hold up the legs bent at the hip joint. Since the two surgeons sit opposite, a second monitor facilitates the assistant's actions. However, a single monitor works as well. In that case the assistant acts are reversed and might appear clumsy. The nurse should be able to follow the procedure on the monitor.

Trocar Positioning

We belong to the minority of pediatric surgeons starting laparoscopy by insertion of the Veress needle and the first trocar blindly. Both are advanced through the umbilicus (Fig. 2). Even in newborns a 10-mm laparoscope may be advanced through the umbilicus. The picture is brilliant but the resultant scar is unnecessarily large. A 5-mm laparoscope suffices.

After the laparoscope is inserted and a first overview is obtained, a further 5-mm trocar is brought into the right lower abdomen. This trocar serves for the working instruments of the surgeon (forceps, scissors, etc.). He then needs a further trocar (again 5 mm) for counteracting with his left hand. It is left to his preference whether this trocar shall be placed in the right or the left abdomen. He is better off with his two trocars to the right and one on the left for the assistant. The assistant holds the camera and lifts up the colon via the left-sided trocar and forceps.

Specific Instrumentation

There are instruments available with small diameters. Of course trocars would be chosen accordingly. Currently there is no clip applier available with a diameter of less than 5 mm. No specific instruments are necessary. Only standard instruments are required: scissors, forceps (both combined with diathermia), suc-

Fig. 2. Trocar placement

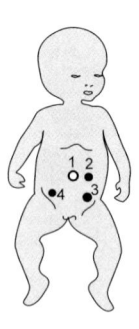

tion/irrigation, clips. The perineal part of the procedure is carried out with conventional instruments for open surgery.

Technique

As in open surgery, the extent of dilatation is first identified and the level of proximal resection is determined. The bowel wall is grabbed and biopsies are taken with scissors. The lesions are oversewn.

The colon is hold up at a convenient place in the rectosigmoid and the mesocolon is coagulated and transected close to the bowel wall until a window is created (Fig. 3)

Usually the very first steps are uncertain. With the window opened the anatomical situation becomes clear immediately. The transsection is advanced proximally and distally. In young children it can be accomplished without scissors and clips. The blood vessels are so small that simple coagulation suffices.

The peritoneal reflection between bladder and rectum is incised, in older children with scissors, in newborns simply by cautery. The rectum is mobilized circumferentially very close to the bowel wall. Anterior dissection is carried down only a few centimeters out of fear of subsequent functional losses. Posterior dissection, in contrast, follows the rectum all the way down. Herewith, it is difficult to judge the extent of dissection by laparoscopy alone. A finger placed at the perineum from outside while advancing a forceps from inside provides a feel for the remaining distance. Dissection is finished with a posterior distance of 1 cm. The anterior distance may be several centimeters.

This completed, a forceps is inserted through the anus. The forceps grabs the bowel wall and pulls it backwards through the anus as if wanting to create an anal prolapse. The tip of the instrument can be checked by laparoscopy. Usually the first moments of eversion are tedious and the pulling requires support from additional perianally placed Allis clamps. Simultaneous, a laparoscopic forceps pushes down from above (Fig. 4a).

After the first few centimeters of bowel are developed into the perineum, the maneuver becomes easier. The sites of biopsy can clearly be seen by laparoscopy. Eventually the whole segment of bowel to be resected is exposed. All laparoscop-

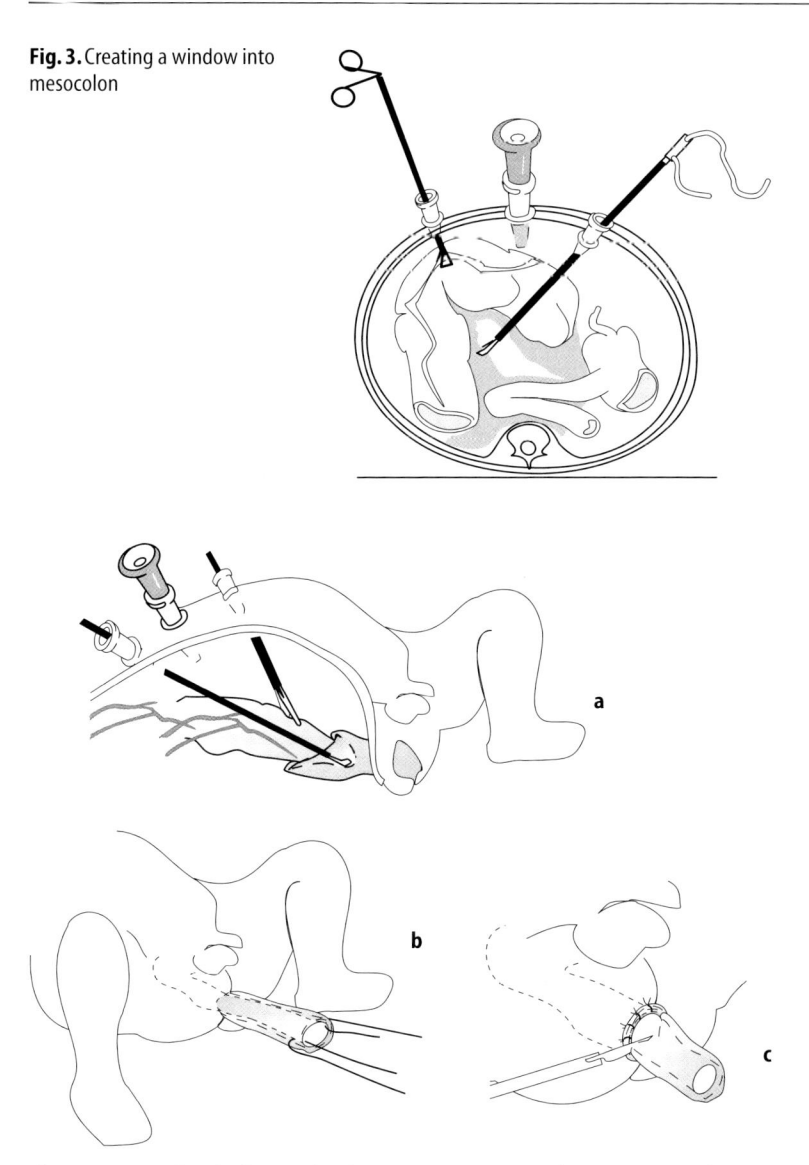

33 Treatment of Hirschsprung's Disease by Laparoscopic Dissection...

Fig. 3. Creating a window into mesocolon

Fig. 4 a-c. a Bowel pushed into pelvis. **b** Perineum with everted bowel. Bowel held by stay sutures. **c** Transsection and anastomosis

ic instruments including the laparoscope are removed. The abdomen is desufflated. The cannulae are left in place.

The surgeons turn to the perineum. The bowel is pulled down and the perineum is counteracted until the mucocutaneous line is seen posteriorly. The everted bowel is secured by stay sutures and transected by cautery close to the skin posteriorly (Fig. 4b,c).

Immediatedly thereafter the two bowel layers are reanastomized step by step using interrupted sutures. The inner layer represents the oral side of the anastomosis. A biopsy is taken from the inner wall and checked for ganglia distribution. The anastomosis is completed in the meanwhile until the result of histology is available. If necessary, the abdomen is insufflated again, bowel dissection is resumed and a new anastomosis is executed. During the whole procedure the everted bowel is under traction. As soon as the last suture is cut, the bowel and its anastomosis recedes into the pelvis. An immediate digital examination reveals a level of anastomosis higher than expected. The level even rises over the next few weeks. Therefore, when in doubt, a new anastomosis should be created.

A last inspection of the abdomen is carried out to ensure that there is no torsion, and that no tension at the bowel pulled down. We do not know whether the peritoneum needs to be closed up again.

The abdomen is finally desufflated and instruments and cannulae are removed. The fascia is approximated only where a 10-mm trocar was placed. The sites of 5-mm trocars are closed with a few skin sutures.

We usually place a large rectal tube in the assumption that the tube might protect the anastomosis. This is unconfirmed. The foreign body might even do harm.

Postoperative Care

The urinary catheter is left for 24–36 h. Removing the catheter earlier might necessitate placement of a new one. The nasogastric tube is left in place as well for 24–36 h. Thereafter liquids are started and the child quickly advanced to regular diet within 3 days. The antibiotics are given for 4 days. The children may lay on their back or belly and they may ambulate or be carried around ad libitum as soon as they tolerate it or wish to do so.

Personal Experience

Thirteen children were operated upon. Except for two with intestinal neuronal dysplasia all children were diagnosed to have Hirschsprung's disease. The age at surgery was between 5 weeks and 13 years (mean 3 months). One child had a transversostomy and another an ascendostomy at the time of laparoscopy. All others had been managed by enemas. The average surgery time was 2.7 h (range 2–4). The levels of anastomosis, as determined weeks after surgery digitally by rectal examination, were 2.5 cm (range 1–6).

In three children an anastomotic stricture developed. They had, much to the dissatisfaction of the parents, to be treated by bougienage. In two children the anastomosis has obviously been placed in the transitional zone. Both children suffer from constipation. They probably shall require reoperation.

It was our impression that postoperative recovery was quicker and that there was less pain medication requirement than after conventional colon resection.

Discussion

The limited number of patients available to us does not yet allow to statistically prove our preliminary impression that postoperative recovery is quicker after laparoscopy [3]. We did not have previous experience with the Swenson technique (the Rehbein procedure is generally preferred in Germany).

With the open Swenson technique, pelvic dissection is tedious, especially in small children. Laparoscopic techniques facilitate this. The laparoscope can be advanced as closely as desired all the way down, a feat never achievable with open surgery.

We are uncertain as to whether recommend the laparoscopic approach in cases the necessity of a reoperation should arise. Certainly there are only few adhesions to be expected.

Years later, rectal strictures occurred in 6.2% of Swenson's own cases. They were his most frequent complication [5]. The first ones of our anastomoses were all performed horizontally. Only later we learned that oblique anastomoses yield less strictures.

Primary anastomosis without colostomy seems more adequate in Hirschsprung's disease. We had adopted this attitude already before the advent of laparoscopy and this has been shared by others [1]. Laparoscopic techniques now perfect this approach.

References

1. Carcassonne M, Morisson-Lacombe G, LeTourneau JN (1982) Primary corrective operation without decompression in infants less than three months of age with Hirschsprung's disease. J Pediatr Surg 17:241–243
2. Holschneider AM (1982) Hirschsprung's disease. Hippokrates, Stuttgart / Thieme-Stratton, New York
3. Hoffmann K, Schier F, Waldschmidt J (1996) Laparoscopic Swenson's procedure in children. Eur J Pediatr Surg 6:15–17
4. Swenson O, Bill AH (1948) Resection of rectum and rectosigmoid with preservation of the sphincter for benign spastic lesions producing megacolon. Surgery 24:212–220
5. Swenson O (1982) Swenson's procedure. In: Holschneider AM (ed) Hirschsprung's disease. Hippokrates, Stuttgart; Thieme-Stratton, New York, p 155

Part III
Abdomen

Liver and Biliary Tree

CHAPTER 34

Endoscopic Surgery for Liver Hydatid Cysts

F.J. Berchi

Introduction

Although liver tumors and cysts are generally uncommon conditions in children, in certain parts of the world e.g. Spain, cystic lesions particularly that of the hydatid disease are not infrequently encountered. Several procedures have been described for the surgical treatment of hydatid liver cysts (from puncture of the cyst to liver resection or liver transplant). My preferred surgical treatment is the laparoscopic partial pericystectomy [1] which is the subject of this chapter.

Preoperative Workup

It is absolutely crucial for the surgeon to make an accurate diagnosis, exclude the presence of hydatid disease elsewhere in the body, evaluate the patient's clinical status, and memorize the segmental anatomy of the liver.

All patients must have preoperative routine blood tests, liver function analysis, and clotting screen. Serological tests, and hydatid markers and titers include: immunoprecipitants, immunoenzymatic tests, radioimmunology, interferon-α/β and conventional serological study, indirect hemoagglutinin and enzyme-linked immunosorbent assay [2–5]. Ultrasonography and computed axial tomography are the most accurate noninvasive diagnostic measures.

Informed consent is necessary and should include both laparoscopic technique and conversion to an open procedure if and when appropriate. It is also important to inform the patient and family about the complications of surgery particularly that of the perioperative intra-abdominal dissemination of hydatid fluid/scolices and anaphylactic reaction [1–3].

Specific Instrumentation

In addition to a camera, monitor, insufflator, suction irrigation apparatus, and a set of conventional instruments for conversion to an open technique when required, the following instruments are necessary:

- Three cannulae/trocars (5–12 mm)
- Two atraumatic grasping forceps
- One dissecting scissors
- Telescope of 0° or 30° (usually 10 mm)
- Specimen retrieval bag
- Tru-Cut needle or a conventional intravenous cannula and needle
- Veress needle
- 10% and 20% saline solutions
- Jackson drain
- Five culture test tubes

Technique

The technique involves general anesthesia with full muscle relaxation. Broad spectrum prophylactic antibiotics are administered at the time of induction and a nasogastric tube is inserted. The patient is positioned supine at the end of the operating table with the surgeon standing between the legs and the assistants/scrub nurse on either side of the operating table (Fig. 1). The operating table should allow fluoroscopic imaging during the procedure when required. A degree of reverse Trendelenburg tilt and a cushion/towel roll under the lower thoracic spine facilitates laparoscopic access.

A sub-umbilical (10-mm) primary cannula is placed using an open technique. A pneumoperitoneum is created using CO_2 and the second (5- or 10-mm) and third (12-mm) cannulae are inserted in the right and left upper quadrants respectively (Fig. 2). Occasionally a fourth cannula may be required. A 14-gauge conventional intravenous catheter or a Veress needle is introduced into the abdominal cavity for continuous irrigation of the surface of the liver and cyst with 10% saline (Fig. 2). After preliminary laparoscopic exploration, the liver is inspected and the cyst is identified. A percutaneous transhepatic (never directly

Fig. 1. Position of patient, crew, and equipment

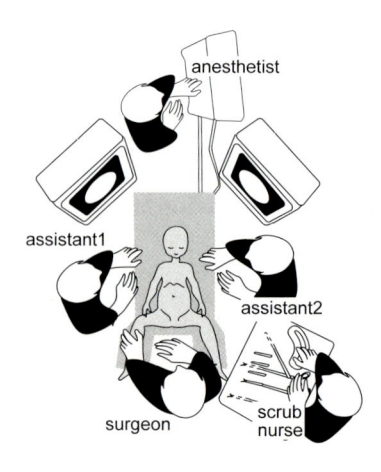

34 Endoscopic Surgery for Liver Hydatid Cysts

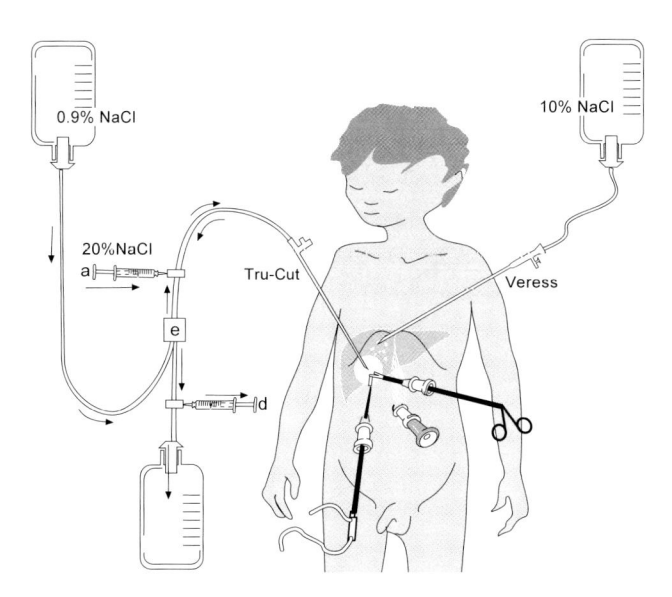

Fig. 2. Postion of the cannulae and irrigation/aspiration needles and lines

into the cyst) Tru-Cut type needle is inserted into the cyst which is then connected to a two way suction/irrigation device and two 20-ml syringes (Fig. 2).

First aspirate the contents of the cyst by a 20-ml syringe and send the sample for analysis (viable and dead scolex, proto-scolex, hooks, inflammatory cells and detritus). Inject 20 ml hypertonic 20% saline and leave for 10 min. Aspirate the contents for the second time via the syringe and send the sample for analysis (check the viability of scolex). This procedure of injection and aspiration is repeated five times. Once the cavity is completely cleared, using diathermy aided scissors, an incision is made directly over the cyst and the germinal layer of the cyst is removed. Care must be taken to keep the germinal layer intact if at all possible. Using a retrieval bag, the specimen is extracted via a cannula or cannula site (Fig. 3). (Meticulous hemostasis is essential and bile leak may be stopped by direct suturing with or without fibrin glue. If desired an omental patch may be used to obliterate the cavity left by the cyst. The abdominal cavity is irrigated with normal saline and every effort should be made to aspirate all the irrigation fluid. This maneuver can be facilitated by tilting the operating table in all four directions (head and right side of the operating table up and down). Finally, a Jackson drain is placed into the cavity via the right upper quadrant cannula site Fig. 4), the pneumoperitoneum is evacuated and the fascial/muscle defects are closed with sutures.

Fig. 3. Laparoscopic opening of the cyst with removal of the endocyst

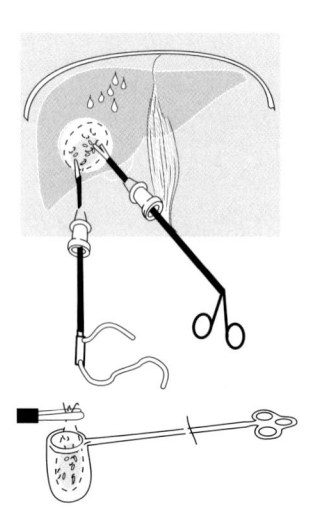

Fig. 4. Drainage of the remaining cavity

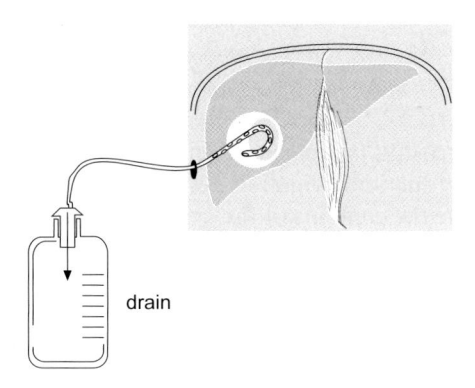

Postoperative Care

Pre- and postoperative antiparasite medication consists of mebendazole or albendazole for 30 days and is repeated at 15- to 30-day intervals for 12–14 months and 6–12 times, respectively [2–5]. The drain is removed at 24–48 h and the patient is sent home within a few days. An ultrasound scan of the liver and liver function, serological and hydatid marker tests are repeated at 6-monthly intervals [2, 3].

Personal Experience

We have treated seven children with liver hydatid cyst disease using a laparoscope. One of these children had to be converted to an open technique. This is because the patient had two separate liver cysts, one in segment two which was easily approached laparoscopically, but the other in segment seven posteriorly which could not be visualized laparoscopically. One patient had a biliary leak which resolved spontaneously after 18-day drainage. There were no other complications.

Discussion

Laparoscopic pericystectomy is a safe and effective approach in the surgical management of hydatid liver disease. We regard accessible univesicular cyst as an ideal lesion for this technique. However, multi-vesicular cysts which are usually small, calcified and located near the liver surface can by treated by complete laparoscopic resection using electro-cautery, ultrasonic cavitational device or laser [6].

As in conventional open surgery the complications of this new approach include: difficult access as in posterior and deep lesions; bleeding from the liver or dense adhesions between liver and other intra-abdominal structures; bile leak from the transected liver, site of the cyst or injury to the intra- or extrahepatic ducts; sepsis particularly in infected cyst; anaphylactic reaction or dissemination of disease from contaminated fluid and contents of the cyst.

Unlike adult patients, children very rarely develop intraductal hydatid vesicles. When cholestasis or cholangitis are suspected pre- and perioperative cholangiogram and ultrasound scan should facilitate diagnosis. If disease is demonstrated, a laparoscopic choledochotomy with or without cholecystectomy and removal of the cyst may be carried out provided the surgeon has sufficient expertise. Alternatively, a pre- or postoperative ERCP with sphincterotomy to drain the common bile duct may be performed.

As for the conventional approach, recurrent disease may be treated with a CT guided insertion of catheter, and aspiration and irrigation of the cyst for 1 week [3, 6, 7].

The surgeon must consider conversion to an open technique if preoperative investigations or laparoscopic exploration revealed a deep or posteriorly located lesion, or extensive local or perihepatic inflammation and adhesions. In these situations inaccessibility of the lesion, bleeding and bile leak can impose serious risks during the laparoscopy.

References

1. Assadourian R et al (1980) Traitment de kyste hydatique du foie. Notre attitude actuell. J Chir (Paris) 117:115–117
2. Berchi FJ (1994) Tratamiento laparoscopico del quiste hepatico en la infancia – Congreo Hispano Luso en Coimbra/Portugal, July 1994
3. Berchi FH (1994) Tratamiento endoquirurgico de la hidatidosis hepatica en la infancia. Premio Video-Med, Badajoz/Espana, Nov 1994
4. Chevis RAF (1976) Mebendazole in surgical and non-operative management of hydatid disease. Med J Aust 2:580
5. Heat DD, Chevis RAF (1974) Mebendazole and hydatid cysts. Lact II:218
6. Bret PM et al (1988) Percutaneous aspiration and drainage of hydatid cysts in the liver. Radiology 168:167–620
7. Keskin E et al (1991) Les kystes hydatiques des enfants. J Chir 128:42–44

CHAPTER 35

Laparoscopic Cholecystectomy

G.W. Holcomb III

Introduction

The modern era of laparoscopy began in 1901 when Kelling described the use of an optical instrument to explore the abdominal cavity in dogs [1]. Ten years later Jacobaeus reported using a cystoscope in humans for this purpose [2]. For the next 60 years, laparoscopy was utilized sporadically and primarily for gynecological procedures. In 1971 and 1973 Gans described the first use of this technique in children and coined the term peritoneoscopy [3, 4]. However, again, it was not utilized significantly by most pediatric surgeons until recently. In 1989 the genesis of the laparoscopic revolution was initiated with the report by Reddick and Olsen of laparoscopic cholecystectomy in 25 patients [5] and with Dubois' description in 63 patients [6]. Following these two early reports, minimally invasive surgery has been attempted for and actively supplanted many open operations.

In general, the use of laparoscopy in children has had a more gradual acceptance, likely because many of the advantages in adults such as faster return to work have not been as applicable to children. However, its utilization in the younger age group is becoming more prevalent for many straight-forward procedures such as cholecystectomy, appendectomy and recently also for complex operations such as fundoplication and pull-through procedures for Hirschsprung's disease.

This chapter describes indications for cholecystectomy in children, the preoperative preparation and operative procedure concluding with an analysis of the author's experience.

Indications

The overwhelming indication for laparoscopic cholecystectomy in children is the development of gallstones and related symptoms. Previously, in many centers, it was reported that the majority of patients with gallstones developed them secondary to hemolysis. However, the trend toward nonhemolytic cholelithiasis appears to be increasing in recent years [7–9]. The two most common hemolytic conditions responsible for gallstones are sickle-cell anemia and hereditary spherocytosis. In both conditions, hemolysis is responsible for the increased pigment load with development of pigmented gallstones. A third condition responsible for hemolytic cholelithiasis is thalassemia major. However, the incidence of gallstones in these children appears to be decreasing due to hypertransfusion therapy which blocks the bone marrow so that fragile red blood cells are no longer produced [10].

Nonhemolytic cholelithiasis may develop in children who have previously required distal ileal resection for conditions such as necrotizing enterocolitis or Crohn's disease. In this situation, cholelithiasis likely results from an interruption of the normal enterohepatic circulation with a resulting decrease in the bile salt pool, cholesterol saturation of bile followed by stone formation. Other children may develop cholelithiasis secondary to prematurity, cystic fibrosis, and prolonged fasting with or without the associated use of total parenteral nutrition (TPN). Teenage pregnancy also seems to stimulate gallstone formation. However, in many children, the development of biliary stones is idiopathic.

A less frequent condition in children which requires cholecystectomy is gallbladder dyskinesia. These youngsters usually exhibit nausea with right upper abdominal pain and demonstrate delayed gallbladder emptying on nuclear medicine studies. Several reports have confirmed the relationship between biliary dyskinesia and chronic cholecystitis in adult patients who have required cholecystectomy [11, 12]

Special Concerns in Children

It is important to emphasize several special concerns related to children when performing laparoscopic procedures in this age group. The abdominal wall of the infant and young child is very pliable and great care must be taken when introducing sharp trocars into the abdominal cavity to prevent injury to underlying viscera. It is suggested that, once the stylet has penetrated the peritoneum, the tip should be directed anteriorly away from the viscera to prevent iatrogenic injury. In my earlier experience, it was my opinion that all children, regardless of age, should have the initial cannula inserted using an umbilical cut-down approach to prevent injury with introduction of the sharp trocar, regardless of the availability of a safety shield. However, with the introduction of the Step cannula (Innerdyne Medical, Sunnyvale, CA) it appears that safe access can be obtained in children, certainly in the older ones, using the Veress needle and blunt obturator. With this approach, injury to the underlying viscera is minimized significantly.

Another concern for children is injury to the common bile duct. The common duct can be small and misidentified as the cystic duct, especially in patients with severe inflammation surrounding the gallbladder and triangle of Calot. Therefore, cholangiography is recommended to accurately identify the cystic duct and common duct prior to clip ligation of any structure. At Children's Hospital, Vanderbilt University Medical Center (CH-VUMC), the Kumar clamp and sclerotherapy needle have been used for several years in children[13]. It is a very effi-

Fig. 1. The Kumar clamp has been placed across the gallbladder infundibulum to prevent passage of dye into the body of the gallbladder and promote its flow into the cystic duct. A 23-gauge sclerotherapy needle is inserted into the infundibulum for instillation of contrast. (From [17], with permission)

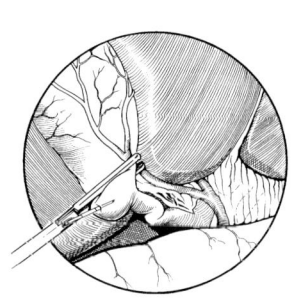

cient method for cholangiography which enables accurate anatomical delineation (Fig. 1). A secondary benefit of cholangiography is identification of unsuspected common bile duct stones; however, the incidence of such findings is infrequent in children [14].

Preoperative Preparation

Although some children, particularly teenagers with gallstones, do present with complications such as acute cholecystitis, biliary pancreatitis, or jaundice related to the stones, most do not. Therefore, for those patients undergoing elective laparoscopic cholecystectomy, it is usually performed as a 23-h admission and does not require hospital entry prior to the procedure. Patients presenting with complications are discussed below.

However, those with sickle-cell disease and cholelithiasis still require greater attention to their underlying hemolytic condition. Often, preoperative transfusion is necessary, but this may be performed as an out-patient 1–2 weeks prior to the cholecystectomy. Preoperative hydration, however, continues to be important and may require admission a day earlier for this purpose.

A thorough preoperative consultation is held with the parents and child, if age appropriate, regarding the nature of the laparoscopic procedure, the associated risks and benefits and the possible need for conversion to an open operation. Depending on the surgeon's experience, conversion to the open procedure may not be likely, but it should always be discussed prior to the laparoscopic procedure. Benefits to the patient include reduced hospitalization and minimal discomfort from the laparoscopic approach compared with the open operation [15]. In addition, a faster return to routine activities such as school or play as well as earlier participation in athletic events is also likely. A cosmetic advantage with smaller scars also exists for this approach.

Operative Technique

Positioning the surgeons and nurses is important and has become standard for both adults and children. The surgeon usually stands to the patient's left with the camera operator to his left. The assistant is usually on the patient's right side opposite the surgeon and camera operator [16].

Before induction of general anesthesia, it is important to ask the anesthesiology team to avoid vigorous insufflation of anesthetic gases into the gastrointestinal tract to prevent gastric and duodenal distention. Overinflation of the alimentary tract, especially in young children, often impairs visualization of the gallbladder during the laparoscopic procedure. Accordingly, following the induction of anesthesia, an orogastric tube is inserted for decompression. A urinary catheter is usually not placed due to the brevity of the procedure, but the bladder can be emptied with a Credé maneuver if desired. The patient is then prepped and draped in standard fashion.

Placement of the ports is individualized according to the patient's age and size. In addition, other modifications may be necessary if previous open surgical procedures have been performed.

Infants

An umbilical cut-down is strongly encouraged in infants to prevent injury to the underlying viscera and intestine with blind puncture using the Veress needle.

Following incision of the umbilical skin and fascia, the cannula is gently manipulated into the abdominal cavity and insufflation initiated. A 3-mm port is placed in the right upper abdomen and a 3- or 5-mm port is inserted in the right inguinal crease region. (Because of the infant's small size, instruments can easily reach the gallbladder in the right upper abdominal quadrant when inserted through the right inguinal crease cannula.) If cholangiography is to be attempted, the author utilizes a Kumar cholangioclamp which requires a 5-mm port and is inserted through the right lower cannula; however, if cholangiography is not necessary, a 3-mm cannula in the right inguinal crease is sufficient. The 5-mm working port is positioned in the left epigastrium (Fig. 2a). By spacing these cannulas in this configuration, there is adequate working space between ports and the operation is more efficient.

Ages 2–8

In children between 2 and 8 years of age, the gallbladder likely can be removed through a 5-mm cannula or incision; therefore, 10-mm cannulas are usually not required. A 5-mm cannula is introduced through the umbilicus. Again, a cut-down approach is suggested, especially in the younger patient, to prevent injury to the underlying structures. A 3-mm port is placed in the right upper abdomen and a 3- or 5-mm cannula inserted in the right inguinal crease region. In older patients cholangiography is usually recommended, and therefore a 5-mm cannula is preferred for the right lower port. A 5-mm cannula is located also in the left middle epigastric region (Fig. 2b).

35 Laparoscopic Cholecystectomy

Fig. 2a–c. Position of cannulas. **a** Placement of the cannulas for laparoscopic cholecystectomy in children under the age of 2 years. With placement of the cannulas in this configuration, adequate working space between ports is established. **b** In children between the ages of 2 and 8 years, an efficient operation is accomplished by placing the cannulas in a similar configuration as shown. **c** In patients between the ages of 9 and 21 years, the ports can be positioned similarly as in adults. The 10-mm port is usually placed in the umbilicus for extraction of the gallbladder

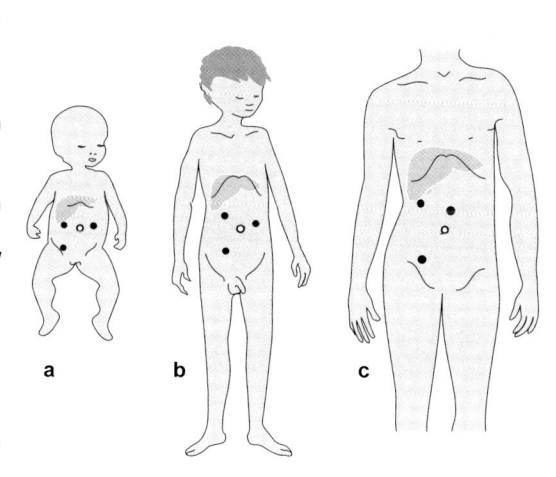

Ages 9–21

In the older patient, placement of the ports resembles the positions used by adult surgeons. Often, a 3-mm port can be used in the right upper abdomen, although with a tense distended gallbladder, usually a stronger grasping instrument is required which may entail the use of a 5-mm right upper abdominal port. The right lower port may be placed in the right inguinal crease in smaller children, but usually situated more superiorly in the older patient. In children these ages, cholangiogram is usually attempted using the Kumar clamp and sclerotherapy needle and may be introduced through the right lower port, although, on occasions, the angle of insertion is better achieved through the right upper abdominal port. In these children, it is usually necessary to use a 10-mm port for removal of the gallbladder, although this can be individualized. The umbilicus is often the best site for placement of the 10-mm incision and it can be inserted using a cut-down or Veress needle technique. The epigastric port is usually situated more toward the midline in the older children as adequate working space is easily achieved in this age group. However, 5-mm clip appliers are readily available which requires a 5-mm incision and cannula (Fig. 2c)

Laparoscopic Cholecystectomy

Following safe introduction of the cannulas, with the telescope inserted through the umbilical port, the patient is placed in reverse Trendelenburg position and tilted to the left to allow the duodenum, colon and small intestine to fall away from the area of dissection. A forceps is introduced through the right lower port, the gallbladder is grasped and rotated superiorly and ventrally over the liver, thereby exposing the infundibulum and cystic duct. A second grasping forceps

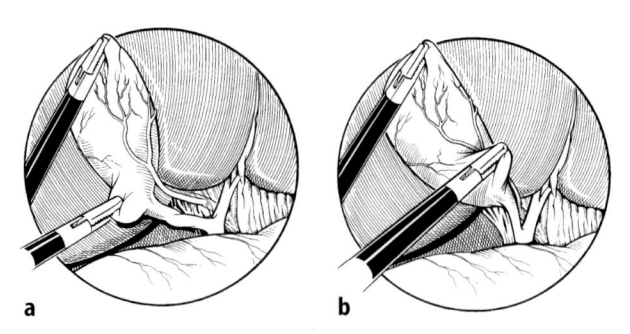

Fig. 3. a Retraction of the gallbladder infundibulum to the patient's right to create a 90° angle between the cystic and common ducts. **b** If the infundibulum is retracted superiorly, the cystic and common ducts become more parallel, which may lead to misidentification of these two structures

is introduced through the right upper port and the gallbladder is retracted laterally to the patient's right. It is important to pull the infundibulum laterally to create more of a 90° angle between the cystic duct and common bile duct. If the infundibulum is pulled superiorly, the cystic and common ducts become more parallel and misidentification of these two structures becomes more likely (Fig. 3).

Using a fine dissecting forceps inserted through the epigastric cannula, dissection should begin on the infundibulum and any adhesions lysed. Taking great care to dissect on the infundibular wall, the cystic duct is identified and dissection then proceeds along the cystic duct toward the common duct. Dissection in the triangle of Calot isolates the cystic duct, common bile duct and cystic artery. At this point, cholangiography is performed to confirm correct identification of the cystic duct. As previously mentioned, the Kumar cholangioclamp is usually inserted through the right lower port, although it may be necessary to introduce this clamp through the right upper port in selected patients. The clamp is placed across the infundibulum, thereby occluding the flow of dye into the body of the gallbladder (Fig. 1). A 23-gauge sclerotherapy needle is introduced through the side arm of the clamp and inserted into the infundibulum. Cholangiography is accomplished using fluoroscopy as this is a more time efficient technique than obtaining static images and allows a dynamic visualization of the biliary tree as the dye is introduced. The cystic duct, common hepatic, and common bile ducts are identified as dye is noted to flow into the duodenum (Fig. 4). Following successful cholangiography, the sclerotherapy needle is removed, the clamp released from the gallbladder and withdrawn from the patient. A grasping forceps is then re-introduced through this port for gallbladder retraction.

The cystic duct is then doubly clipped near the junction of the cystic and common duct. A third clip is placed on cystic duct near the infundibulum to prevent spillage of stones or bile with division of the duct (Fig. 5). The cystic duct is divided between the second and third clips. Similarly, the cystic artery is doubly clipped and divided. Retrograde dissection of the gallbladder from its liver bed is accomplished utilizing the electrocautery (Fig. 6). Either a spatula cautery,

35 Laparoscopic Cholecystectomy

Fig. 4. This cholangiogram was performed using fluoroscopy and shows the contrast material in the cystic, common hepatic, and common bile ducts. The Kumar clamp was placed across the gallbladder infundibulum to prevent dye from distending the body of the gallbladder. The 23-gauge sclerotherapy needle is seen piercing the infundibular wall (*open arrow*). Note the pancreatic duct opacification as well (*closed arrow*)

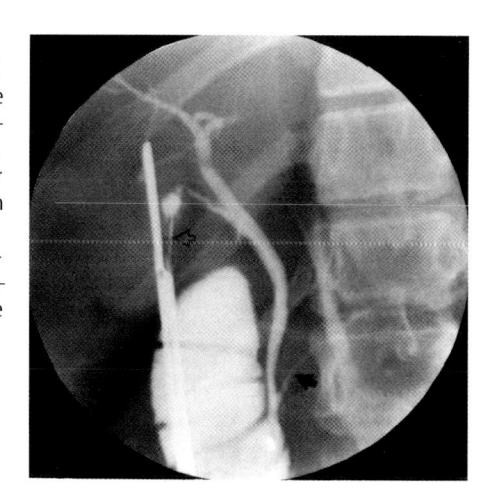

Fig. 5. Two clips have been placed on the cystic duct near the junction of the common duct. A third clip was placed on the cystic duct near the infundibulum with division between the second and third clips. In a similar fashion, the cystic artery is being divided. (From [17], with permission)

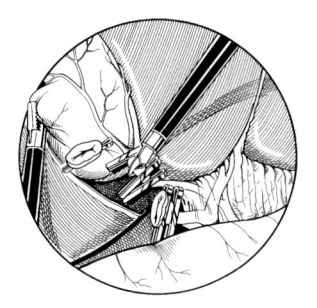

hooked cautery or scissors may be used for this purpose. Prior to almost complete detachment of the gallbladder, the area of dissection and the triangle of Calot are carefully inspected for hemostasis. Once hemostasis is verified, the gallbladder is completely detached from the liver bed and extracted through the umbilicus. As previously mentioned, in infants and young children, it can usually be removed through a 5-mm umbilical incision. In older children, a 10-mm incision is often required. With a very tense or inflamed gallbladder, it may be necessary to enlarge the fascial incision to extract the gallbladder.

Following removal of the specimen through the umbilicus, the telescope is reintroduced, the area of dissection carefully visualized again for hemostasis and as much irrigant as possible is removed. Bupivicaine is instilled into the incisions for postoperative analgesia. The cannulas are then removed. The umbilical fascia is closed with 2-0 or 3-0 absorbable suture and the umbilical skin approximated with interrupted 5-0 plain catgut suture. Attempts are made to close the anterior fascia of the 5-mm incisions with a 3-0 absorbable suture. The skin is then closed with 5-0 absorbable suture.

Fig. 6. The gallbladder is dissected from it's liver bed in a retrograde fashion utilizing the electrocautery. Either a spatula cautery, hook cautery or scissors may be used for this purpose. (From [17], with permission)

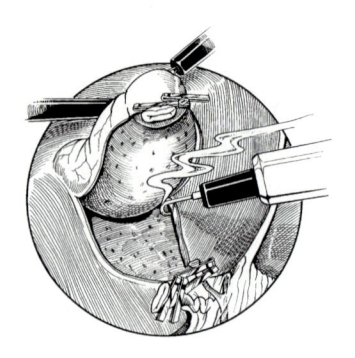

Postoperatively, a clear liquid diet is initiated and oral analgesics administered as needed. Occasionally, an intravenous narcotic is required once or twice, but oral analgesics are usually sufficient. The patients are often discharged the following morning and return for a postoperative examination in 2 weeks. An occasional patient may be discharged the day of the surgery.

Choledocholithiasis

Complications related to cholelithiasis include acute cholecystitis, choledocholithiasis and biliary pancreatitis. Ultrasound examination is the best and most cost-efficient initial modality to evaluate suspected choledocholithiasis. If documented, and assuming there is not an indication for an emergency biliary decompressive procedure, a brief period of supportive care is warranted. Management of choledocholithiasis in the laparoscopic era has gradually evolved into what presently appears to be three possible strategies for the patient with suspected choledocholithiasis:

- A preoperative endoscopic retrograde cholangiopancreatogram (ERCP) confirms the presence of common duct stones. If present, retrieval of the stones at ERCP and/or endoscopic sphincterotomy/papillotomy are possible with decompression of the biliary tree. If successful, the patient may then undergo laparoscopic cholecystectomy. If this approach is utilized, a nasobiliary catheter should be positioned by the endoscopist for intraoperative cholangiography at the time of laparoscopic cholecystectomy. Clips are placed on the cystic duct and, prior to division of the cystic duct, operative cholangiography is performed via the nasobiliary catheter to confirm the correct anatomy (Fig. 7).
- Laparoscopic cholecystectomy and laparoscopic cholangiography are performed in the standard fashion. If residual stones remain in the common duct, laparoscopic choledochal exploration and retrieval of the stones are performed, assuming an experienced laparoscopic surgeon is available. If not experienced in laparoscopic exploration of the common duct, the laparoscopic procedure may be terminated following cholecystectomy and a postoperative ERCP with sphincterotomy/papillotomy performed. The only disadvan-

Fig. 7. This operative cholangiogram was performed using a nasobiliary catheter (*open arrow*) which was inserted at the time of endoscopic retrograde cholangiopancreatography. The cholangiogram was performed following clip ligation of the cystic duct, but prior to division of this duct. As can be seen, a fairly long cystic duct stump is visualized (*closed arrow*), and clip ligation of the duct was then performed closer to the common bile duct. (Reprinted with permission [15])

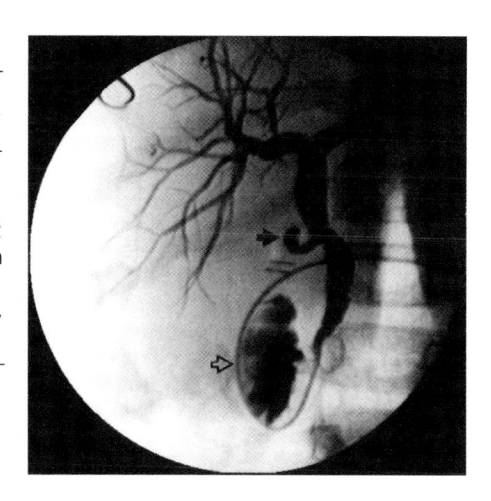

tage of this approach is the dilemma about how to proceed if the ERCP is not successful in clearing the common duct. Another option would be conversion to an open operation for choledochal exploration.
- If neither an experienced laparoscopic surgeon nor endoscopist is available, an open cholecystectomy and choledochal exploration is the third option for this problem.

The author favors preoperative ERCP with sphincterotomy for patients with strongly suspected or documented choledocholithiasis by ultrasound. Experience with this option has been recently reported [14]. The major advantage with this approach is knowing prior to the laparoscopic cholecystectomy whether laparoscopic common duct exploration is likely to be required. However, the major disadvantage is the possibility of unnecessary performance of an ERCP in a few patients when no stones are found.

Finding unsuspected choledocholithiasis in children undergoing elective cholecystectomy is unusual. In a recently presented report of 131 patients with cholelithiasis not suspected of having common duct stones, only one was found to have choledocholithiasis with laparoscopic cholangiography [14].

Personal Experience

The first pediatric laparoscopic cholecystectomy was performed by the author in June 1990. Since then, 72 children have undergone laparoscopic cholecystectomy. Sixty-six had an elective procedure with a mean hospitalization of 1 day (Table 1). Six patients received laparoscopic cholecystectomy following admission to the hospital for complications such as acute cholecystitis, choledocholithiasis and biliary pancreatitis. The laparoscopic procedure was performed 4 days (mean) following admission and the patients were discharged 2 days (mean) postoperatively.

Table 1. Children undergoing elective laparoscopic cholecystectomy at Children's Hospital, Vanderbilt University Medical Center (n=66) 1990–1996

Ages	25 months–18 years
Mean age	11.3 years
Male/female	26/40
Hemolytic disease	13
Sickle cell disease	9
Hereditary spherocytosis	2
Pyruvate kinase deficiency	2
Operative time (mean)	102 min
Cholangiography	52
Kumar clamp	44
Cystic duct incision	6
Nasobiliary catheter	2

In the elective group of 66 patients, laparoscopic cholangiography was attempted in 60 patients and successful in 52. Techniques for cholangiography included cystic duct incision and catheter placement (6), Kumar cholangiography (44) and nasobiliary catheter cholangiography (2) following ERCP. In this series, no complications have occurred. No patient has developed a wound infection, a cystic duct stump leak, hemorrhage requiring transfusion or need for re-operation. In addition, there were no injuries to the abdominal viscera related to introduction of the ports. Also, there were no injuries to the common bile duct.

References

1. Kelling G (1901) Über Oesophagoskopie und Kolioskopie. Munch Med Wochenschr 49:21–24
2. Jacobaeus HC (1911) Kurze Übersicht über meine Erfahrungen mit der Laparo-thorakoskopie. Munch Med Wochenschr 5:2017–2019
3. Gans SL, Berci G (1971) Advances in endoscopy of infants and children. J Pediatr Surg 6:199–234
4. Gans SL, Berci G (1973) Peritoneoscopy in infants and children. J Pediatr Surg 8:399–405
5. Reddick EJ, Olsen DO (1989) Laparoscopic laser cholecystectomy: A comparison with minilap cholecystectomy. Surg Endosc 3:131–133
6. Dubois F, Berthelot G, Levard H (1989) Cholecystectomie par coelioscopie. Presse Med 18:980–982
7. Reif S, Sloven DG, Lebenthal E (1991) Gallstones in children. Am J Dis Child 145:105–298
8. Holcomb GW Jr et al (1980) Cholecystitis, cholelithiasis and common duct stenosis in children and adolescents. Ann Surg 191:626–635
9. Bailey PV et al (1989) Changing spectrum of cholelithiasis and cholecystitis in infants and children. Am J Surg 158:585–586

10. Borgna-Pignatti C et al (1981) Cholelithiasis in children with thalassemia major: an ultrasonographic study. J Pediatr 99:243–244
11. Brugge WR et al (1986) Gallbladder dyskinesia in chronic acalculous cholecystitis. Dig Dis Sci 31:461–467
12. Misra DC et al (1991) Results of surgical therapy for biliary dyskinesia. Arch Surg 126:957–960
13. Holzman MD et al (1994) An alternative technique for laparoscopic cholangiography. Surg Endosc 8:927–930
14. Newman KD, Powell DM, Holcomb GW III (1997) The management of choledocholithiasis in children in the era of laparoscopic cholecystectomy. J Pediatr Surg 32:1120–1123
15. Holcomb GW III et al (1994) Laparoscopic cholecystectomy in infants and children: modifications and cost analysis. J Pediatr Surg 29:900–904
16. Holcomb GW III (1993) Laparoscopic cholecystectomy. Semin Pediatr Surg 2:159–167
17. Holcomb GW III (1994) Diagnostic laparoscopy: equipment, technique and special concerns in children. In: George W, Holcomb GW III (eds) Pediatric endoscopic surgery. Appleton and Lange, Norwalk

Part III
Abdomen

Spleen

CHAPTER 36

Laparoscopic Splenectomy

W.R. Thompson, E. Parra-Davila

Introduction

Splenectomy remains an important therapeutic option in children with a variety of hematological and immunological disorders. For conditions in which the immunological or filtering functions of the spleen lead to anemia, thrombocytopenia or altered white cell function removal of the spleen is often desirable. Pain related to capsular stretch, cyst formation abscess and torsion can also be addressed surgically. Potential disadvantages of the procedure include surgical and anesthetic morbidity, abdominal wall scarring, and the lifelong risk of postsplenectomy sepsis. These concerns have appropriately limited indications for splenectomy to cases in which medical therapy is impractical or no longer effective.

In an attempt to reduce the morbidity related to surgery, minimally invasive techniques have been applied in the pediatric population. Laparoscopic splenectomy offers the opportunity for less postoperative discomfort, less restriction of activity, shorter hospitalization and near elimination of wound complications. Laparoscopic splenectomy was first reported in animal models in 1990. The procedure was rapidly introduced into clinical practice, with the first adult patients reported in 1992 (Thibaulat et al. 1992). Pediatric series have appeared only recently. The surgeon, pediatrician and hematologist should be aware of the comparisons between the open and laparoscopic approaches in order to knowledgeably advise their patients who require splenectomy.

Knowledge of splenic vascular anatomy is critical to success of the minimally invasive approach (Poulin and Thibault 1993). Figure 1 shows the two common types of arterial distribution. Proximal branching is more common and is associated with a lobulated capsule. The upper pole vessel may be difficult to visualize. It must be controlled separately if the artery is interrupted distal to the bifurcation. Proximal control of the vessels at the mid portion of the pancreas greatly reduces the potential for hemorrhage and speeds the operation. Several clinical series indicate that laparoscopic removal of the spleen can be safely and effectively accomplished without jeopardizing long held surgical tenets (Beanes et al. 1995; Farah et al. 1997; Gigot et al. 1996, Hicks et al. 1996; Rothenberg 1996)

Fig. 1a,b. Dominant patterns of splenic vasculature. Proximal branching of the main vessels is more common and is associated with capsular lobulation

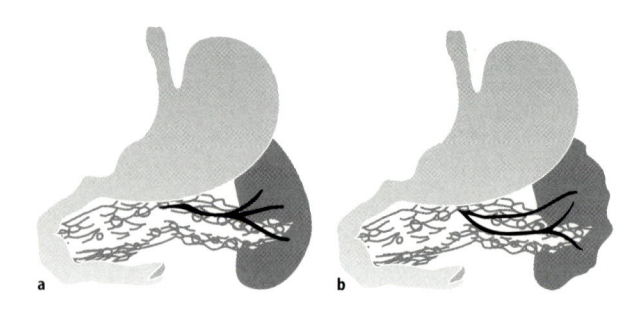

Indications

Examples of conditions for which laparoscopic splenectomy may be useful are listed below:
- Immune thrombocytopenic purpura
- Hereditary spherocytosis
- Sickle cell disease
- Thalassemia
- Hemolytic anemia
- Felty's syndrome
- Wiskott-Aldrich syndrome
- Myeloid Metaplasia
- Leukemia
- Hodgkin's lymphoma
- Primary and secondary hypersplenism
- AIDS-related thrombocytopenia
- Gaucher's disease
- Ectopic spleen
- Splenic cyst
- Sarcoidosis

Relative contraindications include:
- High risk for general anesthesia
- Coagulopathy or history of excessive bleeding
- Massive splenomegaly
- Portal hypertension
- Splenic abscess
- Posttraumatic rupture

Open splenectomy is preferable when extensive collateral vascularization is encountered or when the patient's general condition makes abdominal insufflation and prolonged anesthesia hazardous.

Preoperative Workup

When appropriate indications for splenectomy have been established, including failure of response to medical therapy, additional steps should be taken in preparation for the procedure. These include measures to optimize coagulation status and prevent infectious complications. In selected patients a preoperative search for accessory spleens may be prudent:
- Type and crossmatch for one unit of autologous or donor blood
- Investigate coagulation status. If indicated by diagnosis or history bleeding time, platelet count, PT and PTT should be ordered.
- Patients with immune thrombocytopenia may receive high-dose IgG (400 mg/kg daily for 4–5 days) or intravenous steroids before the procedure. The resulting temporary boost in platelet count may obviate the need for perioperative platelet transfusion.
- Polyvalent pneumococcal, *Haemophilus*, and meningococcal vaccines should be administered to reduce the risk of overwhelming postsplenectomy sepsis. Vaccination is recommended at least 2 weeks prior to the procedure.
- Routine perioperative antibiotics should be used.
- If the patient has received prolonged steroid therapy perioperative steroids should be administered to prevent stress related adrenal insufficiency.
- Transfusion of platelets is seldom necessary if platelet count is 20,000/ml or greater and platelet function is normal. If bleeding time is relatively normal transfusion can usually be avoided. If oozing is noted intraoperatively platelets can be administered at that time. However, if routine platelet transfusion is planned they should be given immediately prior to induction of anesthesia in order to minimize the risk of laryngeal hematoma during insertion of the endotracheal tube.
- Splenic artery embolization may be considered in obese patients.

Preoperative Preparation

As is true with most advanced laparoscopic procedures, splenectomy is greatly facilitated by careful attention to operating room set up.

Positioning Patient. After induction of general anesthesia, an orogastric tube is placed and the bladder is decompressed with a Foley catheter or via the Credé maneuver. The patient is positioned supine, with the left side elevated 30°–45° (Fig. 2a). A "bean bag" positioning pad is useful in maintaining a stable posture while the table is rotated to optimize exposure. The patient is secured to the table with straps or heavy tape as well. The left arm should be supported as well to prevent hyperextension of the shoulder. The legs are placed together, gently flexed. Intermittent compression stockings should be considered for patients at increased risk for deep vein thrombosis. For the alternative "lateral" technique the same principles apply, with the exception of modified right lateral decubitus

Fig. 2a,b. Position of the patient, and ports. **a** Patient and port positions for supine approach. The left side is moderately elevated. Operating ports allow perpendicular orientation of the instruments at the hilum. **b** Patient and port positions for lateral approach. The patient is placed in a true lateral decubitus position. The flank port is placed after internal mobilization of the splenic flexure

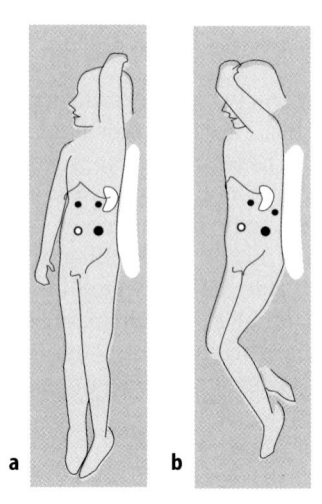

position (Fig. 2b). Wide skin preparation and secure sterile drapes are required, since conversion to open splenectomy may be required.

Position of Surgeon and Staff. The operating team is positioned to allow clear view of the field and monitors. The surgeon, the laparoscope, the splenic hilum and the monitor should form a straight line. Assistants and scrub technicians should not interfere with bimanual operation by the surgeon. Suggested room setup is demonstrated in Fig. 3.

Position of Monitor and Cables. The primary monitor is placed near the patient's left shoulder, perpendicular to the surgeon. Light cords, camera cables and insufflation tubing can be passed off the table together along the most cephalad portion of the field. This provides the least restriction of movement to the surgeon and all important camera operator. A second monitor may help the assistant and technician see more easily but is mandatory only if cholecystectomy is to be performed as well (Fig. 3).

Position of Ports. Laparoscopic splenectomy can usually be completed with four ports (Fig. 2 a). Suggested port positions for the lateral approach are shown in Fig. 2b. With either approach, at least one large port is required for extraction of the specimen. A 12-mm port is preferred since it can be used for clip applier, stapler and extraction. A 10-mm camera port is helpful in larger patients or when equipment requires more light delivery to provide a good image.

Specific Instrumentation. A selection of good dissectors, graspers and scissors is required for delicate dissection around large vessels. Needle drivers and tying devices should also be on the field. Both 0° and 30° laparoscopes should be available, though often only one is required. High pressure irrigation and good suction are useful, particularly in the event of hemorrhage and for extraction of large clots. A 5-mm fan retractor allows safe displacement of the colon and stom-

Fig. 3. Position of the crew and equipment. The surgeon, the telescope, the splenic hilum and the monitor form a straight line

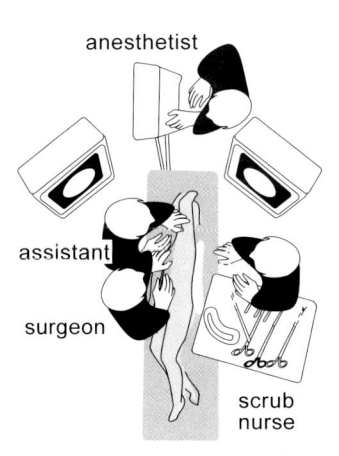

ach. A clip applier or linear stapler is required to divide large vessels, potentially the only disposable instruments required. The ultrasonic scalpel may also be useful for division of short gastric vessels and peritoneal attachments, although cautery works well in most cases. A strong specimen bag large enough to accommodate the spleen is necessary. Commercially available bags are available and should be evaluated in advance. Finally, a morcellator to break up the spleen into pieces small enough to extract through the 12-mm port site is necessary. A specific device which is powered and vacuum assisted is available. However, finger fracture and extraction with ring forceps is simple and effective.

Technique

The abdomen is insufflated through an incision at the umbilicus using open or closed insertion technique. A pressure of 15 mmHg should be well tolerated in most children. Good muscle relaxation is critical to allow easy ventilation and provide sufficient space within the abdominal cavity for exposure. The abdomen must be carefully explored to evaluate for other pathology and the presence of accessory spleens. Special attention to the omentum, gastrocolic ligament and splenocolic ligament is required.

Two major approaches have emerged for division of splenic vasculature and peritoneal attachments. The supine approach and lateral approach are best described separately.

Supine Approach

Application of the classical open surgical sequence to laparoscopic splenectomy is often referred to as the supine approach. The splenic artery and vein are controlled proximally and early in the procedure. With the table in reverse Trendelenburg and the left side elevated dissection begins. The spleen is exposed by

Fig. 4. Sequence of mobilization in the supine approach: *1*, division of the gastrosplenic ligament and short gastric vessels; *2*, interruption of the main splenic artery and vein; *3*, division of peritoneal attachments and hilum

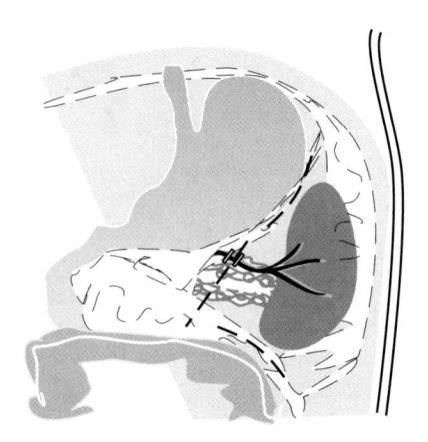

downward traction on the colon and medial retraction of the greater curvature of the stomach. Gravity holds the colon inferiorly. The lesser sac is entered through the gastrocolic ligament about the midpoint of the greater curvature. The branches of the left gastroepiploic and short gastric vessels are divided to completely separate the stomach and spleen. These vessels can be divided between clips but cautery or ultrasonic harmonic scalpel is quicker and equally secure. A fan retractor inserted through the left upper quadrant port is used to elevate the stomach and open the lesser sac.

The splenic artery pulsation is identified along the superior margin of the pancreas. Using Maryland dissectors the splenic artery is carefully exposed and clipped. The vein is located just inferior and deep to the artery. It is dissected and clipped in an identical manner (Fig. 4). It is not necessary to divide the vessels. With the short gastric and splenic vessels interrupted, the spleen is "dead on the vine" and can be safely handled with little risk of bleeding from the capsule or hilum. Similar to the gastrosplenic ligament, the hilum can be divided between clips, with cautery or by the ultrasonic scalpel. A simple ligature around the final vessel may provide an additional measure of comfort. The peritoneal attachments are divided with the hilum as exposure allows. The fan retractor is used to manipulate the spleen, providing traction.

Sequential division of hilar vessels without proximal interruption of blood-flow is sometimes described but this can be tedious and is often associated with bleeding from the hilum or splenic capsule. A linear cutting stapler facilitates this approach.

Lateral Approach

The lateral approach differs in that the patient is placed in a true lateral decubitus position. More importantly, division of the splenic vasculature occurs much later in the procedure. Exposure is excellent with small to moderate sized spleens because the stomach and colon fall away by gravity and require no retraction (Park et al. 1997).

After placement of anterior ports, the splenic flexure of the colon is mobilized and a 5-mm port placed midway between the iliac crest and the 12th rib under direct vision. After a search for accessory spleens is conducted the spleen is partially mobilized (Fig. 4). The peritoneal attachments, the splenorenal ligament and splenocolic ligament are divided leaving the organ suspended by only a 1-cm cuff of lateral peritoneal reflection. Through the lumbar port, the peritoneum is grasped to retract the spleen medially. Dissection of the splenic hilum is approached from the lower pole and continued in a cephalad progression. Branches of the artery and vein are divided between clips or with the linear cutting stapler. Because early branching is common a separate lower pole vessel is often encountered. Division of the hilum allows entry to the lesser sac and exposure of the short gastric vessels. When these vessels are divided, the spleen can be manipulated into the specimen bag. It may be helpful to leave some upper pole attachments of the splenophrenic ligament while manipulating the bag.

Extracting the Spleen

Most surgeons find that placing the detached spleen into a specimen bag is the most challenging and frustrating part of the laparoscopic procedure. Patience and persistence is required. With small soft spleens, a bag with a supporting ring at its mouth and an attached handle allows the surgeon to "scoop" the organ. However, the size and strength of these bags is limited. Larger, stronger bags require a more complex technique. Perhaps the most successful approach is to place the spleen in the pelvis and position the bag in the splenic bed. It may be introduced through one of the larger port sites after temporary removal of the port. Partially filling the bag with irrigation fluid reduces surface tension and helps keep the bag open during manipulation. Graspers are then used to hold the anterior and posterior walls of the bag's mouth widely separated. With the bag in proper position, the table is placed in Trendelenburg position. The spleen can then be grasped by its hilum or capsule and placed into the bag. An umbilical tape tied loosely around the middle portion of the spleen aids in manipulation of softer organs.

Figure 5 depicts optimal positioning of the specimen bag. The graspers on the bag are used to pull the bag over the spleen and to keep its mouth open. With the drawstring closed the bag is then pulled through the port site. The bag is opened and the spleen extracted in fragments with a specially designed morcellator or with ring forceps after digital fracture. Good upward tension on the bag is critical to keep the spleen near the port site and prevent damage to the bag from forceps or morcellator blades. If digital fracture of the spleen is used the fascia may need to be enlarged to 12 mm to allow introduction of the index finger. The capsule should be fractured in pieces 2–3 cm wide. Several cycles of alternating digital fracture and extraction are required for most spleens and frequent suctioning of blood released from the spleen should be anticipated. Figure 6 demonstrates extraction after digital morcellation.

Fig. 5. The spleen is placed in a specimen bag using the hilum or an umbilical tape as a handle

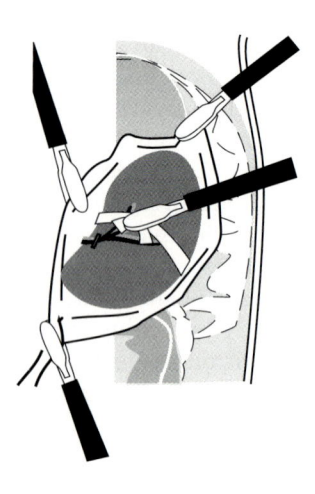

Fig. 6. The spleen is extracted with ring forceps after finger fracture of the capsule

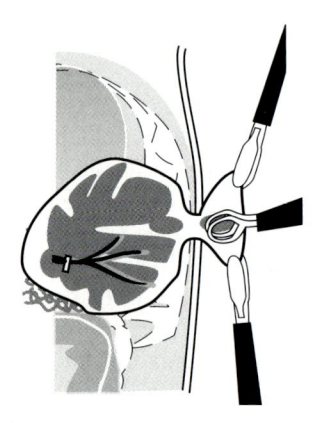

After irrigation and confirmation of hemostasis, carbon dioxide is evacuated and the port sites are closed. The orogastric tube is removed prior to extubation.

Helpful Hints

- The gastrosplenic ligament is placed on tension by anterior retraction of the stomach.
- The splenocolic ligament is exposed by downward traction on the colon.
- Gentle caudal retraction on the tail of the pancreas exposes hilar vessels.
- Anticipate branches of the splenic vessels
- The retrieval bag should be opened toward the telescope and triangulated.
- Grasp the spleen by firm connective tissue or place a tape around it to provide a handle.
- Change table position and angle as often as necessary to take advantage of gravity in retraction and manipulation of the spleen.

- When combined cholecystectomy is planned, it should follow the splenectomy since compromise of port position is possible with the simpler procedure.

Postoperative Care

Though infiltration of bupivicaine at the port sites may reduce the need for postoperative analgesia, intravenous narcotics are useful for the first 24 h. Admission is prudent for all patients since postoperative hemorrhage would have devastating consequences. Early ambulation, incentive spirometry and adequate hydration are important, particularly in patients with sickle cell disease who are prone to "chest syndrome" from atelectasis and intrapulmonary sickling.

Daily oral penicillin prophylaxis is recommended, particularly in children. The patient and his family should be aware of concerns regarding postsplenectomy sepsis. Risk in patients with nonmalignant hematological conditions is 2% or less. Death rate for affected patients is 2%–10%.

Personal Experience

Both descriptive and comparative series of laparoscopic splenectomy in pediatric patients yield remarkably consistent results. In exchange for somewhat greater cost and longer operating times, improved cosmesis, decreased pain and shorter hospitalization are achieved. Our own series demonstrated significant prolongation of both operating and anesthesia times, with means between 2 and 3 h. Estimated blood loss was similar, 74 ml in the laparoscopic group and 78 ml in the open group. The duration of postoperative analgesia and postoperative hospital stay were significantly shorter in the laparoscopic group. Patients in the laparoscopic group had 32 h less of postoperative analgesia and were discharged 1.4 days earlier than those who underwent open splenectomy ($p<0.005$ and $p<0.01$, respectively). Of the patients in the laparoscopic group 93% resumed regular diet during the first 2 postoperative days while only 25% of patients in the open group were able to do so. The overall complication rate was similar, 31% in the laparoscopic group and 40% in the open group. The most common complications were pulmonary (pneumonia, atelectasis, chest syndrome). The need for transfusion was less in the laparoscopic group. No infections occurred (Farah et al. 1997).

Mean spleen weight was 218 g compared to average adult spleen weight of 150 g. Weight in the laparoscopic group is certainly understated since a significant amount of blood is removed with suction during extraction and not sent to pathology. The specimens in the laparoscopic group were deemed adequate for pathological interpretation.

Although the mean operating room charges were higher in the laparoscopic group (primarily related to increased time), total hospital charges were not significantly different between the groups. Cost can be reduced by use of reusable instruments. Hematological results were comparable, though fewer accessory spleens were identified in the patients undergoing laparoscopic splenectomy.

Discussion

Compared with open splenectomy, laparoscopic splenectomy requires more operating room time but is associated with similar cost, blood loss and complication rates. The minimally invasive approach appears to be superior with regard to duration of postoperative analgesia, length of hospital stay and return of bowel function. Cosmetic superiority of the laparoscopic approach is obvious, particularly when cholecystectomy is also contemplated. Attention to details of patient positioning and operative approach greatly simplify the procedure.

Though hematological results have been excellent, long-term follow-up is required to determine whether laparoscopic exploration is equivalent in detection of significant accessory spleens. Both scintigraphy and CT may be useful in selected patients. CT is 75% sensitive with accessory spleens over 10 mm in diameter. Scintigraphy is less sensitive but is inexpensive and may guide exploration. Careful visualization of the omentum and ligaments must be a part of each laparoscopic splenectomy.

In patients for whom a modest prolongation of the procedure is acceptable, laparoscopic splenectomy is an attractive option. However, since the risk of serious infection is not reduced by variation of technique, splenectomy should be avoided if other treatment alternatives are available or if the underlying disorder has little impact on the patient's quality of life.

References

Beanes S et al (1995) A comparison of laparoscopic versus open splenectomy in children. Am Surg 61:908–910

Farah RA et al (1997) Comparison of laparoscopic and open splenectomy in children with hematologic disorders [see comments]. J Pediatr 131: 41–6

Gigot JF et al (1996) Laparoscopic splenectomy in adults and children. Experience with 31 patients. Surgery 119(4):384–389

Hicks BA et al (1996) Laparoscopic splenectomy in childhood hematologic disorders. J Laparoendosc Surg 6 [Suppl 1]:S31–S34

Park A, Gagner M, Pomp A (1997) The lateral approach to laparoscopic splenectomy. Am J Surg 173:126–130

Poulin EC, Thibault C (1993) The anatomical basis for laparoscopic splenectomy. Can J Surg 36:585–590

Rothenberg SS (1996) Laparoscopic splenectomy using the harmonic scalpel. J Laparoendosc Surg 6 [Suppl 1]:S61–S63

Thibaulat C et al (1992) Laparoscopic splenectomy: operative technique and preliminary report. Surg Laparosc Endosc 2:248–253

Part III
Abdomen

Diaphragm

Laparoscopic Repair of Diaphragmatic Conditions in Infants and Children

D.C. van der Zee, N.M.A. Bax, J-S. Valla

Introduction

The diaphragm, which is the muscular septum between thoracic and abdominal cavity, can be approached either by the thoracic or the abdominal route. Usually, in conventional open surgery, the thoracic approach is better for right-sided diseases because the liver is in the way if a transabdominal approach is used; a transabdominal approach is preferred for anterior and left-sided conditions. Even after the recent advances in endoscopic surgery, this rule has not been changed or superseded. The thoracoscopic approach has been described for the diagnosis and treatment of right-sided diaphragmatic disorders (Yamashita et al. 1996). We present here the laparoscopic approach for anterior and left-sided diaphragmatic disorders in children, such as congenital or traumatic hernia or eventration.

Left-Sided Hernia

Indications

Congenital diaphragmatic hernia often presents as a neonatal emergency with respiratory distress due to lung hypoplasia. Sometimes symptomatology is much milder and occasionally symptoms start only after a long, relatively symptom-free interval (Anderson 1986; Schimpl et al. 1993; Weber et al. 1991). Therapy consists of respiratory and hemodynamic support and closure of the defect. In neonates it is often advantageous to restore the dome of the diaphragm (Bax and Collins 1984), but in older children this is usually not necessary. With the development of pediatric minimal invasive techniques, these techniques may be applicable in children with delayed presentation of congenital diaphragmatic hernia (Newman et al. 1995; Van der Zee and Bax 1995) and who have no pulmonary restriction and are therefore less sensitive for the consequences of CO_2 uptake. On the other hand neonates with respiratory distress and lung hypoplasia are not candidates for the laparoscopic approach as CO_2 uptake during laparoscopy may be detrimental for the child with pulmonary hypertension and return to fetal circulation.

Preoperative Workup

The children usually have a symptom-free interval and more often than not the respiratory distress is initially attributed to a pulmonary infection. X-ray of the thorax, however, demonstrates the existence of a diaphramgatic hernia. There may or may not be a hernia sac present. In children with a delayed onset of symptoms the stomach usually retains its normal position, as may be seen by the normal position of the gastric tube. Ultrasound may indicate the presence of the spleen in the hernia. The further contents usually consist of small and large intestines. Contrast studies generally are not necessary. All children should receive a nasogastric tube for decompression. Blood-gas sampling is mandatory to determine the general circulatory and respiratory condition of the child. Only children who are stable in cardiorespiratory terms are candidates for a laparoscopic approach.

Technique

The patient is placed on a short table in a supine position with a tilt under the left side (Fig. 1). The legs of the patient are placed in a frog position and held by a turned-up table sheet that prevents the patient from sliding from the table when tilting the table. The surgeon stands at the lower end of the table with the assistant on his left and the scrub nurse on his right. The monitor is at the left upper side of the patient (Fig. 2). The first 5-mm trocar is placed through the inferior umbilical fold using an open procedure. CO_2 is insufflated into the abdominal cavity with a maximum of 0.5 l/min flow and 6 mmHg pressure under close anesthesiological monitoring. When it is ascertained that CO_2 insufflation has no negative effect on the child's circulation and respiration, a 5-mm endoscope is introduced. The second trocar is placed under direct vision in an imaginary line of incision in the left subcostal space and the third trocar placed under the xiphoid (Fig. 1), and the table is turned in a more right lateral and reversed Trendelenburg position. The spleen, when not in the defect, has no diaphragmatic attachments and is easily displaced medially, giving clear access to the defect. The defect is usually ovoid in shape.

Fig. 1. Left-sided diaphragmatic hernia. Position of the patient and of the cannulae. The patient is placed on a short table in a supine position with a tilt under the left side. Slight reversed Trendelenburg. The first cannula to hold the scope is inserted in an open way through the inferior umbilical fold. The working cannulae are placed subcostally, one on the left, and one under the xyphoid.

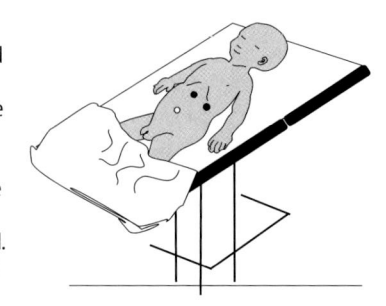

37 Laparoscopic Repair of Diaphragmatic Conditions in Infants and Children

Fig. 2. Left-sided diaphragmatic hernia. Position of the patient, crew, and equipment

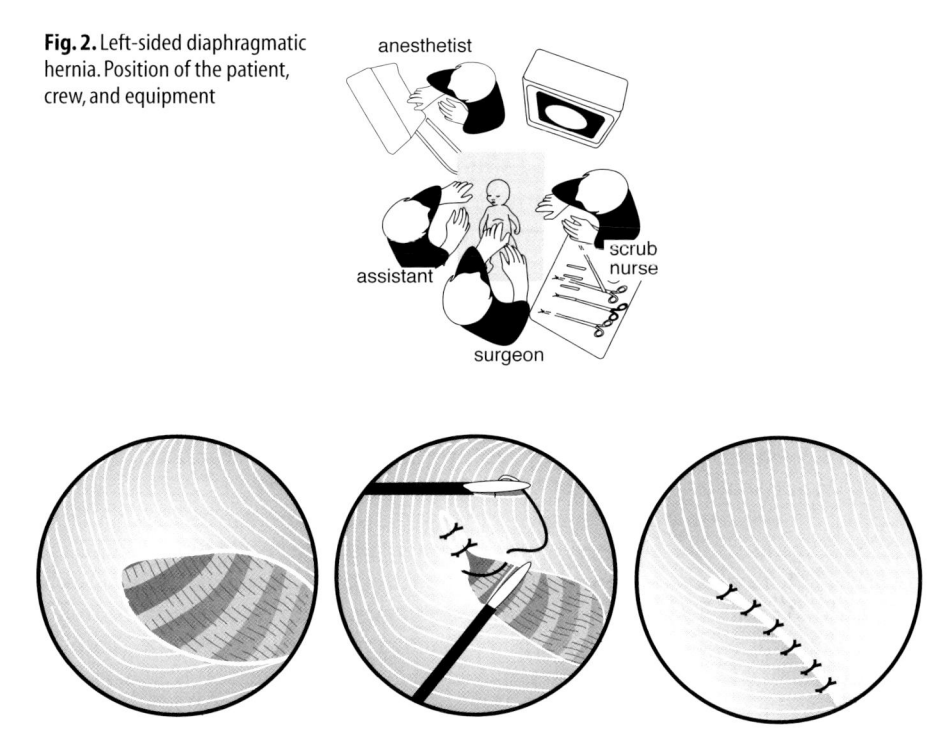

Fig. 3. Endoscopic view of a left-sided diaphragmatic defect. Closure with interrupted sutures, knotted intra-abdominally

Under close monitoring of respiratory conditions the intestines can be retrieved from the thoracic cavity using two forceps. When the spleen is in the defect it can be pulled out of the thorax, taking care not to tear the capsule. When a hernia sac is present, a small opening is made to create a pneumothorax to allow the diaphragm to come down. After incision of the peritoneal reflection of the defect, the diaphragmatic hernia can be closed with interrupted nonabsorbable sutures, using the internal knot-tying technique (Fig. 3). In case of a larger defect, a patch can be used. Trocars are retrieved under direct endoscopic vision and the defects are closed with absorbable sutures and the skin with adhesive bands. Retained air is aspirated from the left thoracic cavity.

Personal Experience

In four instances we have approached a left-sided Bochdalek defect via the laparoscopic route. In two children, aged 4 and 6 months, we were able to close the defect laparoscopically, without the use of a patch. In two other children we converted to an open procedure. One child was only 3 weeks old and proved to be too small to have the procedure performed laparoscopically. Although the child endured the procedure well, the abdominal cavity was too small for both retrieving the intestines and leaving sufficient space for the working instruments to present the defect for closure. After conversion, half of the intestines were still in the thoracic cavity. The defect was closed with the use of a patch. The second child was a five-month-old boy where, in addition to small and large intestine, the spleen was in the thoracic cavity attached to the retroperitoneal reflection of the peritoneum. Although the spleen could be brought into the abdominal cavity we were unable to divide the peritoneal reflection, which lay directly behind the spleen. The spleen is vulnerable and laceration should be avoided. After several attempts the procedure was converted and the spleen could be liberated and the defect closed directly.

Discussion

The laparoscopic approach for repair of congenital diaphragmatic hernia is definitely not suitable for pulmonary compromised neonates, but in the somewhat bigger and older infant with delayed onset of symptoms it may provide a new approach of minimal invasive repair of diaphragmatic defects. The procedure is, however, not simple and requires great manual dexterity on the part of the surgical team. We only have experience with left-sided defects approached from the ventral abdominal side. A left-lateral approach gives a better exposure (Fig. 4). Choosing a laparoscopic approach requires insufflation of the abdominal cavity with CO_2, which causes an ipsilateral pneumothorax through the diaphragmatic defect when no hernia sac is present. When using only low pressures of maximal 5 mmHg the risk of adverse effects is minimized. The laparoscopic approach has the advantage of easy reposition of intestines into the abdominal cavity. When the child is small and the intestines have been in the thoracic cavity since or before birth, however, retrieval into abdomen may render difficulties in those cases where the abdominal cavity is (too) small. The repositioning of the spleen may also sometimes be more difficult, while lesions and bleeding should be avoided at all costs. The closure of the defect, especially when there is little tissue left around the posterolateral aspect of the defect, may be easier from the abdominal side. Most defects in patients with delayed onset of symptoms may be closed directly. Closure with the use of a patch, however, is possible. This technique can also be used in cases of posttraumatic diaphragmatic hernia (Ugazzi and Chirigoba 1996).

Fig. 4. Left-sided diaphragmatic defect. Alternative position of the patient and the cannulae. The patient has a more left lateral decubitus position. The cannulae are inserted according to the triangle principle: the working cannulae subcostally in the anterior and posterior axillary line, the scope more distally

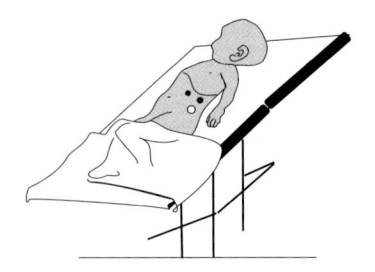

Anterior Hernia Through Foramen of Morgagni

Preoperative Workup

The retrosternal hernia is a rare congenital defect, constituting 2%–5% of all diaphragmatic hernias. Symptomatology is often mild, and the hernia is often discovered when an air-fluid level is noted in the anterior lower mediastinum on routine chest X-ray. Associated malformations are frequent.

Technique

The position of the patient, crew and equipment is the same as in laparoscopic fundoplication with the table in reversed Trendelenburg position. A 0° telescope is used. Typically, a hernia sac is present and contains either omentum or transverse colon, occasionally stomach or liver. The herniated viscera are reduced. The defect is exposed; it can be in the midline or on either side. The hernia sac is resected, taking great care not to injure the pleura or pericardium. The anterior part of the diaphragmatic defect is sutured to the undersurface of the sternum and the posterior rectus sheath using nonabsorbable sutures. Most of these sutures are placed employing a Keith needle as described by Newman et al. (1995): after localizing the fascia edges with a 23-gauge needle that is passed from the skin into the peritoneal cavity, small (3 mm) skin incisions are made and the Keith needle is passed through the fascia and controlled intra-abdominally under direct vision (Fig. 5). A mattress suture is passed in the Keith needle, which is taken out of the abdominal cavity and exits through the same small skin incision. The suture is then tied while inspecting the closure from inside. The skin is closed with adhesive bands.

Personal Experience

In two children aged 3 and 8 years, one with Down syndrome, we were able to close the defect laparoscopically. No complications arose. The two patients have been followed-up for 2 years and are doing well.

Discussion

The late presenting pediatric Morgagni hernia is usually a benign condition (Berman et al. 1989). Incarceration of bowel is extremely unusual. Operative repair is easily performed laparoscopically (Newman et al. 1995). The only specific risk is perforation of pericardium, which has not been observed in our limited experience.

Fig. 5. Closure of an anterior hernia (Morgagni). The position of the patient, crew, and equipment is the same as in laparoscopic fundoplication. A 0° scope is inserted through the umbilicus. One working cannula is placed in the right hypochondrium and another one in the left hypochondrium. The hernial sac is resected. The anterior part of the diaphragm is sutured to the undersurface of the sternum and posterior rectus sheath using nonabsorbable sutures. These sutures are placed with the help of a Keith needle

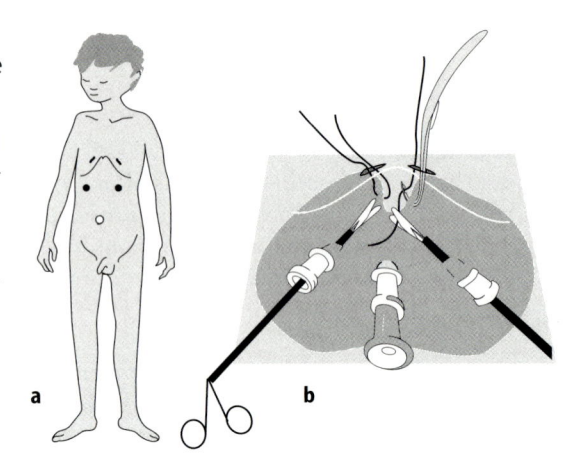

Conclusion

Laparoscopic repair of left and anterior diaphragmatic defects is principally possible in the somewhat older child with no respiratory distress. However, the safety and welfare of the child should have first priority, and laparoscopic repair of the defect should not be pursued at all costs.

References

Anderson KD (1986) Congenital diaphragmatic hernia. In: Welch KJ, Randolph JG, Ravitch MM, O'Neill JA Jr, Rowe MI (eds) Pediatric surgery, 4th edn. Year Book Medical Publishers, London, pp 589–601
Bax NMA, Collins DL (1984) The advantages of reconstruction of the dome of the diaphragm in congenital posterolateral diaphragmatic defects. J Pediatr Surg 19:484–487
Berman L et al (1989) The late presenting pediatric Morgagni hernia: a benign condition. J Pediatr Surg 24:970–972
Newman L III et al (1995) Laparoscopic diagnosis and treatment of Morgagni hernia. Surg Laparosc Endoscop 5:27–31
Schimpl G, Footer R, Saner H (1993) Congenital diaphragmatic hernia presenting after the newborn period. Eur J Pediatr 152:7658–768
Ugazzi M, Chirigoba A (1996) Laparoscopic treatment of incarcerated post-traumatic diaphragmatic hernia. J Laparoendosc Surg 6 [Suppl]:83–88
Van der Zee DC, Bax NMA (1995) Laparoscopic repair of congenital diaphragmatic hernia in a 6 month old child. Surg Endosc 9:1001–1003
Weber TR et al (1991) Congenital diaphragmatic hernia beyond infancy. Am J Surg 162:643–646
Yamaschita JI et al (1996) Thoracoscopic approach to the diagnosis and treatment of diaphragmatic disorders. Surg Lap Endosc 6:485–488

Part III
Abdomen

Inguinal Hernia

Contralateral Groin Exploration During Inguinal Hernia Repair

K.E. Georgeson

Introduction

A recent survey indicated that 90% of North American pediatric surgeons explore the contralateral groin in children presenting with a unilateral hernia under 1 year of age, and 80% explore the contralateral groin in children under 2 years of age [1]. The reported incidence of patency of contralateral open groin exploration is around 40% [2, 3]. However, the incidence of later development of a symptomatic hernia after unilateral hernia repair is only 10%–20% [4]. It is apparent that many unnecessary open groin explorations are performed which do not benefit the patient. Potential complications of negative open groin exploration include malposition of the testicle (5%), scrotal hematoma, injury to the vas or vessels (1%–2%), and wound infection [4].

Indications

The rapid and safe laparoscopic exploration of the contralateral groin is now practiced by many pediatric surgeons. Laparoscopic exploration reduces the potential for the complications of negative open groin exploration. Laparoscopic contralateral groin exploration can be performed whenever considering open contralateral groin exploration.

Preparation

The patient is positioned on the operating table for standard inguinal hernia repair. The bladder should be emptied using Credé's maneuver prior to skin preparation.
  The instruments that are needed for laparoscopic contralateral groin exploration are:
- Scope 0°, 1.2 mm 1×
- Blunt needle cannula, 16 gauge 1×
- Venous access catheter, 14 gauge 1×
- 2-0 silk tie, 1×

Technique

Three techniques have been utilized. All three techniques are briefly described here. The hernia repair should proceed as usual to the point where the sac on the symptomatic side is dissected free. A small catheter is introduced into the open hernia sac. A suture is tied snugly around the sac and catheter, and a pneumoperitoneum is developed through the catheter. The patient is then placed in a steep Trendelenburg position to shift the small bowel out of the pelvis. A 14-gauge intravenous catheter is introduced through the abdominal wall above the contralateral groin in the anterior axillary line at the level of the umbilicus (Fig. 1). The catheter is directed toward the internal ring. A 1.2-mm scope is passed through the 14-gauge catheter after the needle stylet has been removed. The internal ring is visualized in a direct line (Fig. 2). The scope can be advanced into a visualized sac. The length of the patent processus is then measured during withdrawal of the scope. The presence of a patent processus longer than 0.5 cm is indication for open repair of the opposite groin.

Alternative techniques for exploration of the contralateral groin include placing a trocar and telescope through the umbilicus after insufflation of the peritoneum through the dissected sac. A third technique utilizes placement of a reusable trocar through the sac of the hernia being repaired with insufflation of the peritoneal cavity through this trocar. A 70° or 110° scope is then passed through the trocar and advanced transversely across the lower abdomen. The contralateral internal ring is visualized with the angled scope.

The author prefers to utilize the first technique. Using this direct, in-line method of visualization, only 21% of 108 patients under age 2 had a patent processes vaginalis identified [5]. Using the technique of viewing the groin through the umbilicus or the contralateral groin yields an incidence of approximately 40% visualized patency of the asymptomatic groin. This difference in incidence of visualized patency between the three techniques may be due to the partially obscured view of the internal ring when viewed from an angle.

Occasionally a patient has a small symptomatic hernia, which makes introduction of a catheter or trocar through the symptomatic sac difficult. In this case, it is better to abandon the procedure than to try to force the introduction of the cannula.

Fig. 1. The trocar site is located in the anterior axillary line on the contralateral side at the level of the umbilicus

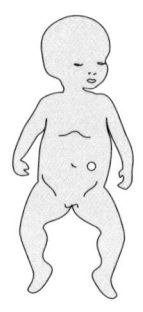

Fig. 2. CO_2 is infused through a small cannula introduced through the symptomatic hernia sac. A 14-gauge needle catheter is inserted in the anterior axillary line at the level of the umbilicus. The needle is removed and a 1.2-mm laparoscope is passed through the indwelling catheter giving a direct view of the contralateral internal ring

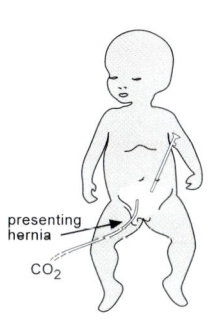

Personal Experience

There have been no complications in patients explored so far at The Children's Hospital of Alabama. One premature infant with a 1-cm tract, which was deemed a negative exploration, developed a symptomatic hernia 6 months later. We now explore all premature children with a patent processus vaginalis of any depth. Average time for exploration was 4 min.

Conclusion

Laparoscopic contralateral groin exploration prevents unnecessary open groin exploration in about 75% of patients.

References

1. Wiener ES et al (1996) Hernia survey of the section on surgery of the American Academy of Pediatrics. J Pediatr Surg 31:1166–1169
2. Holcomb GW III, Morgan WM III, Brock JW III (1996) Laparoscopic evaluation for contralateral patent processus vaginalis: part II. J Pediatr Surg 31:1170–1173
3. Wulkan ML et al (1996) Laparoscopy through the open ipsilateral sac to evaluate presence of contralateral hernia. J Pediatr Surg 31:1174–1177
4. Surana R, Puri P (1993) Is contralateral exploration necessary in infants with unilateral inguinal hernia? J Pediatr Surg 28:1026–1027
5. Fuenfer MM, Pitts RM, Georgeson KE (1996) Laparoscopic exploration of the contralateral groin in children: an improved technique. J Laparoendosc Surg 6:S1–S4

**Part III
Abdomen**

Shunts and Catheters

CHAPTER 39

Laparoscopic Approach to Ventriculoperitoneal Shunts

N.M.A. Bax, D.C. van der Zee, W.P. Vandertop

Introduction

Historically, hydrocephalus has been treated by shunting cerebrospinal fluid from the brain into many different body cavities and organs. Nowadays, the most commonly inserted system is the ventriculoperitoneal shunt which consists of a silicone catheter placed inside the brain's ventricle and connected to a valve and a longer tube which is brought beneath the skin of the head, neck, and anterior chest wall, into the peritoneal cavity.

Shunt complications are numerous and caused by either mechanical failure, infections or functional failure (Drake and Saint-Rose 1995). The most frequent cause of shunt dysfunction is mechanical failure (obstruction in 56% and fracture in 15%; Sainte Rose et al. 1991). The risk for a patient to experience shunt failure is highest in the first few months after surgery, ranging from 25%–40% at 1-year follow-up. Thereafter the risk remains 4%–5% per year (Drake and Saint-Rose 1995). Blind placement of either the proximal, ventricular catheter, or the distal, peritoneal, part of the shunt probably predisposes for more mechanical complications than when both parts are inserted under endoscopic guidance. Laparoscopic techniques may be useful in two different areas: firstly, the insertion under laparoscopic view of the peritoneal part of the shunt without mini-laparotomy and secondly, diagnosis and treatment of intra-abdominal shunt problems.

Laparoscopic-Assisted Insertion of the Peritoneal Part of the Shunt

Introduction

Blind placement of either the ventricular or peritoneal part of the shunt predisposes for more complications than when both parts are inserted under endoscopic control. The technique of the endoscopic insertion of the ventricular catheter is described elsewhere in this volume (see Grotenhuis and Vandertop, "Indications, Techniques and Results of Pediatric Neuroendoscopy"). The present chapter deals with the endoscopic insertion of the peritoneal part.

Indication

Schievink praised the laparoscopic assisted placement of the peritoneal part of the shunt in the event of previous intra-abdominal surgery (Schievink et al. 1993). In such a situation, laparoscopy allows the catheter to be placed in an adhesion-free area or alternatively, adhesions can be divided laparoscopically. However, even when no previous abdominal surgery has taken place, a laparoscopic approach may be superior (Armbruster et al. 1993; Basauri et al. 1993; Box et al. 1996; Cuatico and Vannix 1995; Schievink et al. 1993). It does not only avoid a minilaparotomy with its related pain and potential complications, but also allows for an exact positioning of the catheter.

Contraindication

One should be aware that the increase in intra-abdominal pressure as a result of the CO_2 pneumoperitoneum causes a concomitant increase in intracranial pressure (Este-McDonald et al. 1995; Josephs LG et al. 1994; Uzzo et al. 1997). This negative influence of laparoscopy can be kept to a minimum by using low intra-abdominal pressures, for example, 5 mmHg, which is sufficient when optimal muscle relaxation is provided. Alternatively, when the ventricular catheter is inserted first, the intracranial pressure can be monitored and if necessary some cerebrospinal fluid can be removed (Uzzo et al. 1997).

Preoperative Workup

The indication and workup for insertion of a ventriculoperitoneal shunt is the responsibility of the pediatric neurosurgeon involved. In general, a progressive noncommunicating hydrocephalus is the most frequent indication. In the event of previous intra-abdominal surgery, ultrasound of the abdomen may be useful to determine an adhesion free area for insertion of the first cannula.

Preoperative Preparation

Apart from prophylactic antibiotics (flucloxacillin, 25 mg/kg intravenously at the induction of anesthesia), no special preparation is required.

Technique

The patient is positioned in such a way that both the frontal or occipital region of the head and the abdomen can be approached at the same time, which means a supine position of the patient with the head turned contralateral to the side to be operated upon. The neurosurgeon stands next to the head of the patient on the side to be operated and looks at an opposite monitor (Fig. 1). The laparoscopist stands at the same side of the patient next to the abdomen and looks at a second monitor in front. The neurosurgeon and pediatric surgeon assist each

39 Laparoscopic Approach to Ventriculoperitoneal Shunts

Fig. 1. Position of the patient, crew, and equipment

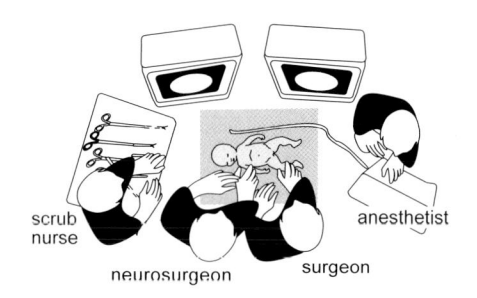

Fig. 2. Position of the VP drain and cannula sites. The cannula for the scope is introduced through the inferior umbilical fold. A secondary cannula is inserted in the right hypochondrium for a grasper to position the drain in the abdomen. The peritoneal part of the drain is passed subcutaneously in a retrograde fashion through a tunneling device from the left hypochondrium to the right neck. Insertion into the abdomen is achieved with the Seldinger technique and appropriate peel-away system

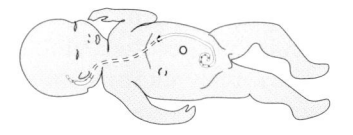

other. The scrub nurse stands to the left of the neurosurgeon. The anesthetist stands at the lower end of the table.

It is best to have two different camera circuits. This is not only more convenient but, more importantly, also better from the point of view of asepsis. A 6-mm cannula is inserted in an open way through the umbilicus, or in a different area in the event of periumbilical scarring (Fig. 2). CO_2 is insufflated at a maximal pressure of 5 mmHg and a flow of 2–5 l/min depending on the age and size of the patient.

Firstly, the inguinal region is inspected for patency of the processi vaginales. If these processi are still open, they should be closed as the likelihood of getting hydroceles and hernias is high (Grosfeld and Cooney 1974; Moazam et al. 1984). We still close open processi vaginales in a classical, open way, but this may also be performed laparoscopically when enough expertise is available. Next, a second small trocar is inserted in the right upper or right lower quadrant for a grasping forceps (Fig. 2). With this forceps the end of the catheter can be grasped at a later stage.

A small incision is made in the left (or right) upper quadrant and a long tunneling device with trocar is introduced from that incision, subcutaneously along the anterior chest wall and neck up to the right (or left) frontal or occipital area, where the ventricular part of the shunt has been inserted (Fig. 2). Through the small incision in the left (or right) upper quadrant a needle is inserted into the abdomen under endoscopic control. Over a guide wire a peel-a-way system of appropriate size is inserted. The distal catheter of the shunt is fed into the tunneling device till its end reaches the left upper quadrant. The tunneling device is removed and the catheter inserted into the abdominal cavity via the peel a way system. The end of the catheter is now grabbed and approximately 40 cm of catheter is pulled into the abdomen to allow for growth of the patient. The distal end is nicely positioned in the lower abdomen. The peel-a-way system is removed and the wound is closed with one subcuticular absorbable stitch and an adhesive strip to the skin. Meanwhile the neurosurgeon assembles the ventricular part of the shunt. Now that the shunt is complete cerebrospinal fluid runs freely into the abdominal cavity, which can be witnessed through the laparoscope. The laparoscope is withdrawn, and the fascia closed with a resorbable stitch. The skin is approximated with an adhesive strip.

If intra-abdominal adhesions are present, they can be cut, but this usually necessitates the insertion of another cannula for an additional working instrument. Extensive adhesiolysis should be avoided as these adhesions recur, possibly sandwiching and therefore blocking the catheter.

Laparoscopic Diagnosis and Treatment of Shunt-Related Intra-abdominal Complications

Indications

The use of laparoscopy for intra-abdominal complications related to the ventriculoperitoneal shunt has been advocated for almost 20 years (Lemay et al. 1979; Morgan 1979; Rodgers et al. 1978). These complications can be divided into:
- Infection
- Blockage
  - Due to omentum
  - Due to encystation
  - Due to disconnection or fracture
- Bowel obstruction
- Perforation (stomach, bowel, bladder, vagina, umbilicus, scrotum)

Contraindication

One should be aware that an increase in intra-abdominal pressure causes an increase in intracranial pressure. A low pneumoperitoneum pressure should therefore be used e.g. 5 mm Hg. Trendelenburg position which also causes an increase in intracranial pressure should also be avoided as much as possible.

Technique

The patient lies supine on the operating table. If the valve needs to be explored at the same time then the patients head should face the opposite side of the region to be operated upon. When the system has been implanted into the abdomen along the patient's right side, the surgeon should stand at the patient's left side with a monitor opposite him (Fig. 1). The first 6-mm cannula is inserted as described earlier and a classical pneumoperitoneum is created. During inspection the presumed problem is identified.

Peritonitis

Laparoscopy allows differentiation between shunt infection and other causes of peritonitis of which appendicitis is the most frequent one. In the event of peritonitis due to an infected system, material for culture is taken. One can leave the system in place and try to treat the condition with antibiotics. Alternatively, the distal end of the shunt can be exteriorized through a small hole in the abdominal wall. In a later phase at least the distal end of the catheter will need replacement.

Blockage

Omentum. If the catheter is blocked by omentum, this can easily be lysed laparoscopically with a grasper.

Encystation. If encystation has taken place, this diagnosis is usually made preoperatively by ultrasound or other imaging techniques. Such a cyst can be well approached laparoscopically (Kim et al. 1995). Unroofing of the cyst and repositioning of the tip of the catheter in the remaining abdominal cavity is all that is required. In addition, except for a cannula for the laparoscope two more cannulae for instrumentation are usually required.

Disconnection or Fracture. If shunt disconnection or fracture has occurred, the distal part of the catheter can either be removed laparoscopically, or alternatively the peritoneal part of the shunt can be replaced in a laparoscopically assisted way (Guzinsky 1982; Lemay et al. 1979; Schrenk et al. 1996).

Perforation of the Distal End

Such perforation can occur anywhere. If such a perforation occurs, the distal end of the catheter is amputated laparoscopically after which the distal end can be pulled out. Obviously the peritoneal part of the shunt needs replacement. Depending on which structure has been perforated the perforation needs closure or not.

Bowel Obstruction

If a small bowel obstruction is caused by an intra-abdominal catheter, laparoscopic repositioning of this catheter and lysis of eventual adhesions solve the problem unless the bowel is gangrenous in which case the operation should be converted (see also van der Zee and Bax, "Laparoscopic Approach of Intestinal Obstruction in Children").

Discussion

The combination of neuroendoscopy with laparoscopy optimizes the placement of ventriculoperitoneal shunts and undoubtedly reduces complications, related to shunt malpositioning. In the long-term it might even reduce the frequency of shunt revisions by diminishing the incidence of distal obstruction. Moreover, by using an almost no-touch technique, the infection rate may further decline. Other advantages are the avoidance of a minilaparotomy. Thus less pain, less adhesions, a smaller scar and less wound related complications. In shunt related intra-abdominal problems, laparoscopy can be a very valuable tool not only in the diagnostic but also in the therapeutic field.

Essential for this type of surgery is of course a good collaboration between the neurosurgeon and pediatric surgeon.

References

Armbruster C et al (1993) Laparoscopically assisted implantation of ventriculoperitoneal shunts. J Laparoendosc Surg 3:191–192
Basauri L, Selman JM, Lizana C (1993) Peritoneal catheter insertion under laparoscopic guidance. Pediatr Neurosurg 19:109–110
Box JC et al (1996) A retrospective analysis of laparoscopically assisted ventriculoperitoneal shunts. Surg Endosc 10:311–313
Cuatico W, Vannix D (1995) Laparoscopically guided peritoneal insertion of ventriculoperitoneal shunts. J Laparoendosc Surg 5:309–311
Drake JM, Sainte-Rose C: The shunt book. Blackwell Science, New York, 1995
Este-McDonald JR et al (1995) Changes in intracranial pressure associated with apneumic retractors. Arch Surg 130:362–365
Grosfeld JL, Cooney DR (1973) Inguinal hernia after ventriculoperitoneal shunt for hydrocephalus. J Pediatr Surg 9:311–315
Josephs LG et al (1994) Diagnostic laparoscopy increases intracranial pressure. J Trauma 36:815–818
Kim HB, Raghavendran K, Kleinhaus S (1995) Management of an abdominal cerebrospinal fluid pseudocyst using laparoscopic techniques. Surg Endosc 5:151–154
Lemay J-L et al (1979) Laparoscopic removal of the distal catheter of ventriculoperitoneal shunt (Ames valve) Gastroint Endosc 25:162–163
Moazam F, Glenn JD, Kaplan BJ (1984) Inguinal hernias after ventriculoperitoneal shunt procedures in pediatric patients. Surg Gynecol Obstet 159:570–572
Morgan WW Jr (1979) The use of peritoneoscopy in the diagnosis and treatment of complications of ventriculoperitoneal shunts in children. J Pediatr Surg 14:180–181
Rodgers BM, Vries JK, Talbert JL (1978) Laparoscopy in the diagnosis and treatment of malfunctioning ventriculo-peritoneal shunts in children. J Pediatr Surg 13:247–253
Sainte-Rose C et al. (1991) Mechanical complications in shunts. Pediatr Neurosurg 17:2–9
Schievink WI et al (1993) Laparoscopic placement of ventriculoperitoneal shunts: preliminary report. May Clin Proc 68:1064–1066

Schrenk P et al (1996) Laparoscopic removal of dislocated ventriculoperitoneal shunts. Report of two cases. Surg Endosc 8:1113–1114

Uzzo RG, Mininberg DT, Poppas DP (1997) Laparoscopic surgery in children with ventriculoperitoneal shunts: effects of pneumoperitoneum on intracranial pressure: Preliminary experience. Urology 49:753–757

CHAPTER 40

Laparoscopic Insertion of Peritoneal Dialysis Catheters in Children

C.K. Yeung, K.F. Yip

Introduction

Peritoneal dialysis (PD) was first described for the treatment of children with acute renal failure nearly half a century ago [1]. Since then PD has been well established as an effective renal replacement therapy in children both for tiding over an episode of acute severe renal insufficiency, or as maintenance therapy in patients with end-stage renal disease (ESRD) waiting for renal transplantation [1–3]. In countries with extreme shortage of donor organs, such as Hong Kong, patients with ESRD often need to wait for many years for a suitable organ for transplant and hence are completely dependent on a secure and reliable system of dialytic therapy for life maintenance. Compared with hemodialysis, peritoneal dialysis has many advantages for use in children. Firstly, the peritoneum of children is more suitable as a dialysis membrane because of the bigger surface area to weight ratio, which is nearly double that of adults [4]. Secondly, peritoneal dialysis results in less metabolic complications, including both acute electrolyte disturbances and chronic disorders such as aluminum deposition after prolonged hemodialysis, and is not associated with the disequilibrium syndrome. It also obviates the need for difficult vascular access and the complex machinery required for hemodialysis and incurs a much lower running cost, thus making it more affordable to most patients' family. Furthermore, it is more acceptable to the young patients because it avoids repeated painful punctures as well as immobility during treatment.

Indications for PD

Peritoneal dialysis is the most frequently employed dialytic modality in the treatment of acute renal insufficiency in children [5–7]. The candidates under this category are mostly children suffering from an acute episode of major renal insult. For instance, children may develop acute tubular necrosis after profound hypovolemic shock as in multiple injuries, with or without preexisting renal disease. The generally accepted criteria for initializing peritoneal dialysis in children includes: (a) severe acute electrolyte imbalance (serum potassium > 7.0 mmol/l); (b) uncontrollable acidosis; (c) fluid overload not controlled with diuretics and fluid restriction; (d) symptomatic uremia with encephalopathy, pericarditis. Since PD is convenient, safe, cheap, and reversible, it is generally recommended that peritoneal dialysis therapy should be started as soon as it is needed in patients with acute renal insufficiency.

Early attempts in using intermittent peritoneal dialysis techniques in the management of children with chronic renal insufficiency was hampered by the necessity to reinsert the PD catheter before each treatment. The development of a "permanent" PD catheter, first introduced by Palmer [8], and later perfected by Tenckhoff and Schecter [9], however, has made long-term peritoneal dialysis a much more feasible and effective form of renal replacement therapy for children with ESRD. The recent advances in continuous ambulatory peritoneal dialysis (CAPD) has further revolutionized dialytic therapy for children [10–13]. CAPD is particularly suitable for use in the pediatric patients because of its excellent biochemical control in a near steady state, greatly reduced restrictions on dietary and fluid intake, and freedom from repeated needle puncture as is necessary for hemodialysis. Furthermore, CAPD allows most patients to receive dialysis at home and hence decreases dramatically the frequency of hospitalization. Over the past two decades, the successful implementation of a CAPD and home peritoneal dialysis program in most countries has greatly improved the quality of life of ESRD patients and their families alike. Most children can now attend school regularly and have normal activities. Understandably, there has been a very rapid growth of CAPD as the maintenance therapy of choice for children with ESRD throughout the world over the last decade [14].

Techniques of Insertion of a PD Catheter

Blind Insertion Versus Open Techniques

For patients with acute renal failure, the choice between a percutaneously placed temporary catheter and a "permanent" peritoneal catheter inserted surgically is somewhat arbitrary under an emergency situation. However, if it can be anticipated that dialysis therapy will be necessary for over 3–4 days then surgical catheter placement would be preferable because of an increased risk of peritonitis associated with the use of temporary catheters for over 72 h [15]. For very unstable infants in the intensive care unit, surgical placement of the catheter can even be performed at the bedside under local anesthesia [16]. Recent abdominal surgery is not an absolute contraindication to PD. Infants with vesicostomies or other urinary diversions, for example, in patients with posterior urethral valves and bilateral renal dysplasia, can also be successfully treated with peritoneal dialysis [17].

A secure, reliable and trouble-free PD catheter is of vital importance for the success of continuous peritoneal dialysis in patients with ESRD. Various kinds of peritoneal catheters have been invented for dialysis. Tenckhoff introduced the double-cuffed soft silicone tube for dialysis in the middle 1960's [9], and this has since been widely accepted as the standard catheter for prolonged continuous peritoneal dialysis. In his original description, Tenckhoff inserted the PD catheter by a blind trocar technique [9]. This was, however, associated with a very high incidence of complications including leakage of dialysate and catheter malpositioning. Most centers have therefore now adopted an open surgical approach for catheter insertion. This is usually performed via a minilaparotomy either through a midline or a paramedian incision. Despite this technical modification catheter blockage as a result of either improper placement or omental occlusion is still a very commonly encountered and often annoying problem. Blockage of catheter can occur in 15%–20% of cases in most adult series and with a much higher incidence of up to 50% in pediatric patients [3, 15, 18–21]. Successful placement of the PD catheter into an optimal position in the pelvis helps to reduce the incidence of early catheter failure. In addition, removing a substantial proportion of the omentum has been shown to reduce the rate of catheter blockage significantly and therefore many surgeons have advocated to include omentectomy as a routine procedure during insertion of PD catheters, particularly in infants and young children [19–22]. Despite its popularity, the open surgical method for peritoneal catheter insertion has several drawbacks. Firstly, proper positioning of the catheter in the pelvis free from encasement by omentum or other viscera is often difficult to accomplish via a small minilaparotomy wound. Similarly, effective omentectomy can rarely be achieved with such an approach. In addition, with the open surgical method adhesiolysis of intraperitoneal adhesion bands for patients with previous peritonitis is usually impossible without a formal laparotomy.

Laparoscopic-Assisted Insertion of PD Catheter

Indications

Because of the aforementioned limitations with PD catheters inserted with open surgical method, laparoscopically guided placement of peritoneal catheters were introduced in the late 1980's and have been shown to give more long-lasting and trouble-free dialysis [23–28]. The laparoscopic technique is especially applicable for placement of PD catheters in patients with previous abdominal surgery, or with history of repeated catheter blockage or peritonitis. In addition, previous studies have reported inguinal hernias developing in 12%–42% of infants and young children undergoing peritoneal dialysis [29, 30]. Because of this many surgeons have advocated routine bilateral inguinal exploration and ligation of any patent processus vaginalis at the time of Tenckhoff catheter insertion [21, 31, 32]. Particularly in infants and young children, therefore, the internal inguinal orifices can be carefully inspected with the laparoscopic insertion technique and prophylactic ligation of any patent processus vaginalis can be performed to avoid the annoying but common complication of hernia formation immediately after the commencement of peritoneal dialysis.

Contraindications

There is no absolute contraindication to laparoscopic PD catheter insertion. However, for those patients with marginal cardiopulmonary function, special precautions may be necessary during the procedure, and close intraoperative monitoring of the physiological changes is mandatory.

Preoperative Workup

Before the operation, the catheter exit site and the course of the subcutaneous tunnel must be carefully thought out and chosen in consultation with the patient as in standard PD catheter insertion using the open method. The catheter exit site should not encroach on the line where the child usually wears his or her belt. For young infants the exit site should be placed high above the diaper line to minimize risk of contamination. Patients with vesicostomies should have the catheter exit site as far from the stoma as possible.

Special preoperative precautions are necessary for patients with ESRD. A preoperative chest X-ray is necessary to exclude silent chest infection, and to detect any significant pleural effusion or evidence of congestive heart failure associated with renal insufficiency. An electrocardiogram should be performed to look for evidence of hyperkalemia or ventricular hypertrophy. Blood for biochemistry including electrolytes and blood gases should also be taken.

Operative Techniques

There are various techniques of laparoscopic-assisted insertion of Tenckhoff catheters described in the literature, which can be categorized as follows:

Laparoscopic-Guided Percutaneous Catheter Insertion. Percutaneous insertion of Tenckhoff catheter is performed under simple peritoneoscopic visual guidance. Major organs and vessels can be inspected during the procedure. However, the Veress needle is inserted blindly and has therefore potential risks of visceral and vascular injuries. Furthermore, manipulation of the catheter and omentectomy is difficult with this simple technique.

The Y-Tec System. A small size peritoneoscope is inserted blindly using an introducing needle with organ protective device. Pneumoperitoneum is created, and a peritoneoscope is advanced into the pelvic cavity. A guide wire is placed into the pelvis through the peritoneoscope. Catheter is inserted over the guidewire with Seldinger technique. This method is especially applicable for catheter replacement inside a previously infected peritoneal cavity. However, the initial blind insertion of needle before introduction of pneumoperitoneum can still be associated with potential hazards. Furthermore the technique cannot tackle intraperitoneal adhesive bands which can give rise to problems in the future.

Laparoscopic-Assisted Insertion of a PD Catheter. This is perhaps the most popular method of PD catheter insertion under laparoscopic assistance. After general anesthesia, urethral catheterization is performed for intraoperative monitoring of urine output and for decompression of the urinary bladder to facilitate the operative procedure. Skin is prepared with antiseptics from nipple to thigh level and draped to expose the abdomen from the xiphoid process to just above the pubis. Prophylactic antibiotics are given before skin incision as a single dose of second generation cephalosporin. A supraumbilical port is first introduced with an open technique for the initial pneumoperitoneum and insertion of telescope to minimize visceral injury especially in patients with previous abdominal surgery and with marked intraperitoneal adhesions. The peritoneal cavity is carefully inspected. Adhesiolysis can be performed under laparoscopic guidance. A separate, small 2- to 3-cm incision is then made down to the peritoneum as the entry point of the PD catheter. The PD catheter is introduced through a small peritoneal incision and advanced downwards just beneath the anterior abdominal wall to a clear space in the pelvic cavity under direct laparoscopic vision. The peritoneum is then closed around the catheter with a purse-string suture which is passed through the base of the cuff of the Tenckhoff catheter at several points to anchor the catheter in position and to secure a more watertight closure. Another purse-string nonabsorbable suture is placed through the rectus muscle and anterior rectal sheath. A subcutaneous tunnel is then created and the catheter brought out through a separate exit site that has been marked preoperatively. An additional 3.5-mm port may or may not be needed for a grasping instrument to adjust the catheter position. The supraumbilical port is then taken out and the greater omentum is exteriorized as much as possible through the umbilical wound and excised with a bipolar electrocautery extracorporeally. About 15–20 ml/kg of normal saline is then infused through the catheter and then drained immediately to ascertain proper catheter position and function before completion of the procedure and reversal of anesthesia. Peritoneal dialysis can usually be started 24–48 h after catheter placement.

Laparoscopic Insertion of Peritoneal Catheter. This has now evolved to become our own method of choice as near total omentectomy can be more easily and effectively performed under laparoscopic vision and hence further minimizing the chance of subsequent catheter occlusion and treatment failure. Peritoneal catheters for both acute and chronic dialysis are inserted using the same technique in our hospital. In order to optimize the ergonomics of surgical instruments and make efficient use of all the port sites to avoid unnecessary incision, the surgical procedure must be well planned, and the technique is described in greater details. The surgeon stands on the patient's right side with the monitor placed across the table just opposite to him. The assistant stands on the surgeon's right hand side, and the scrub nurse on the opposite side of the table next to the monitor (Fig. 1).

After the patient is put under general anesthesia and placed in a supine position, the bladder is catheterized. Once again the abdominal port is inserted under direct vision with open Hasson's method. A 1.5- to 2-cm-long transverse infraumbilical incision is made. The rectal sheath is incised transversely followed

Fig. 1. Operating room layout showing position of surgeons, anesthetist, scrub nurse, and monitor

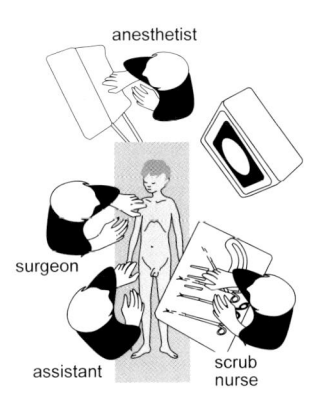

by the peritoneum and a 2-0 polyglactin purse-string suture is placed around the opening for maintaining the pneumoperitoneum subsequently. A 10-mm port with adapter for instruments of either 5 or 10 mm is then inserted and secured by tying the purse-string suture. Pneumoperitoneum is created with carbon dioxide and maintained at a pressure of 12 mmHg. The peritoneal cavity is inspected with a videoscope. A 5-mm incision is created on the right lower quadrant of the abdominal wall. This becomes the future exit site of the Tenckhoff catheter and hence should avoid the iliac bony prominence. Through the 5-mm incision a 5-mm port with air-vent channel is inserted under videoscopic guidance. Another 5-mm port is then inserted at the right upper quadrant under videoscopic guidance to avoid the liver and gallbladder (Fig. 2). A 5-mm videoscope is inserted through the lower abdominal port. Thorough laparoscopic inspection of the peritoneal cavity is then performed. The internal inguinal openings are inspected particularly for patent processus vaginalis. Any intra-abdominal adhesion bands can be divided and released with graspers and electrocautery. A 5-mm ultrasonic scalpel or bipolar forceps is introduced via the infraumbilical port for near-total omentectomy to minimize catheter occlusion. Another 5-mm grasper is inserted via the upper abdominal port. Omentum is controlled by the grasper with the surgeon's left hand, and near-total omentectomy can be performed using the ultrasonic scalpel or bipolar forceps with the surgeon's right hand (Fig. 3). All redundant omental tissue can be excised and hemostasis achieved using the ultrasonic scalpel alone without a change of instrument, thereby shortening the operative time remarkably. After completion of the omentectomy the ultrasonic scalpel is replaced by a grasper and the omental tissue can be easily removed via the infraumbilical port.

A double-cuffed Tenckhoff catheter is then flushed and trimmed to suitable length. The 10-mm infraumbilical port and the polyglactin purse-string suture are removed and the Tenckhoff catheter is introduced via the peritoneal opening which is then closed with a nonabsorbable purse-string suture incorporating the base of the inner cuff. The rectal sheath is then closed with interrupted nonabsorbable sutures just above the top of the cuff. Pneumoperitoneum is re-introduced via the air vent in the lower abdominal port. The videoscope is now moved

Fig. 2. Position of the ports: 10-mm port infraumbilically, 5-mm port in the right iliac fossa, and 5-mm port in the right upper quadrant

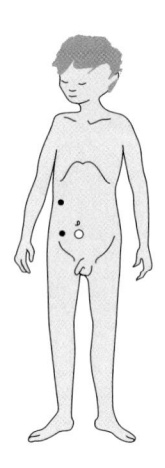

Fig. 3. Omentectomy with the ultrasonic scalpel

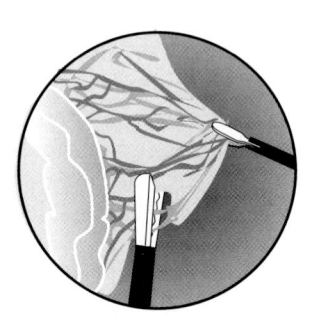

Fig. 4. Manipulation of the peritoneal dialysis catheter under videoscopic control into the pelvis

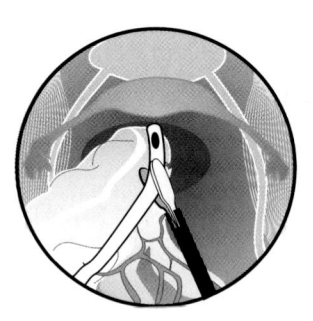

to the upper abdominal port and the grasper is introduced via the lower abdominal port. The catheter is manipulated with the grasper under videoscopic guidance and guided into a clear space in the pelvis so that it lies in the rectovaginal pouch in females and in the rectovesical pouch in males (Fig. 4).

After the procedure the abdominal ports are removed. A subcutaneous tunnel is created between the infraumbilical and lower abdominal incisions. The catheter is brought out via the lower abdominal incision with the outer cuffed em-

Fig. 5. Completion of procedure. The right lower abdominal wound is used as the exit site of the peritoneal dialysis catheter

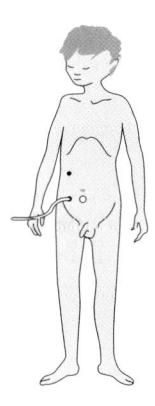

bedded in the subcutaneous tissue about 2.5 cm from the exit site of catheter. The catheter is anchored and the upper abdominal incision is closed with subcuticular absorbable sutures (Fig. 5). Free two-way flow via the Tenckhoff catheter is tested with about 15–20 ml/kg of normal saline and the catheter is then flushed with 2000 U heparin to ensure patency. Patients with evidence of patent processus vaginalis on laparoscopic inspection also have inguinal exploration and herniotomy with ligation of the processus vaginalis during the same operation.

Postoperative Care

Patients who do not require extensive adhesiolysis are allowed oral diet once they recover full consciousness postoperatively. Vital signs are observed overnight, and abdominal signs are monitored. If necessary, peritoneal dialysis can be started immediately after the procedure with frequent, low-volume exchanges at 25%–30% of full volume cycles; although we would usually recommend waiting for 24–48 h after catheter placement before commencement of dialysis. Patients can be discharged home if oral diet is tolerated well and the catheter is functioning satisfactorily.

Complications of Laparoscopic PD Catheter Insertion

Data from the literature have indicated that PD catheters inserted under laparoscopic guidance were associated with longer survival and significantly less complications. In a recent review, the overall incidences of catheter blockage, pericatheter leaks, peritoneal sepsis and exit site infection were significantly higher for PD catheters placed either blindly or by open surgical method than for catheters placed under laparoscopic guidance [27]. A prospective study by Pastan et al. comparing CAPD catheters inserted by laparoscopic and open surgical methods has also shown significantly better survival (89% with a median follow-up of 251 days) for laparoscopically placed catheters than catheters inserted by open methods (57% with a median follow-up of 102 days), although the incidences of exit site infection and catheter leaks were similar between the two groups [28].

We have employed the laparoscopic peritoneal catheter insertion technique with omentectomy using a ultrasonic scalpel or bipolar forceps as described above in our hospital in four children (3 boys) aged 8–14 years with ESRD. All four patients dialyzed successfully with a total follow-up of 41.5 months (median follow-up: 12.5 months). There was only 1 episode of transient catheter blockage which responded to flushing. One patient developed early leakage which settled with a temporary switch to low-volume dialysis. Two patient developed peritonitis (3 episodes) during dialysis treatment, all of which responded to antibiotics treatment. One catheter was complicated by mild exit site infection. No catheter had been removed for infection or mechanical failure.

Although uncommon, complications specific to the laparoscopic procedures may need special consideration when deciding on the choice of surgical approach. These include:

- Exaggerated physiological response to abdominal distension and splinting of the diaphragm due to pneumoperitoneum, for example, hypercapnia, reduction in tidal volume and cardiac arrhythmias, which may be particularly salient in a small infant with ESRD. Careful intraoperative monitoring, routine endotracheal intubation with muscle paralysis and rigorously keeping the intra-abdominal pressure to below 10–12 mmHg is of crucial importance in preventing these complications.
- Veress needle/trocar injuries and surgical emphysema. These are usually due to incorrect or extraperitoneal placement of the trocar or Veress needle and can be safely avoided by inserting the primary port using an open Hasson method, and all other subsequent ports under direct laparoscopic vision.
- Electrocautery complications: These are mostly related to the use of monopolar diathermy and/or inadvertent coagulation of adjacent structures outside the view of endoscopic vision, and are largely preventable by limiting to the use of bipolar electrocautery units or the ultrasonic scalpel only, and to ensure that the active tip of the diathermy unit should always be in full view and away from any metal cannula or instruments.
- Visceral injuries: These include bowel perforations, bladder and ureteral injuries and major vessel injuries, etc., most of which are related to poor endoscopic vision, inadvertent electrocautery or trocar injuries and can therefore be largely avoidable by sticking to the safety precautions as outlined previously.

Laparoscopic Replacement of Problematic Peritoneal Catheters

Peritoneal catheters that are complicated by repeated septic episodes or mechanical failures including catheter occlusion, breakage or leakage, often need to be replaced. The laparoscopic procedure for peritoneal catheter replacement is essentially similar to that for primary insertion except that a supraumbilical incision is usually used for insertion of the new catheter to avoid the previous infraumbilical site. Any intraperitoneal adhesions can be released under laparoscopic vision. A new peritoneal catheter can then be placed as described above in a free space in the peritoneal cavity identified laparoscopically. Catheters with intermittent partial blockage due to malpositioning can also be repositioned to a more optimal free peritoneal space under laparoscopic guidance. An infected or blocked catheter should be removed.

Conclusions

A reliable catheter is the key to success for peritoneal dialysis therapy and therefore perfection of the surgical technique for PD catheter insertion is essential. Laparoscopic-assisted insertion of peritoneal dialysis catheter has been shown to provide significantly better catheter survival and trouble-free dialysis in other series. The technique also allows simultaneous partial to near-total omentectomy which has been proven to be crucial in preventing postoperative catheter occlusion especially in children. In addition, the approach allows clear inspection of the inguinal orifices for prophylactic ligation of patent processus vaginalis, a particularly useful step in infants and young children to avoid hernia formation after the commencement of peritoneal dialysis. We have described a simple technique for laparoscopic insertion of Tenckhoff catheter. Although the experience is admittedly preliminary, the complete absence of catheter occlusion during dialysis therapy in our small series is encouraging. Further application and evaluation of the technique is warranted.

Reference

1. Bloxsum A, Powell N (1948) The treatment of acute temporary dysfunction of the kidneys by peritoneal irrigation. Pediatrics 1:52–57
2. Feldman W, Baliah T, Drummond KN (1968) Intermittent peritoneal dialysis in the management of chronic renal failure. Am J Dis Child 116:30–36
3. Potter DE, McDaid TK, Ramirez JA (1981) Peritoneal dialysis in children. In: Atkins RC, Thomson NM, Farrell PC (eds) Peritoneal dialysis. Churchill-Livingstone, New York, pp 356–361
4. Esperanca MJ, Collins DL (1966) Peritoneal dialysis efficiency in relation to body weight. J Pediatr Surg 1:162–169
5. Lloyd-Still JD, Atwell JD (1966) Renal failure in infancy, with special reference to the use of peritoneal dialysis. J Pediatr Surg 1:466–475
6. Lugo G, Ceballos R, Brown W (1969) Acute renal failure in the neonate managed by peritoneal dialysis. Am J Dis Child 118:655–659
7. Chan JCM (1978) Peritoneal dialysis for renal failure in childhood. Clin Pediatr 17:349–354
8. Palmer RA, Quinton WE, Gray JF (1964) Prolonged peritoneal dialysis for chronic renal failure. Lancet 1:700–702
9. Tenckhoff H, Schechter H (1966) A bacteriologically safe peritoneal access device. Trans Am Soc Artif Int Org 14:181–186
10. Balfe JW, Irwin MA (1980) Continuous ambulatory peritoneal dialysis in children. In: Legrain M (ed) Continuous ambulatory peritoneal dialysis. Excerpta Medica, Amsterdam, pp 131–136

11. Kohaut EC (1981) Continuous ambulatory peritoneal dialysis: a preliminary pediatric experience. Am J Dis Child 135:270-271
12. Potter DE, McDaid TK, McHenry K (1981) Continuous ambulatory peritoneal dialysis (CAPD) in children. Trans Am Soc Artif Int Org 27:64-67
13. Salusky IB et al (1982) Continuous ambulatory peritoneal dialysis in children. Pediatr Clin North Am 29:1005-1012
14. Alexander SR, Honda M (1993) Continuous peritoneal dialysis for children: a decade of worldwide growth and development. Kidney Int 43 [Suppl 40]:S65-S74
15. Day RE, White RHR (1977) Peritoneal dialysis in children: review of 8 years' experience. Arch Dis Child 52:56-61
16. Borzotta A, Harrison HL, Groff DB (1983) Technique of peritoneal dialysis cannulation in neonates. Surg Gynecol Obstet 157:73-74
17. Alexander SR (1983) Pediatric CAPD update - 1983. Perit Dial Bull 3 [Suppl]:S15-S22
18. Lewis MA, Nycyk JA (1992) Practical peritoneal dialysis - the Tenckhoff catheter in acute renal failure. Pediatr Nephrol 6:470-475
19. Nicholoson ML et al (1991) The role of omentectomy in continuous ambulatory peritoneal dialysis. Perit Dial Int 11:330-332
20. Pumford N, Cassey J, Uttley WS (1994) Omentectomy with peritoneal catheter placement in acute renal failure. Nephron 68:327-328
21. Clark KR et al (1992) Surgical aspects of chronic peritoneal dialysis in the neonate and infant under 1 year of age. J Pediatr Surg 27:780-783
22. Orkin BA, Fonkalsrud EW, Salusky IB (1983) Continuous ambulatory peritoneal dialysis catheters in children. Arch Surg 118:1398-1402
23. Watson DI, Paterson D, Bannister K (1996) Secure placement of peritoneal dialysis catheters using a laparoscopic technique. Surg Laparosc Endosc 6:35-37
24. Copley JB et al (1996) Peritoneoscopic placement of Swan neck peritoneal dialysis catheters. Perit Dial Int 16 [Suppl 1]:S330-S332
25. Hughes CR, Angotti DM, Jubelirer RA (1994) Laparoscopic repositioning of a continuous ambulatory peritoneal dialysis (CAPD) catheter. Surg Endosc 8:1108-1109
26. Ash SR, Handt AE, Bloch R (1993) Peritoneoscopic placement of the Tenckhoff catheter: further clinical experience. Peritoneal Dial Bull 3:8-12
27. Ash SR (1990) Chronic peritoneal dialysis catheter: effects of catheter design, materials, and location. Semin Dial 3:39-46
28. Pastan S et al (1991) Prospective comparison of peritoneosopic and surgical implantation of CAPD catheters. Trans Am Soc Artif Int Org 37:M154-M156
29. Tank ES, Hatch DA (1986) Hernias complicating chronic ambulatory dialysis in children. J Pediatr Surg 21:41
30. Grosfeld JL (1989) Current concepts in inguinal hernia in infants and children. World J Surg 13:506-515
31. Matthews DE, West KW, Rescorla FJ (1990) Peritoneal dialysis in the first 60 days of life. J Pediatr Surg 25:110-116
32. Stone MM, Fonkalsrud EW, Salusky IB (1986) Surgical management of peritoneal dialysis catheters in children: five-year experience with 1,800 patient-month follow-up. J Pediatr Surg 21:1177-1181

**Part III
Abdomen**

Complications

CHAPTER 41

Complications in Laparoscopic Surgery in Children

N.M.A. Bax, D.C. van der Zee

Complications Related to the Pneumoperitoneum

Consequences of an Increased Intra-abdominal Pressure

A raised intra-abdominal pressure has not only respiratory and hemodynamic consequences, which are addressed elsewhere in this volume (see Sfez, "Basic Physiology and Anesthesia"), but also consequences for the intracranial pressure which is increased concomitantly (Este-McDonald et al. 1995; Josephs et al. 1994) and for splanchnic perfusion, which is decreased (Diebel et al. 1992a,b; Eleftheriadis et al. 1996; Hashikura et al. 1994). Especially in the event of a preexistent elevation of intracranial pressure, for example, in trauma, one should be careful to create a pneumoperitoneum. The raised intra-abdominal pressure results in venous stasis in the lower part of the body (Beebe et al. 1993) and predisposes for thromboembolism especially in combination with a reversed Trendelenburg (Caprini and Arcelus 1994). The above described effects, however, do only occur at higher pressures. Below a pressure of 6 mmHg no significant alterations are noted. It is therefore of utmost importance to limit pressure. This does not have to interfere with available space provided that optimal muscle relaxation is given. Mechanical abdominal wall lifting is an alternative.

Consequences of the Use of Gas

Gas in General

Gas Embolism. The use of gas predisposes for gas embolism. Most cases, however, do not seem to be related to the pneumoperitoneum as such but rather to direct intravascular insufflation caused by a misplaced Veress needle (Lee 1994). Nevertheless it does occur (Cottin et al. 1996; Cooperman 1995). The matter of possible intracardiac right to left shunting and therefore gas embolism to the arterial system is in most publications not addressed. In massive embolism, however, air has also been found on the left side of the heart (Black et al. 1991; Butler and Hill 1979). The mechanism for this most likely is that the formamen ovale is not completely closed, even not in adults, and can open up in the event of pulmonary hypertension. Whether a cardiac septal defect should be considered as a contraindication for a pneumoperitoneum is not clear at present. Newborns have a ductus arteriosus which can open up under certain conditions, for example, acidosis, fluid overload, hypoxia.

Subcutaneous Emphysema, Pneumothorax, Pneumomediastinum, Pneumopericardium. When gas is used, it may escape along the trocar sites and cause subcutaneous emphysema. If the pleura or pericardium is damaged or if congenital channels between the abdomen and the chest are present, a pneumothorax, pneumomediastinum or pneumopericardium may develop. Whether organ function is impaired depends largely on the pressure used. We rarely use a pressure in excess of 8 mmHg. An insufficient working space usually means that muscle relaxation has worn off.

Hypothermia. The use of large flows of gas, leads easily to hypothermia (Bessell et al. 1995). Warming up of the CO_2 before entering the body does not help much as most of the body heat is lost by saturating the gas with H_2O. It is our experience that hypothermia in children is less of a problem during laparoscopy than during open surgery. This has undoubtedly to do with the fact that an open abdomen in a small child leads to a far greater heat loss than when that same abdomen is approached laparoscopically. Moreover in children a pressure of 8 mmHg, in combination with optimal muscle relaxation, usually suffices. Moreover we try to avoid leakage as much as possible.

Specific Gas

CO_2, N_2O and helium can be used. N_2O can lead to combustion and is therfore not used. Helium is an inert gas, leading to much less metabolic changes than CO_2. The danger of helium for causing embolism has been stated not be greater than for CO_2 (Rademaker et al. 1995).

In contrast to N_2O and helium, CO_2 leads to hypercapnia, local acidosis, and hemodynamic alterations. Moreover retained CO_2 may be a significant cause of postoperative shoulder tip pain (Shrivastav and Nadkarni 1992; Jackson et al. 1996) and removal of retained CO_2 is an important preventive measure. Recently it was shown that the use of warm CO_2 greatly reduced the level of the postoperative shoulder tip pain (Korell et al. 1996; Semm et al. 1994). The duration of the operation is also correlated positively with the level of postoperative shoulder tip pain (Korell et al. 1996). Whether CO_2 as such, its total amount, and its temperature and the length of the laparoscopic procedure are the only factors involved remains to be proven. There could also be a correlation with the level of the intra-abdominal pressure used, and perhaps also with the initial flow. A higher flow might stretch the central diaphragmatic tendon more than a lower flow. The item of postoperative shoulder tip pain after laparoscopy seems to be underestimated. Apart for the inconvenience for the patient, it has been shown that it reduces pulmonary function (Di Massa et al. 1996).

Complications Related to Access

Inadvertent Injury of Intra-abdominal Structures

Major complications may result from puncture injuries by the Veress needle or trocar (Minz 1977). Stomach, colon and bladder injuries lacerations (Angle and Young 1995; Chamberlain and Carron Brown 1978; Spinelli et al. 1991) as well as major vessels injuries (Bacourt and Mercier 1993; Chamberlain and Carron Brown 1978; Nordestgaard et al. 1995; Peterson et al. 1982; Savill and Woods 1995; Seidman et al. 1996) have been described. Minor injuries undoubtedly often occur as puncture of the liver, omentum, and bowel, and most of them pass by unnoticed. In the multicentre enquiry of the Royal College of Obstetricians and Gynaecologist in 1978, a morbidity of 4% was reported and a mortality of 8 per 100,000 (Chamberlain and Carron Brown 1978). Of the four deaths one was caused by gas embolism, one by bowel perforation and two by cardiac arrest. In a more recent French multicentre study among gynaecologists there was one death in 7,604 laparoscopic procedures and 2.67 complications per thousand requiring laparotomy (Chapron et al. 1992). For major laparoscopic procedures 4.46/thousand required laparotomy versus only 0.42/thousand in the case of minor procedures. Vascular injuries were responsible for 38% of the laparotomies, and intestinal injuries for 52%. Natali (1996) reviewed 21 forensic medical complications of vascular injuries associated with endoscopic surgery. Three fourths of the cases occurred after 1990 and the fatal ones were usually related to bleeding caused by the inflation trocar. Usually the surgeon involved was well trained in this type of surgery!

Many of the complications of inadvertent puncture of organs or blood vessels can be avoided by using an open introduction technique for the first trocar as has been originally described by Hasson (1974). In a series of 330 cases of laparoscopic surgery, Nuzzo et al. (1997) did not see any complication related to trocar insertion. We feel that the open technique should always be used in children. However, even with the open technique inadvertent opening of the bowel can happen as has been described (Sadeghi-Nejad et al. 1994) and as recently occurred in our institution. Fortunately the mistake in our patient was recognised and the hole was closed without further consequences. Shielded trocars give a false feeling of safety as the shield is made of hard synthetic material. The edge of the shield is quite sharp and mechanical damage as a result may occur if underlying tissue is struck. Especially in small children the abdominal wall is tough and pushing hard on a trocar with sudden loss of resistance may injury the intra-abominal contents or even the opposite wall.

If an open infraumbilical technique is used, one should always remember that an omphaloenteric duct or urachus may be present and that these structures may be entered (McLucas and March 1994). We encountered once a long omphaloenteric duct, which ended blindly in the umbilicus but which was completely open just underneath the abdominal wall.

Port Site Bleeding

Severe bleeding from a secondary port site hole has been described on several occasions (Riza and Deshmukh 1995; Lewis 1995). We also have had such an experience. This complication is rare. In order to prevent port site bleeding, secondary ports should be inserted at places were no major abdominal wall vessels are known to run. Moreover secondary ports should always be removed under vision. It seems a good idea to insert a blunt instrument through the trocar before removal of the trocar a to remove the instrument only after inspection of the hole, as has been advocated by Lewis (1995).

Port Site Herniation

Intra-abdominal contents can herniate through the previous port site holes (Bourke 1977; Farney 1996; Fear 1968; Kadar et al. 1993; Plaus 1993; Sauer and Jarrett 1984; Shif and Naftolin 1974; Spier et al. 1993; Stringer et al. 1995). A relationship with the diameter of the port used and the likehood of herniation is undoubtedly present and all holes having contained a port of 10 mm or more should be closed. Herniation through smaller holes, however, has been described in children (Bloom and Ehrlich 1993) and this has also been our experience. Even when using 6-mm ports, we try to close the anterior abdominal wall fascia in thin children. In obese children this is difficult and perhaps not necessary.

Port Site Metastasis

Port site metastasis is a well known complication after endoscopic surgery both in the chest and in the abdomen (Andersen and Steven 1995; Ash et al. 1995; Bacha et al. 1996; Berends et al. 1994; Cirocco et al. 1994; Childers et al. 1994; Fry et al. 1995; Jorgesen et al. 1995; Walsh and Nesbitt 1995).

This poses serious questions behind the use of endoscopic surgery in malignant conditions. Intrapleural or intraperitoneal chemotherapy may avoid this complication but randomised studies have not been reported yet (Jacquet and Sugarbaker 1996).

Complications Related to Instrumentation

Inadvertent Injury

Inadvertent injury of intrathoracic or intra-abdominal structures during the endoscopic surgery itself has been reported on several occasions. Specific injury during specific operations may occur as common bile duct injury during cholecystectomy or ureteral injury during hysterectomy, but inadvertent bowel injury during laparoscopic surgery of any type has been reported most frequently. Especially during the initial years of laparoscopic surgery, warnings were expressed in relationship with the use of monopolar electrosurgery. Unrecognised tissue injury may occur as a result of an insulation break, capacitive coupling, or direct coupling (Grosskinsky et al. 1993; Voyles and Tucker 1992). Such injuries seem to occur infrequently. Preventive measures include avoiding the use of electrosurgery when the noninsulated end is not fully in view, confirmation of the integrity of the instruments for coagulation, and avoidance of activation of the system when the instrument is not in contact with tissue. Bipolar electrosurgery is certainly safer but is not really ready today to be used for cutting.

Dropped Clips and Staples

In endoscopic surgery the use of clips and staples is much simpler and faster than intracorporeal suturing and knotting. Clips and part of the staples may be lost within the body cavity (Huntington and Klomp 1995; Rawson et al. 1996). Complications caused by lost clips and staples have been documented but the incidence is not known (Huntington and Klomp 1995). In any case it seems wise to remove dropped clips and staples whenever possible.

Dropped Stones

Spillage of stones during laparoscopic cholecystectomy has been as high as 20% (Cooperman 1995). Most surgeons leave these stones behind as morbidity seems to be low. Occasionally, however, problems such as abscess formation (Carlin et al. 1995; Tzardis et al. 1996), chronic pelvic pain (Pfeifer et al. 1996) and pseudoaneurysm formation of the hepatic artery (Porte et al. 1996) have been reported. It is possible that retained material after perforated appendicectomy is responsible for the higher intra-abdominal abscess rate after laparoscopic appendicectomy (Tang et al. 1996).

Tissue Rupture and Spillage During Removal

Removal of large specimens still poses a problem in endoscopic surgery. If such a specimen ruptures specific complications may arise, for example, implantation of tumour cells or implantation of normal cells, for example, spleen cells during splenectomy. In one of our patients having a splenectomy for severe hemolytic disease, the hemolysis persisted postoperatively and the patient died. At autopsy several splenic implants on the serosa and peritoneum were seen.

Postoperative Nausea and Vomiting

It seems that laparoscopy and laparoscopic surgery predisposes for postoperative nausea and vomiting (Cooperman 1995; Iitomi et al. 1995; Philips 1992; Stanton 1991; Watcha and White 1992). Koivusalo et al. (1997) showed that abdominal wall lifting in combination with a low total amount of CO_2 resulted in less postoperative drowsiness and emetic sequelae than in a comparable group of patients receiving classic CO_2 pneumoperitoneum and thus a much higher total amount of CO_2. Stretching of the peritoneum and surrounding structures, for example, the diaphragm, however, could have been co-responsible. More research is needed to clarify the problem of postoperative nausea and vomiting, which is annoying for the patient and results in longer hospital stay and increased costs (Carroll et al. 1994; Green and Jonsson 1993).

Complications Related to a Specific Operation

Early Complications. Important bleeding during an endoscopic operation may occur but this can usually be controlled endoscopically at least when enough experience is available. The conversion rate for a specific procedure should be considered as an index of peroperative complications. Specific complications, for example, intra-abdominal abscess after appendicectomy are dealt with in the specific chapters.

Insufficient Operation. Whether the laparoscopic approach has poor, the same, or better long-term results has not been sufficiently investigated yet for most procedures. A higher failure rate after an endoscopic approach should be considered as a complication.

Personal Experience

We present here our total experience since we started with laparoscopic surgery. This means that our learning curve is included.

Patients

In the period from 1992 to November 1997, 532 laparoscopic procedures were performed. Of these 160 were purely diagnostic, the remaining 372 therapeutic. About 30% of the patients were less than 1 year of age.

Among the diagnostic procedures there were 85 laparoscopies for abdominal pain, 34 for taking a biopsy of the liver, 26 for cryptorchidism. Among the therapeutic procedures there were 83 antigastroesophageal reflux procedures, 23 gastrostomies, 75 pyloromyotomies, 65 appendectomies, 22 rectosigmoidectomies, 22 gonadal interventions, 14 procedures for intestinal malrotation, 14 cholecystectomies or cholecystotomies, and 12 splenectomies.

Complications Related to the Pneumoperitoneum

Major problems related to the pneumoperitoneum did not occur. On a few occasions some subcutaneous emphysema was noted at the end of the procedure. In long-standing procedures, low diuresis was noted. We do not have the impression that children approached laparoscopically lose more heat than children approached by formal laparotomy.

In one neonate with intestinal malrotation, the laparoscopic operation had to be abandoned shortly after insertion of the cannulae because of a persistently high intra-abdominal pressure without obvious reason. In one patient undergoing antireflux surgery the laparoscopic operation needed to be converted as a result of severely distended bowel loops.

Complications Related to the Access

No major vascular complications have occurred related to the insertion of cannulae, except for one patient who developed postoperatively a bleeding from a secondary cannula site. The patient required a blood transfusion and repeat laparoscopy but no laparotomy.

Two bowel perforations occurred as a result of cannula insertion. In one patients, this happened during the open insertion of the first cannula, in another patient during the insertion of a second cannula. Both perforations were noticed immediately. In the first patient the hole was closed and the laparoscopic procedure continued. In the second patient the operation was converted and the hole closed.

Port site herniation has occurred in five patients. Three out of the five hernias developed at the site of a previous epigastrial cannula. In four out of the five a 6-mm cannula had been used and the resulting fascia been had not been closed at the end of the procedure. Port site infections were seen in 6 patients, requiring antibiotics in one patient.

No oncological surgery has been carried out laparoscopically yet, so we cannot comment on possible port site metastasis.

Complications Related to Instrumentation

Inadvertent perforation during intra-abdominal instrumentation occurred in one patient with intestinal obstruction. There was gross contamination of the peritoneal cavity and despite immediate conversion and cleaning, the patient developed a wound infection. We have not seen complications related to dropped clips, staples or stones yet.

Removal of the spleen after complete laparoscopic freeing has been a problem. The sac in which the spleen was enveloped ruptured twice during extraction and another patient, with ongoing hemolysis after splenectomy, proved to have splenosis at autopsy.

Complications Related to a Specific Operation

Bleeding. Intraoperative bleeding let to conversion on 2 occasions, once during an antireflux procedure (at laparotomy the bleeding had stopped) and once during splenectomy. Uncontrollable bleeding occurred after a laparoscopic liver biopsy in a patient with rapidly progressive liver failure and severe coagulation disturbances and the patient died.

Perforation. Mucosal perforation during pyloromyotomy occurred in 4 out of 75 procedures. In all 4 patients the operation was converted. Mucosal perforation also occurred during a Heller's myotomy for achalasia, but this was repaired laparoscopically. In another patient diagnosed to have achalasia, perforation also occurred but this patient proved to have a cartilage containing congenital stenosis at conversion. In one patient who had a rectosigmoidectomy for Hirschsprung's disease one of the biopsy sites leaked postoperatively resulting in peritonitis. The patient was relaparoscoped the hole closed and the peritoneal cavity cleaned. Another patient with Hirschsprung's disease developed pelvic peritonitis. No clear perforation was found but to be on the safe side a diverting ileostomy was performed.

Insufficient Operation. Only insufficiency of the operation in the short term is addressed here. In one out of 83 patients undergoing laparoscopic antireflux surgery the wrap was too tight and corrective open surgery needed to be performed. Four out of 75 patients who had a laparoscopic pyloromyotomy needed a second pyloromyotomy. In one patient with Hirschsprung's disease, more bowel needed to be removed in a second operation.

Cetrimide Toxicity. In the laparoscopic treatment of hydatid disease of the liver, the intraperitoneal use of cetrimide in order to kill inadvertent spillage of scolices has been advocated (Khoury et al. 1996). We followed this suggestion in a 2-year-old child with chronic granulomatous disease and suspected hydatid disease of the liver. Unfortunately the child did not wake up after the procedure and died, most likely as a result of the intraperitoneal use of cetrimide. We think that cetrimide should not be used at all intraperitoneally (Bax et al. 1997).

Discussion

From our experience we can conclude that we have not seen major complications related to the CO_2 pneumoperitoneum and that relatively few complications were related to the access itself. Open insertion of the first cannula does not necessarily mean that no complications will occur as in one of our patients the bowel was picked up at the umbilicus and was entered. Fortunately this complication was noted immediately and was corrected. Since we have seen a number of incisional hernia's with the use of 6-mm cannulae, we have decided to close the fascia of these port sites as well the more so when the cannula has been introduced in the midline epigastrium.

Especially patients with obstruction are prone for iatrogenic perforation as the distended bowel is inflamed and friable and as the working space is rather limited. One should be extremely careful in these patients and use rather blunt than pointed instruments. Instruments with a very small diameter are more dangerous than the somewhat lager instruments.

During splenectomy it is important to avoid spillage of splenic tissue into the abdominal cavity as this leads to splenosis. This means careful dissection without entering the spleen and removal of the spleen in a sac. As the spleen is removed through a small hole in the abdominal wall, the spleen must be morcelated. Great care should be exerted in avoiding rupture of the sac.

Despite one of our patients died of ongoing bleeding after a laparoscopically taken liver biopsy, we still believe that liver biopsy is a good indication for a laparoscopic approach even when the coagulation status is not optimal. Of course the coagulation status should be optimised preoperatively and argon electrocoagulation should be available to control the bleeding from the puncture hole.

From our experience we learned that all laparoscopic extramucosal biopsy sites should be oversewn in order to prevent unexpected leakage.

We realise that we have a rather high complication rate in pyloromyotomy.

We conclude that it is important to register all complications meticulously as this may indicate causes and therefore prevention.

References

Andersen JR, Steven K (1995) Implantation of metastasis after laparoscopic biopsy of bladder cancer. J Urol 153:1–1048

Angle HS, Young SB (1995) Conservative management of incidental cystostomy at laparoscopy. A report of two cases. J Reprod Med 40:809–812

Ash AK et al (1995) Laparoscopy and spread of ovarian cancer (letter). Lancet 346:709–710

Bacha EA, Barber W, Ratchford W (1996) Port-site metastasis of adenocarcinoma of the fallopian tube after laparoscopically assisted vaginal hysterectomy and salpingo-oophorectomy. Surg Endosc 10:1102–1103

Bacourt F, Mercier F (1993) Plaies de l' aorte abdominale au cours des laparoscopies. Chirurgie 119:457–461

Bax NMA et al (1997) Cetrimide overdose. Surg Endosc 11:967–968

Beebe DS et al (1993) Evidence of venous stasis after abdominal insufflation for laparoscopic cholecystectomy. Surg Gynecol Obstet 176:443–437

Berends FJ et al (1994) Subcutaneous metastases after laparoscopic colectomy (letter). Lancet 344:58

Bessell JR et al (1995) Hypothermia induced by laparoscopic insufflation. A randomized study in a pig model. Surg Endosc 9:791–796

Black M et al (1991) Paradoxic air embolism in the absence of an intracardiac defect. Chest 99:754–755

Bloom DA, Ehrlich RM (1993) Omental evisceration through small laparoscopy port sites. J Endourol 7:31–32

Bourke JB (1977) Small intestinal obstruction from a Richter's hernia at the site of insertion of the laparoscope. Br Med J 2:1393–1394

Butler BD, Hill BA (1979) The lung as a filter for microbubbles. J Appl Physiol 47:537–543

Carroll NV et al (1994) Costs incurred by outpatient surgical centers in managing postoperative nausea and vomiting. J Clin Anesth 6:364–369

Caprini JA, Arcelus JI (1994) Prevention of postoperative venous thromboembolism following laparoscopic cholecystectomy. Surg Endosc 8:741–747

Carlin CB, Kent RB Jr, Laws HL (1995) Spilled gallstones-complications of abdominal-wall abscesses. Case report and review of the literature. Surg Endosc 9:341–343

Chamberlain GVP, Carron Brown JA (1978) Report of the Confidential Enquiry into Gynaecological Laparoscopy. London, Royal College of Obstetricians and Gyneacologists
Chapron C et al (1992) Complications de la coeliochirurgie gynécologique. Étude multicentrique à partir de 7,604 coelioscopies. J Gynecol Obstet Biol Reprod Paris 21:207–213
Childers JM et al (1994) Abdominal wall tumor implantation after laparoscopy for malignant conditions. Obstet Gynecol 84:765–769
Cirocco WC, Schwartzman A, Golub RW (1994) Abdominal wall recurrence after laparoscopic colectomy for colon cancer. Surgery 116:842–846
Cooperman AM (1995) Complications of laparoscopic surgery. In: Arregui ME, Fitzgibbons RJ Jr, Katkhouda N, McKernan JB, Reich H (eds) Principles of laparoscopic surgery. Basic and advanced techniques. Springer, Berlin Heidelberg New York, pp 71–77
Cottin V, Delafosse, Viale JP (1996) Gas embolism during laparoscopy. Surg Endosc 10:166–169
Diebel LN, Dulchavsky SA, Wilson RF (1992a) Effect of increased intraabdominal pressure on mesenteric arterial, intestinal mucosal blood flow. J Trauma 33:45–49
Diebel LN et al (1992b) Effect of increased intraabdominal pressure on hepatic arterial, portal venous, and hepatic microcirculatory blood flow. J Trauma 33:279–283
Di Massa A, Avella R, Gentili C (1996) Respiratory dysfunction related to diaphragmatic shoulder pain after abdominal and pelvic laparoscopy. Minerva Anesthesiol 62:171–176
Eleftheriadis E et al (1996) Splanchnic ischemia during laparoscopic cholecystectomy. Surg Endosc 10:324–326
Este-McDonald JR et al (1995) Changes in intracranial pressure associated with apneumic retractors. Arch Surg 130:362–365
Farney TL (1996) Laparoscopically induced hernia. Letter to the editor. Surg Endosc 10:865
Fear R (1968) Laparoscopy: a valuable aid in gynecologic diagnosis. Obstet Gynecol 31:297–309
Fry WA et al (1995) Thoracoscopic implantation of cancer with fatal outcome. Ann Thorac Surg 59:42–45
Green G, Jonsson L (1993) Nausea: the most important factor determining the length of stay after ambulatory anaesthesia. A comparative study of isoflurane and/or propofol techniques. Acta Aneathesiol Scand 37:742–746
Grosskinsky CM et al (1993) Laparoscopic capacitance: a mystery measured. Experiments in pigs with confirmation in the engineering laboratory. Am J Obstet Gynecol 169:1632–1635
Hashikura Y et al (1994) Effects of peritoneal insufflation on hepatic and renal blood flow. Surg Endosc 8:759–761
Hasson HM (1974) Open laparoscopy: a report of 150 cases. J Reprod Med 12:234–238
Huntington TR, Klomp GR (1995) Retained staples as a cause of mechanical small bowel obstruction. Surg Endosc 9:353–254
Iitomi T et al (1995) Incidence of nausea and vomiting after cholecystectomy or laparoscopy. Masui 44:1627–1631
Jackson SA, Laurence AS, Hill JC (1996) Does post-laparoscopy pain relate to residual carbon dioxide? Anaesthesia 51:485–487
Jacquet P, Sugarbaker P (1996) Wound recurrence after laparoscopic colectomy for cancer: new rationale for intraoperative intraperitoneal chemotherapy. Surg Endosc 10:295–296
Jorgesen JO, McCall JL, Morris DL (1995) Port site seeding after laparoscopic ultrasonographic staging of pancreatic carcinoma. Surgery 117:118–119
Josephs LG et al (1994) Diagnostic laparoscopy increases intracranial pressure. J Trauma 36:815–818 (see comments 818–819)
Kadar N et al (1993) Incisional hernias after major laparoscopic gynecologic procedures. Am J Gynecol 168:1493–149
Khoury G, Jabbour-Khoury S, Bikhazi K (1996) Results of laparoscopic treatment of hydatid cysts of the liver. Surg Endosc 10:57–59

Koivusalo AM, Kellokumpu I, Lingren L (1997) Postoperative drowsiness and emetic sequelae correlate to total amount of carbon dioxide used during laparoscopic cholecystectomy. Surg Endosc 11:42–44

Korell M et al (1996) Pain intensity following laparoscopy. Surg Laparosc Endosc 6:375–379

Lee A (1994) General anaesthesia for laparoscopic surgery. In: Paterson-Brown S, Garden J (eds) Principles and practice of surgical laparoscopy. Saunders, London, pp 23–38

Lewis JE (1995) A simple technique for anticipating and managing secondary puncture site hemorrhage. J Reprod Med 40:729–730

McLucas B, March C (1990) Urachal sinus perforation during laparoscopy. A case report. J Reprod Med 35:573–574

Minz M (1977) Risks and prophylaxis in laparoscopy: a survey of 100.000 cases. J Reprod Med 18:269–272

Natali J (1996) Implications médico-légales des traumatismes au cours de la chirurgie video-endoscopique. J Mal Vas 21:223–226

Nordestgaard AG et al (1995) Major vascular injuries during laparoscopic procedures. Am J Surg 169:543–545

Nuzzo G et al (1997) Routine use of open technique in laparoscopic surgery. J Am Coll Surg 184:58–62

Peterson HB, Greenspan JR, Ory HW (1982) Death following puncture of the aorta during laparoscopic sterilization. Obstet Gynecol 59:133–134

Pfeifer ME et al (1996) Ovarian cholelithiasis after laparoscopic cholecystectomy associated with chronic pelvic pain. Fertil Steril 66:1031–1032

Philips BK (1992) Patient's assessment of ambulatory anesthesia and surgery. J Clin Anesth 4:355–358

Plaus WJ (1993) Laparoscopic trocar site hernia. J Laparoendosc Surg 3:567–570

Porte RJ, Coerkamp EG, Koumans RKJ (1996) False aneurysm of a hepatic artery branch and a recurrent subphrenic abscess. Two unusual complications after laparoscopic cholecystectomy. Surg Endosc 10:161–163

Rademaker BM et al (1995) Effects of pneumoperitoneum with helium on hemodynamics and oxygen transport: a comparison with carbon dioxide. J Laparoendosc Surg 5:15–20

Rawson JV, Klein RM, Hodgson J (1996) Dropped surgical clips following laparoscopic cholecystectomy. Surg Endosc 10:77–78

Riza ED, Deshmukh AS (1995) An improved method of securing abdominal wall bleeders during laparoscopy. J Laparoendosc Surg 5:37–40

Sadeghi-Nejad H, Kavoussi LR, Peters CA (1994) Bowel injury in open technique laparoscopic cannula placement. Urology 43:559–560

Sauer M, Jarrett J Jr (1984) Small bowel obstruction following diagnostic laparoscopy. Fertil Steril 42:653–654

Savill LE, Woods MS (1995) Laparoscopy and major retroperitoneal vascular injuries (MRVI). Surg Endosc 9:1096–1100

Seidman DS et al (1996) Delayed recognition of iliac artery injury during laparoscopic surgery. Surg Endosc 10:1099–1101

Semm K et al (1994) Schmerzreduzierung nach pelvi/-laparoskopischen Eingriffen durch Einblasen von körperwarmen CO_2. Geburtshilfe Frauenheilkd 54:300–304

Shif I, Naftolin F (1974) Small bowel incarceration after uncomplicated laparoscopy. Obstet Gynecol 43:674–675

Shrivastav P, Nadkarni P (1992) Prevention of shoulder pain after laparoscopy. Lancet 339:744

Spier LN et al (1993) Entrapment of small bowel after laparoscopic herniorhaphy. Surg Endosc 7:535–536

Spinelli P et al (1991) Laparoscopic repair of full thickness stomach injury. Surg Endosc 5:156–157

Stanton JM (1991) Anaesthesia for laparoscopic cholecystectomy. Anaesthesia 46:317

Stringer NH et al (1995) New closing technique for lateral operative laparoscopic trocar sites. Surg Endosc 9:838–840

Tang E et al (1996) Intraabdominal abscesses following laparoscopic and open appendectomies. Surg Endosc 10:327–328

Tzardis PJ et al (1996) Septic and other complications resulting from biliary stones placed in the abdominal cavity. Surg Endosc 10:533–536

Voyles CR, Tucker RD (1992) Education and engineering solutions for potential problems with laparoscopic monopolar electrosurgery. Am J Surg 164:57–62

Walsh GL, Nesbitt JC (1995) Tumor implants after thoracoscopic resection of a metastatic sarcoma. Ann Thorac Surg 59:2–216

Watcha MF, White PF (1992) Postoperative nausea and vomiting. Its etiology, treatment, and prevention. Anesthesiology 77:162–184

Part IV
Urogenital Tract

CHAPTER 42

Transperitoneal Laparoscopic Nephrectomy

A.S. Najmaldin

Introduction

Laparoscopic nephrectomy was first described by Clayman and associates in 1991 [1]. Since then other surgeons have described successes using the technique of laparoscopy or its modification for nephrectomy, partial nephrectomy, nephroureterectomy, bladder neck suspension, pyeloplasty, excision of renal cyst, renal and ureteric stones, and reimplantation of ureter in adult patients [2, 3]. The application of laparoscopy in paediatric renal surgery, however, has remained largely undiscovered and experience so far is limited to case reports and sporadic short series of patients [4–6]. Most reports describing these techniques, in both adults and children, have attested to a reduction in post-operative pain, hospital stay, chest complications, recovery period, and improved cosmesis when compared with traditional open surgery [2–4, 6, 7].

Laparoscopic nephrectomy can be performed either transperitoneally [4, 5] or extraperitoneally [8, 9], with the former being more widely practised.

Indications and Pre-operative Preparations

At present laparoscopic nephrectomy should be limited to those children requiring a nephrectomy for benign renal diseases including: non-functioning kidneys secondary to reflux nephropathy, multicystic dysplasia, obstruction, nephrolithiasis and vascular ischaemia. Occasionally a nephrectomy may be indicated for protein-losing nephritis or uncontrollable hypertension due to renal or vascular diseases.

The place of laparoscopy in the management of urological cancer has remained limited to adult surgical practice and is highly controversial largely because of concerns about tumour size, seeding and the inability to examine surgical margins of the excised specimen [2, 10, 11].

As is the case with most laparoscopic procedures, there is no absolute contra-indications for the laparoscopic technique in nephrectomy for benign renal diseases in children. However, relative contra-indications may include: severe cardio-pulmonary disease, coagulopathy, severe obesity, previous surgery and scarring and very large/inflamed kidneys.

As for the conventional surgical approach, the successful completion of a laparoscopic nephrectomy requires the consideration of careful and adequate pre-operative radiological and endoscopic investigations. All patients must have informed consent for both laparoscopic nephrectomy and conversion/emergency laparotomy.

Equipment and Instruments

In addition to the essential and basic laparoscopic equipment and a set of instruments for laparotomy in case of emergency or conversion to open surgery, the following instruments are necessary:
- Cannula/trocar ×4 (3.5–12 mm)
- 0° or preferably 30° angled telescope (5–10 mm)
- Atraumatic, preferably curved and insulated, grasping forceps without ratchets ×2 (3.5–5 mm) for manipulation and dissection.
- One atraumatic grasping forceps or Babcock or soft bowel clamp with ratchet (3.5–5 mm) to grasp kidney or ureter
- One pair of insulated, preferably curved, double-jaw action, scissors with a diathermy point (3.5–5 mm). The insulation sleeve should extend to the actual blades.
- One retractor (3.5–10 mm). In most instances a simple rod or grasping forceps with or without ratchet may be adequate for retraction.
- Unipolar diathermy probe (3.5–5 mm). An additional bipolar instrument is an advantage.
- Single channel, two way suction irrigation probe (3.5–5 mm).
- Single-fire or preferably automatic multi-fire clip applicator with appropriate clips (5 or 10 mm).
- Occasionally suture materials or pretied ligatures may be used

Technique

The patient is anaesthetised with endo-tracheal intubation and full muscle relaxation. A small naso-gastric tube is placed and left on free drainage and urinary catheterisation is required only if the bladder is palpable. Theatre layout, position of the patient, surgical team, and the placement of the cannulae are shown in Fig. 1. In general, the child is placed and strapped in the lateral or semilateral position with a sandbag/towels under the contralateral loin/lower chest to allow lateral flexion and the bowel to fall medially under gravity. A slight reverse Trendelenburg tilt improves exposure. A peri-umbilical 5- to 12-mm primary cannula is inserted using an open technique (see Najmaldin and Grousseau "Basic Technique," section "Open Method," this volume). However, a primary cannula placed 2–3 cm lateral to the umbilicus allows better laparoscopic viewing especially in older and obese children. The primary cannula must be

42 Transperitoneal Laparoscopic Nephrectomy

Fig. 1a. Theatre layout for right nephrectomy. *D/D1*, diathermy/high-energy ultrasound/laser. **b** Position of patient (lateral or semilateral) and cannulae. *A*, Periumbilical or lateral primary cannula for insufflation, telescope, instrument and tissue retrieval; *B*, iliac fossa skin crease working cannula for dissecting instrument, large clip applicator, telescope, and tissue retrieval; *B1*, upper-quadrant working cannula; *C*, secondary cannula for retractor and dissecting instrument; *D*, lower abdominal crease line

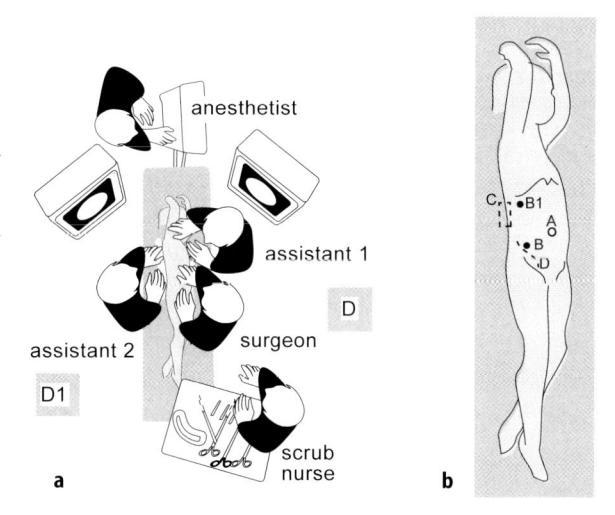

fixed with either a grip-on device or suture to prevent displacement. A pneumoperitoneum is then created using CO_2 (flow rate of 0.2-0.5 l/min, pressure 8-10 mmHg). Although a 0° telescope may provide adequate viewing, a 30° telescope is a better choice. The sites and sizes of secondary 'working' cannulae are dependent on the size of the patient, the size of the instruments to be used, the surgeon's preference and whether the patient requires ureterectomy or bladder surgery at the same time as the laparoscopy.

For nephrectomy one cannula is placed in the upper quadrant, one in the iliac fossa, preferably within the crease line, and a third is placed 2 cm above the iliac crest (mainly for retraction). In children, particularly on the right side, the kidney is usually palpable and often visible. A few centimetres long opening in the peritoneum, lateral to the upper border of the colon and directly over the kidney allows adequate exposure (Fig. 2). A true mobilisation of the colon is not necessary in paediatric patients. The kidney is then mobilised by blunt and sharp dissection using scissors, atraumatic dissecting forceps and diathermy (alternatively ultrasonic scalpel) starting with the lower pole lateral border, then the anterior surface and upper pole and finally the hilar and posterior regions. Mobilisation of the kidney may be facilitated by identification and traction on the renal pelvis and/or upper ureter. The renal capsule/substance can be held 'gently' by soft grasping forceps (or Babcocks or bowel clamps) for the purpose of traction and retraction without the risk of significant bleeding. Early identification and stenting of the ureter are not necessary.

The vessels are exposed usually close to the kidney substance and divided between two proximal and one distal clip. If thought necessary, the vascular pedicle may be further secured with additional suture ligature or pretied suture. In cases of simple nephrectomy, the ureter is clipped or ligated and divided at a convenient level. This specimen is then removed via the largest access cannula or the site of a cannula. A retrieval bag only be necessary if there is a risk of septic

Fig. 2a, b. Laparoscopic view. **a** A small incision directly over the kidney. **b** Mobilization of the kidney. A grasping forceps or retractor is used to retract the superior margin of the peritoneal incision

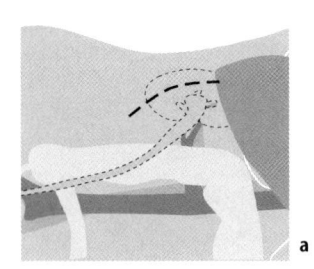

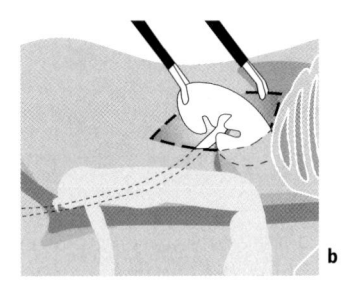

contamination or stone spillage, or the specimen is too large and requires morcellation. In cases of multicystic and hydronephrotic kidneys, the size of the specimen can be reduced by needle aspiration prior to the specimen extraction. The cannula site in the iliac fossa line or even the peri-umbilical region may be extended to extract large specimens if and when necessary. A change of telescope and/or instrument from one cannula to another may facilitate viewing and dissection during the procedure.

In cases of nephroureterectomy, however, the ureter is traced from above as far distally as possible, usually to the pelvic rim and the kidney (attached to the ureter) placed distally alongside the ureter in the retroperitoneal pouch, to be retrieved at a later stage (Fig. 3). The operative field including the adjacent colon, is then checked and the pneumoperitoneum is evacuated. All the cannulae are removed and the fascial incisions greater than 4 mm are closed (if desired the primary cannula may be left in situ until the end of the operation).

The iliac fossa crease-line cannula site is then extended sufficiently, excluding peritoneum, so that the distal ureter can be approached, ligated and divided, and the specimen is removed, all extraperitoneally. The semi-lateral position of the patient, with or without a slight lateral tilt of the operating table, allows both the laparoscopic and open distal ureteric procedures to be carried out without the need for changing the patient's position. If a concomitant bladder or contralateral ureteric procedure is required, the distal ureter is approached and the laparoscopically mobilised specimen is retrieved extraperitoneally through the Pfannensteil incision (the iliac fossa cannula site may be incorporated with the incision to approach the bladder). Alternatively, the procedure of nephro-ure-

Fig. 3a. Mobilization of the ureter from above as far distally as possible. **b** The kidney is placed low in the extraperitoneal pouch. **c** An extended iliac fossa cannula site (or lateral edge of a Pfannensteil incision) allows ligation and division of the distal ureter and removal of the specimen extraperitoneally

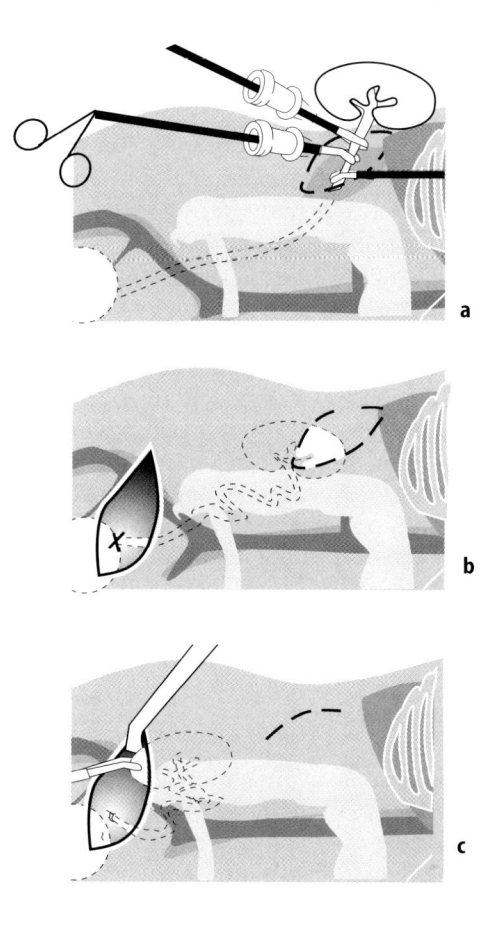

terectomy is performed entirely via the laparoscope. Here five or more cannulae are usually required and the distal ureter may be approached through a small peritoneal incision directly over the distal ureter, adjacent to the bladder.

Post-operative Care

At the end of the procedure the nasogastric tube is removed. In laparoscopic nephrectomy, local infiltration of the cannulae sites with appropriate anaesthetic agent provides adequate, short term pain relief and opiate analgesia is usually not necessary. The patient is ready to go home within 24–48 h postoperatively. However, the requirement for opiate analgesia and recovery time for those children undergoing combined procedures (laparoscopic and open) is usually dependent upon the nature of open procedure performed at the time of the laparoscopy.

Personal Experience

Over a 3.5-year period 22 consecutive children underwent laparoscopic nephrectomy. The indications for surgery were non-functioning or poorly functioning kidneys (less than 6% function on DMSA scan) due to reflux (11), multicystic dysplastic kidney (6), pelvi-ureteric junction obstruction (3), small dysplastic kidney (1) and an obstructive ureterocele (1). There were 13 girls and 9 boys, 9 right and 13 left nephrectomies. The average age was 5.4 years (range 1–15 years). One procedure was converted to an open technique due to faulty camera/light systems. Ten children had a simple nephrectomy (1 combined contralateral pyeloplasty). The remaining 11 children had nephro-ureterectomy. In the latter group, the distal ureter was approached and the laparoscopically mobilised kidney and upper ureter removed extraperitoneally via either an extended right iliac fossa cannula site (4), or the Pfannensteil incision which was made for concomitant bladder surgery (7). The average operating time for laparoscopic nephrectomy alone was 92 min (range 45–160 min). Children who had nephrectomy, with or without open excision of the distal ureter, through a small iliac fossa incision stayed in the hospital for an average of 2 days post-operatively (range 1–4). There were no laparoscopic technique-related complications.

Potential Complications

Although laparoscopic nephrectomy is a minimally invasive procedure, it is an operation nonetheless and the associated risks of the anaesthetic and procedure itself parallel those of established open, conventional procedures.

In collective data from two different adult urological centres (121 laparoscopic nephrectomies, 5% for malignant conditions) the conversion rate to an open technique because of intra-abdominal adhesions or bleeding was 8 %[12, 13]. Other complications in this series included haematoma formation (1), subphrenic abscess formation (1), post-operative bleeding requiring transfusion (2), pulmonary embolism (1) and colonic perforation (1).

At present experience in paediatrics is limited to case reports and sporadic small series of patients. In a combined adult/paediatric series of 230 laparoscopic procedures for urological conditions, (25% children), the incidence of serious peri-operative complications was 2.5% [major bleed 3, 2 of whom required laparotomy, pneumothorax 1, cardiovascular insufficiency 1] [14]. In this series one child developed cannula site incisional hernia.

As other authors in paediatric renal surgery [4, 8]. we have experienced no peri- or post-operative laparoscopic complications. The limitations of the laparoscopic method of nephrectomy are essentially related to the experience of the surgeon. The surgeon must recognise when to abandon the laparoscopic approach and to continue the operation via an open technique. With experience, and appropriate instrumentation and patient selection, the conversion rate to open nephrectomy could be less than 5%.

Discussion

In our experience we have found that in laparoscopic nephrectomy the routine, pre-operative bowel operation and peri-operative bladder catheterisation and ureteric stenting as reported previously by both adult [10, 11] and paediatric [4, 15] surgeons are unnecessary. In children the bladder is usually empty and easily expressible if full, therefore catheterisation is reserved for those who require an adjunct surgical procedure that necessitates a urinary catheter in position or monitoring of urine output. The ureter is readily identifiable because children have little retroperitoneal fat. Also, complete mobilisation of the kidney and upper two thirds of the ureter can be performed via a few or several centimetres long peritoneal incision directly over the lower part of the kidney without the need to mobilise the colon, thereby reducing the risk of, if any, post-operative adhesion formation. Most paediatric nephrectomy specimens are either small in size or cystic and decompressible, therefore they can be removed via the cannula, cannula site, or slightly extended cannula site incision. Morcellation is probably never required and a retrieval bag may be used only if there is a risk of infective contamination or stone spillage which are rare occurrences in paediatric practice.

The conventional open surgery approach to nephrectomy and nephroureterectomy involves one or two incisions respectively. In adult patients, prospective [7, 16] and retrospective [2, 17] comparisons between laparoscopic and conventional open nephrectomies have shown that the cost of surgery and post-operative opiate analgesic requirements, chest complications, hospital stay and time required to return to normal activities are reduced in the laparoscopic patients. Similar observations have been reported in paediatric patients [4]. However, the time required for laparoscopic surgery, at least initially, is significantly longer.

Traversing the peritoneal cavity may be a disadvantage in transperitoneal laparoscopic nephrectomy. Preliminary studies, however, indicate that transperitoneal and retroperitoneal approaches for laparoscopic nephrectomy produce equivalent outcomes in terms of morbidity and post-operative hospital stay [8].

Conclusions

Transperitoneal laparoscopic nephrectomy can be performed safely and successfully in the majority of paediatric benign conditions. The technique combines well with an open approach to the distal ureter and/or bladder surgery. However, meticulous attention to the details and instrumentation cannot be over emphasised.

References

1. Clayman RV et al. Laparoscopic Nephretcomy (letter). N Engl J Med 324:1370–1371
2. Kerbl K, Clayman RV (1994) Advances in laparoscopic renal and ureteral surgery. Eur Urol 25:1–6

3. Janetschek G (1995) Laparoscopic interventions in urology. Wien Klin Wochenschr 107:70–76
4. Ehrlic RN, Gerschman A, Fuchs G (1994) Laparoscopic renal surgery in children. J Urol 151:735–739
5. Najmaldin A (1994) Laparoscopy. Curr Opin Urol 4:316–320
6. Peters CA (1996) Laparoscopy in pediatric urology: challenge and opportunity. Semin Pediatr Surg 5:16–22
7. Eden CG et al (1994) Laparoscopic nephrectomy results in better post-operative pulmonary function. J Endourol 8:419–423
8. Guillonneau B et al (1996) Laparoscopic versus lumboscopic nephrectomy. Eur Urol 29:288–291
9. Gaur DD (1992) Laparoscopic operative retroperitoneoscopy: use of a new device. J Urol 148:1137–1139
10. Kerbl K et al (1993) Laparoscopic nephrectomy: current status. Arch Esp De Urol 46:581–584
11. Coptcoat MJ et al (1992) Laparoscopic nephrectomy – the king's experience. Min Invas Then 1 [Suppl]:325
12. Eraky I et al (1994) Laparoscopic nephrectomy: an established routine procedure. J Endoureol 8:275–278
13. Weber HM, Hormann M (1997) Sixty transperitoneal laparoscopic nephrectomies – a personal series. J Endoureol 11 [Suppl 1]:S126
14. Janetschek G (1995) Laparoscopic interventions in urology. Wien Klin Wochenschr 107:70–76
15. Emmert GK, Eubanks S, Ling LR (1994) Improved technique of laparoscopic nephrectomy for multicystic dysplastic kidney. Urology 44:422–424
16. Wilson BG et al (1995) Laparoscopic Nephrectomy: initial experience and cost implications. Br J Urol 75:276–280
17. Doublet JD et al (1996) Retroperitoneal nephrectomy: comparison of laparoscopy with open surgery. World J Surg 20:713–716

CHAPTER 43

Videosurgery of the Retroperitoneal Space in Children

J-S. Valla

Introduction

After the extraordinary expansion of video surgery in the natural cavities (abdomen, thorax) we are today at the birth of other mini-invasive approaches into virtual spaces. The first step of the operation consists in creating a working space from a virtual space with the help of gas insufflation. The virtual space is usually a well-known anatomical detachment area. The second step consists in introducing into this created space, with the help of trocars, some laparoscopic devices in order to realise the intervention. The goal is to reduce to the maximum parietal aggression, and the lumbotomy has a justified reputation as an impairing approach for muscles and nerves.

All surgical specialities actually develop such mini-invasive approaches into virtual spaces: general surgery suggests a preperitoneal approach for hernia repair, an axillary approach for lymph node removal in case of breast cancer; vascular surgery suggests a retroperitoneal approach for aortic and iliac surgery; plastic surgery suggests some new techniques for frontal lifting. Urology does not stand idly by: the mini-invasive techniques are proposed for approaching the retropubic space in order to perform an uterocervico cystopexy; the lumbar area is entered in order to perform renal and adrenal surgery. In classical paediatric urology the renal and ureteral approach is realised along a retroperitoneal path, except for Wilms' tumour and trauma: these indications represent only 10%–20% of cases according to the data. So it appeared logical to develop this mini-invasive retroperitoneal approach. As did other paediatric urologists [3, 6, 8, 11, 18, 21, 28, 29], we performed our first two cases of laparoscopic nephrectomy by a transperitoneal approach; these two attempts rapidly convinced us that the retroperitoneal approach is better suited than the transperitoneal approach for the treatment of benign lesions.

So the advent of laparoscopic surgery has revived the historical debate between the trans- and retroperitoneal approach to the retroperitoneal organs. In traditional surgery (and except for the indications mentioned above) this debate has been closed for a long time, since the advantages of the retroperitoneal approach over the intraperitoneal approach are obvious. We maintain that it is the same in mini-invasive surgery.

From an historical point of view, retroperitoneal gas insufflation was first used by radiologists in order to perform retroperitoneography. The visual exploration, without insufflation also called lumboscopy, was developed until 1969 by several surgeons, such as Bartel and Wurtz (cited in [5]). A modified mediastinoscope allows taking biopsies and cutting sympathetic nerves, but the lack of insufflation and therefore the lack of real working space for several devices combined with the limited view only allows for minor operations. The lumboscopy with gas insufflation was described in an animal model in 1976 by Roberts [27] and in humans by Wikham [30], who first realised an ureterolithotomy in 1979. This technique was only expanded upon in 1992, following the works of Gaur [12–14] and Kerbl [20].

Indications

There are three contraindications for retroperitoneoscopy:
- Wilms tumour for obvious oncological grounds
- Renal trauma due to the bad view into the perirenal hematoma if trauma is recent or perirenal fibrosis if trauma is old
- Previous retroperitoneal surgery because parietal fibrosis could jeopardise a new retroperitoneal insufflation

In children which procedures are feasible using this technique? First of all nephrectomy: total nephrectomy without ureterectomy might be indicated for multicystic dysplastic kidney, for destructed kidney by obstructive uropathy and for small kidney with hypertension. We do not discuss here the value of removing multicystic dysplastic kidneys, but this congenital malformation represents an excellent indication for beginning to gather experience with lumboscopic surgery because the dissection is easy and hemostasis problems are negligible. Kidneys destructed by obstructive uropathy are generally bulky, but after emptying by puncture, they collapse and become easy to grasp and handle because of the thinness of the cortex. Small kidneys with arterial hypertension do not pose particular technical problems. Kidneys destructed by pyelonephritis are generally of small size, stuck to the spinal column, and sometimes difficult to pull away from the surrounding structures. The presence of vesico-ureteral reflux demands a total ureterectomy down to the bladder level. In case of xanthogranulomatous pyelonephritis, the nephrectomy is famous for its difficulty; several examples of failure have been described [1, 10, 26]. The only case of our series operated by retroperitoneoscopy was a success, but this indication must be considered only with a well-trained team. In the same manner, a partial nephrectomy is a more difficult procedure than a total nephrectomy: partial nephrectomy is indicated when pathological ureteral duplication has destroyed one part of the kidney, with the upper pole nephrectomy in case of ureterocele or ectopic ureter being more frequent than lower pole nephrectomy in case of reflux. In both cases, a total ureterectomy is necessary. Others kidney diseases could be approached by retroperitoneoscopy. An example is the unilocular cyst: the unroofing is easy to do by retroperitoneoscopy.

The whole upper urinary tract could be seen and dissected by retroperitoneoscopy from the renal pelvis down to the bladder: the main indication is the lithotomy when endoscopic management or extracorporeal shock wave lithotripsy has failed or is contraindicated.

Several cases of pyelo-ureteral junction resection by laparoscopy have been reported in adults or adolescents. This indication can be justified at this age but is difficult to defend in infancy because treatment of pyelo-ureteral obstruction is usually indicated around or before 1 year of age. Classical surgery uses a small posterior approach and optical magnification (microscopic lenses) of a higher quality than the laparoscope.

The treatment of a varicocele by dividing the spermatic vessels is easy to perform by retroperitoneoscopy. Finally others rare indications can be considered: retrocaval ureter, ureterolysis for retroperitoneal fibrosis, adrenalectomy for benign tumour, lymph node removal, or removal of a benign retroperitoneal tumor, e.g. lymphangioma.

Preparation

Patients. The parents give their informed consent to the procedure. Children are prepared for surgery as usual without bowel preparation. A preoperative placement of ureteral catheter is useful only in two circumstances: in partial nephrectomy, where the nonpathological ureter is catheterised, and in lithotomy, where the ureteral catheterism allows the urinary tract to be flushed and to be checked for watertightness at the end of the procedure.

Materials. The instrumentation for the retroperitoneoscopic operation is the same as for abdominal laparoscopy. However, the following are useful: narrow and deep Faraboeuf retractors, a trocar with a specific system to avoid its extraction (balloon or umbrella), and a 5-mm clip applier. One or two 5-mm De Bakey clamps are also helpful. We have never used the endoscopic linear stapler.

Technique

Under general anaesthesia, the patient is placed in a lateral kidney position (Fig. 1a) monitored with an oxymeter and a capnometer. A soft bolster is applied underneath the child in order to enlarge the space between the last rib and the iliac crest. The surgeon, assistant and nurse stand at the patient's back as shown in Fig. 2. The video column stands on the other side, the cables are fixed to the inferior part of the operative field at the level of the thigh. The position of the surgeon and his assistant, and the position of the video column may change during the procedure. The installation must be planned accordingly. During the renal time of the procedure, the surgeon is placed between his assistant and nurse,

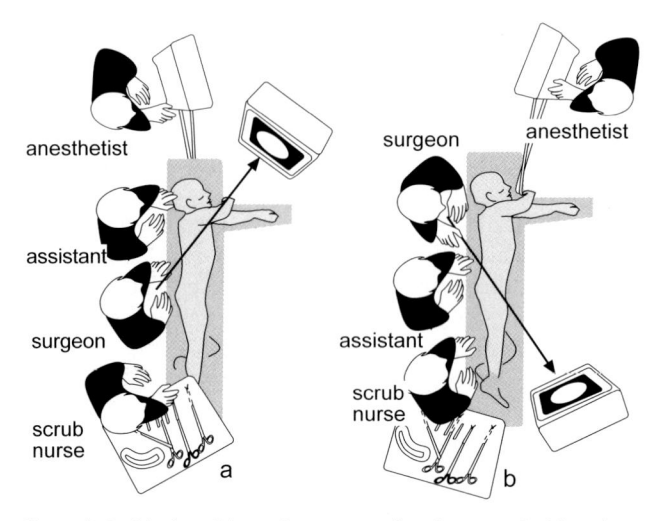

Fig. 1a,b. Positioning of the patient, crew, and equipment. **a** Position of surgeon and staff for the renal step. **b** Position of surgeon and staff for the ureteral step

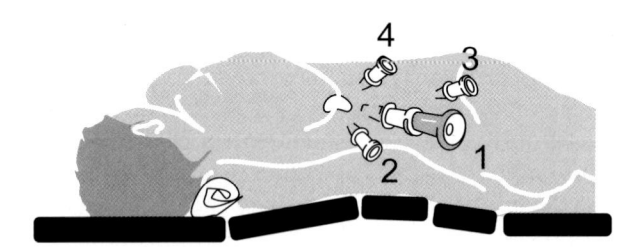

Fig. 2. Position of the trocars. *1*, Optic; *2, 3*, operating instruments; *4*, retractor

and the instruments are pointed toward the diaphragmatic area (Fig. 1a). During the ureteral time, the surgeon stands at the head of the patient, and the instruments are pointed toward the bladder (Fig. 1b).

A plastic bag is fixed to the ventral part of the patient: instruments are put away in this bag: monopolar hook, bipolar forceps, aspiration cannula. The position of the trocars is always the same, as shown in Fig. 2. The area where the trocars can be introduced is very limited in the infant – between its last rib, iliac crest and spine. This means that the trocars are very close to each others.

The four steps are as follows.

Retroperitoneal Approach

The retroperitoneal approach requires good anatomical knowledge; it has recently been reviewed by Himpems [17] for that purpose. The two main land-

43 Videosurgery of the Retroperitoneal Space in Children

Fig. 3. Retroperitoneal approach: the muscular landmarks

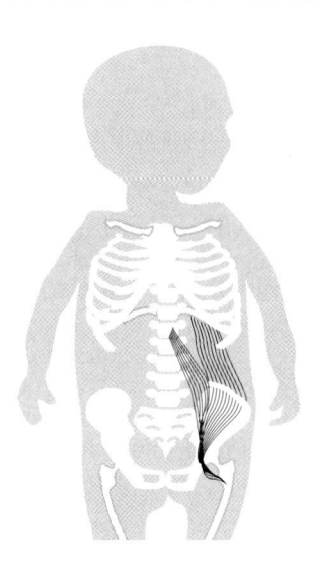

Fig. 4. Retroperitoneal approach under visual control with the help of the 0° 10-mm optic introduced between Faraboeuf retractors

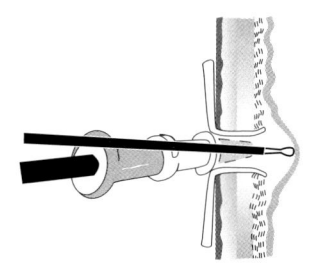

marks are the anterior part of the psoas muscle (Fig. 3) and the lower pole of the kidney, mobile with respiration.

A 15-mm-long skin incision is made at the tip of the 11th rib (or if too long, sometimes at the tip of the 12th) in the midaxillary line. This incision is deepened by blunt dissection down to the retroperitoneal space. Usually, dissecting forceps, Faraboeuf retractors, and Metzenbaum scissors are sufficient. Sometimes it can be useful to perform this dissection with the help of the 0° 10-mm telescope introduced between the retractors and a dissecting peanut grasped with a Kelly forceps which is moved under visual control on the screen (Fig. 4). In children the cutaneous incision is too small to enable finger dissection of the retroperitoneal space but large enough to visualise the two main landmarks. The surgeon must keep the dissection in close touch with the posterior muscular wall to avoid a peritoneal perforation.

Creation of the Working Space

After locating the lower pole of the kidney, a trocar – usually of 10 mm, sometimes 8 or 5 mm – is introduced: an airtight seal is ensured by means of pursestring sutures around the trocar.

A 0° or 30° telescope is introduced, and the insufflation is started between the capsula of the kidney and the perirenal fat with 8–15 mmHg pressure. The working space is progressively created by moving the tip of the telescope, used as a palpator to free retroperitoneal fibrous tissues, behind the kidney, taking great care not to injure the peritoneum. The thick lateral and posterior abdominal wall, closely attached to bony boundaries, cannot be distended by insufflation as well as the anterior abdominal wall; so a sufficient operating space can only be achieved by pushing away peritoneum and intra-abdominal organs. This explains why parietal suspension is worthless during lumboscopy and why good curarisation is essential. After the posterior surface of the kidney is completely freed, two operating trocars (5 or 3 mm) are introduced under visual control: one posterior in the costo-spinal angle, one inferior just above the iliac crest. This inferior trocar must not be placed too close to the iliac crest because the bony relief could restrict the device's mobility. With the help of two atraumatic instruments (palpator or peanut) the anterior surface of the kidney is carefully freed. It is only when the working space is large enough, when the peritoneum is sufficiently pushed away, that it could be possible to introduce, if necessary, a third anterior trocar usually of 3 mm: the instrument introduced through this trocar allows for retraction of the kidney in the upper part of the operative field. It is possible to introduce a Lowe retractor directly, without trocar, in order to expose the posterior part of the renal pelvis.

Performing the Operation: Usually a Nephrectomy

As noted above, several operations can be performed by lumboscopy. We describe only the total and partial nephrectomy.

After its two faces and two poles are completely freed, the kidney is mobilised and pushed to the top; then the renal vessels are dissected via a posterior approach (Fig. 5). They appear vertically in the view field: in order to realise a total

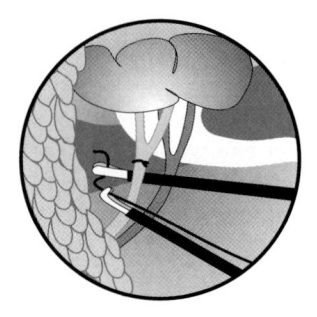

Fig. 5. Right total nephrectomy: the vena cava is clearly visible. The renal vessels are dissected and ligated in the inferior part of the view field

nephrectomy, the renal vessels must be dissected in the inferior part of the field, where there is only one artery and one vein and not too close to the kidney where the vessels divide into several branches. If possible the artery is managed first, by clip or extracorporeal ligature or, if small, by bipolar coagulation.

If the search for renal vessels proves difficult, the ureter may serve as the vital lead; the ureter is easy to discover in the retroperitoneal space, and its dissection up to the kidney leads to the renal vessels.

The ureterectomy could be limited to the lumbar part in case of nonrefluxing ureter and a ligature is not necessary. On the other hand, in case of refluxing or dilated ureter a total ureterectomy is essential. After changing the team position the ureteral dissection is carried out down to the bladder. In a boy this retroperitoneal approach allows a good view of the vas deferent and marks the inferior level for resection. The ureteral ligature is made by pretied ligature or extracorporeal ligature.

In case of partial nephrectomy, the operation begins with the search for the two ureters. The healthy ureter is recognised because of its normal calibre and due to the ureteral catheter. The pathological ureter is huge, tortuous; it is dissected taking great care to preserve the blood supply of the normal ureter. The pathological ureter is then divided and its upper part is freed up to the kidney. The next step is to discover the polar vascular pedicle close to the kidney parenchyma; usually bipolar coagulation is sufficient for hemostasis. The partition between healthy and destructed kidney is possible because of the modification of colour and consistency. The parenchyma section can be performed with monopolar hook or scissors, with ultrasonic scalpel or laser. In our short experience, it has never been necessary to clamp the whole renal vascular pedicle. However, this safety manoeuvre can be carried out, as in classical surgery, with a tourniquet or a laparoscopic De Bakey clamp.

Extraction of the Specimen

The specimen's extraction is of variable difficulty according to its volume. In case of multicystic dysplastic kidney, after puncture of all the cysts, the extraction is very easy; in the same manner in case of small kidney or large kidney with very thin cortex, the extraction can be performed without morcellation. Large specimens (7 cases) can be extracted after enlargement of the 10-mm hole, with or without the use of an endobag and morcellation. Personally we never have used an endobag except for calculus. When a total ureterectomy is necessary, a short inguinal incision allows resecting the ureter close to the bladder and extracting ureter and kidney; this manoeuvre is particularly useful in large children or adolescents (3 cases).

Personal Experience

From 1993 to 1998, a total of 67 children were operated on.

Renal Surgery (n=44)

- 24 boys, 20 girls from 2 months–16 years old, median age 3.7 years (12 cases before 1 year).
- 2 pyelolithotomies in the same patient: a 14-year-old girl with a large (25 mm) cystinic pyelic calculus. The first retroperitoneoscopic approach was easy, the pyelotomy was closed by a 5/0 resorbable running suture without stent, the recovery was uneventful, and the hospital stay was 3 days. Despite medical treatment after 18 months there was a recurrence; a new attempt at a retroperitoneoscopic approach was a failure, and a conversion was necessary; the hospital stay after this open procedure was 11 days.
- 2 unilocar renal cystectomies without conversion and without complication; hospital stay of 2 days.
- 40 nephrectomies:
  – 31 total nephrectomies for multicystic dysplasia (10), kidney destructed by reflux (10) or by obstruction (8), renal vascular hypertension (3), xanthogranulomatous pyelonephritis (1).
  There were no conversions, no major complications, no significant blood loss (no transfusion). Operative incidents involved 13 cases of peritoneal perforation. In no case did peritoneal perforation induce a conversion. There were 4 cases of mild subcutaneous emphysema, no pneumomediastinum, no pneumothorax. The mean operative time was 95 min. No postoperative complications and particularly no paralytic ileus were noted. In 8 cases a small suction drainage was left for 24 h. Pain medication was minimal and no patient needed pharmacological medication for pain after 48 h. One day after surgery solid food was given. All children returned to normal unrestricted activities within 6 days. A clinical and echographic check-up was performed 1 week and 1 month after surgery. The follow-up range was 6 months–4 years.
  – 9 partial nephrectomies:
  8 *upper-pole partial nephrectomies* indicated for upper poles destructed by obstruction (ectopic ureteral duplication). Five patients were under 6 months of age, and three were converted because of lack of space, poor visibility (5 peritoneal perforations) and the fact that it was almost impossible to identify the vascular pedicle of the upper pole. In one case after conversion a small perforation of the posterior part of the duodenum was found and repaired without deleterious effect. The mean operative time for the five nonconverted cases was 150 min. The postoperative course was uneventful exept in two cases where a postoperative urinoma occured at the upper-pole, which disappeared spontaneously in few weeks. The echo-Doppler and IVP control showed good function for the remaining lower pole.
  1 *lower pole partial nephrectomy* for a lower pole destructed by reflux in a eight years old boy, with good result.

Ureteral Surgery (*n*=2)

- A retrocaval ureter in a adolescent boy, initially treated by double J catheter and 2 months later by section, uncrossing, and termino-terminal anastomosis performed by retroperitoneal endoscopic approach with four trocars. Hospital stay 3 days. No complications. Ureteral obstruction was relieved as seen in echographic and IVP control 6 months later.
- One pyeloureteral junction resection in an obese fifteen year old girl; the pyeloureteral anstomosis was not satisfying so this case has to be converted with a good final result.

Varicocele (*n*=20)

- In male adolescents, a retroperitoneal approach to the spermatic vessels is made using only a 11-mm cannula for a telescope with operative channel. Vessels are coagulated with monopolar hook and divided (Palomo technique).
- 19 successes.
- Mean duration 10 min, hospital stay 1 day.
- No recurrence in 19 cases with a median follow-up of 6 months.
- 1 conversion because of the impossibility of identifying the vessels; in this case, the spermatic artery was not divided, and the varicocele recurred 1 year later. Interestingly, only one peritoneal perforation occurred in this age group.
- One postoperative complication was recorded: an ureteral burn injury, due to monopolar coagulation, which required a repair with good final result.

Adrenal Exploration (*n*=1)

- In a 1-month-old boy, with antenatal diagnosis of right adnexal mass, the postnatal biological and radiological examinations were unable to distinguish between adrenal hematoma, neuroblastoma, or other. The procedure began with endoscopic exploration of the retroperitoneal space and when faced with a solid tumour, a conversion was carried out. Removal of the adrenal gland including the tumour was easy. Histology: neuroblastoma N-Mic negative. Good evolution after 1 year of follow-up.

All in all, out of 67 cases, our global results are as follow:
6 (9%) conversions,
19 (28%) peritoneal perforations,
3 (4%) postoperative complications, but only one required a reoperation.

Discussion

Some *technical points* must be discussed.

As for intraperitoneal laparoscopy, the retroperitoneal approach can be performed by either blind or open technique. The blind technique advocated by Mandrassi [23] consists in the introduction of a Veress needle in the retroperitoneal fatty tissue under fluoroscopic or echographic control: then insufflation is started and the first trocar is also introduced by blind technique. This technique seems very dangerous because two sharp instruments with cutting edges are pushed in with only a radiological control. This is not advisable in children. Visual control represents the best guarantee against visceral or vascular injuries; it allows safe introduction of an atraumatic smooth trocar.

The creation of the working space – in other words, the detachment of the parietal posterior peritoneum – can be carried out directly with conventional instruments or with an inflatable balloon as described by Gaur [12]. According to its promoter, the use of a dissecting balloon allows an atraumatic progressive peritoneal detachment and simultaneously hemostasis by compression. We have made use of the balloon technique twice with good results, but its use seems superfluous in children because the peritoneal detachment is easy and bloodless. Its cost and the risk of balloon rupture and latex particle seeding are two others arguments against its use.

The consequences of CO_2 insufflation into the well delimited peritoneal cavity are well known. However, what about a CO_2 insufflation into a nondelimited artificially created fibrofatty space? Experimental and clinical studies provide various answers: according to Wolf [32], retroperitoneal insufflation may diffuse into the subcutaneous tissues, may increase the risk of pneumomediastinum or pneumothorax, and, finally it is responsible for a greater CO_2 resorption than intraperitoneal insufflation. On the other hand, Mandrassi [23] and Guillonneau (personal communication) state that this procedure does not carry any anaesthetic risk. Hemodynamic changes and CO_2 diffusion were identical with the two laparoscopic techniques intra- and retroperitoneal. Our results seem to confirm this: no deleterious effect of retroperitoneal insufflation, no pneumothorax, or pneumomediastinum have been recorded.

The most important part of the discussion must consider the *comparison between retroperitoneal laparoscopy and classical open surgery* and also other mini-invasive techniques such as minor lumbotomy or transperitoneal laparoscopy.

The objective of retroperitoneoscopic surgery is to decrease the damage to the abdominal wall. The intensity of parietal complications and sequelae depend on the length of the cutaneous, muscular, and aponeurotic incision. In open surgery, according to the retroperitoneal disease and surgeon's habits, different kinds of incision are used, more or less large, more or less posterior; these incisions may cut or split the three muscular layers but all cut across the course of the 10th, 11th, and 12th intercostal nerves, which can be injured directly or by retractors. The usual parietal complications, such as hematomas, abscesses, and eventrations, are less frequent in children than in adults. However, in our series of 80 nephrectomies between 1982 and 1992, we have recorded 4 cases of parietal complications which needed a second intervention; this number is quite low but the risk of nerve injury is much higher with conventional surgery, i.e. 17 out of 80 cases in our open series had abdominal wall paresis or paralysis. Since we started using the lumboscopic approach, we have recorded no parietal complications, no abdominal wall paralysis. With open surgery, the wound healing duration varies from 4 to 7 days in infancy, and from 8 to 15 days in adolescents. Finally, the permanently visible scars grow with the child; when a total ureterectomy is needed, a second groin scar is added to the lumbar scar. So the advantages of lumboscopic retroperitoneal nephrectomy seem obvious. They have been proven in adults by Para [25] and Doublet [7], but no comparative study in children is yet available.

Our mean hospital stay of 2.3 days for all kinds of nephrectomy is meaningful. With open surgery via a small posterior incision, it is possible to perform an outpatient nephrectomy [9]. However, indications must be carefully chosen and with this narrow approach, the operative view and the mobility of the surgical devices are reduced, because vision and instruments all enter together through the same little hole; in case of complication, vascular control of the renal pedicle would be hazardous. Furthermore, total ureterectomy down to the bladder is not possible and needs a second incision in the groin area. By the laparoscopic approach, with the same three or four ports, nephrectomy and total uretectomy can be performed with a better view of all the retroperitoneal organs, a view that only a large flank incision can offer. This struggle of lumboscopy against the short incision resembles the controversy between laparoscopic cholecystectomy and cholecystectomy via mini-incision that raged at the beginning of the 1990's: today we know how this confrontation turned out, even if laparoscopic surgery needs specific equipment, specific training, and prolonged operative time for the initial cases.

In adults [1, 2, 10, 31] and in children [6, 8, 11, 18, 19, 21, 28, 29] most of the published data about laparoscopic nephrectomy reported transperitoneal laparoscopic nephrectomies, so why *choose the retroperitoneal approach*? The main advantage of a retroperitoneal course is its more direct and rapid exposure [4,7,16] without peritoneal cavity transgression and without dissection and handling of intraperitoneal structures which could be injured during these manoeuvres. The working space is not obscured by intestinal loops, which must be pulled away by one or two instruments. After every intraperitoneal laparoscopic procedure, there is a risk of shoulder pain, postoperative paralytic ileus, omental evisceration, or intestinal adhesions [24]. The retroperitoneal approach eliminates all these risks; it can be performed easily even after previous abdominal surgery and uses fewer trocars.

The first and the primary disadvantage of the retroperitoneal approach is the lack of a natural cavity: the working space needs to be created and this step creates great difficulty at the beginning of the procedure. The younger the child, the easier this manoeuvre is, but the thinner the peritoneum. Thus great care must be taken during the initial access and insufflation to maintain the integrity of the peritoneum. The learning curve is quite real: out of our first 20 cases, we had 8 cases of perforation; out of our last 20, we had only 4.

Accidental peritoneal perforation induces pneumoperitoneum and reduces the retroperitoneal working space and visibility. If this mistake occurs at the end of the procedure, it is of no importance; if the perforation occurs at the beginning of the procedure it is sometime useful to close it with a purse-string suture or to desufflate the pneumoperitoneum continuously using a needle. An unexpected peritoneal perforation has never been the sole motive for conversion.

The second disadvantage of the retroperitoneal approach is that the working space is smaller than with the intraperitoneal approach and that the trocars are closer to each other because of the short rib to iliac crest distance. These constraints have been expressed by Ehrlich [8] who, out of 17 nephrectomies, tried one retroperitoneal approach "but the limited retroperitoneal working space in this small child procluded introducing other retroperitoneal instruments and, a routine transperitoneal laparoscopic placement was performed."

However with good training, good retroperitoneal insufflation, and good abdominal wall relaxation, this obstacle can be removed for total nephrectomy, but remains cumbersome for partial nephrectomy, as described by Gill [15], Jordan [19] and Winfield [31]. We have tried it in six cases and had to convert in three. Partial nephrectomy, especially in patients under 6 months of age by retroperitoneoscopy, remains an advanced procedure.

Conclusion

The laparoscopic retroperitoneal approach is simple in the child: there is no need for bowel preparation, ureteral catheter, balloon dissection, or an endoscopic stapler. There seems to be no age limit (ten cases under 1 year); the posterior peritoneal detachment is easy but requires great delicacy. This retroperitoneal approach is logical, anatomical and allows fewer trocars to be used, thus reducing the wound aggression to the minimum. Consequently this technique must decrease postoperative pain, wound complications, hospital stay, and scarring. This advantage can be decisive in some children expecting renal transplantation or in whom immunosuppressive therapy delays wound healing. Prospective randomised comparative studies between open and laparoscopic nephrectomy and between two kinds of laparoscopic techniques, intra- and retroperitoneal, are not yet available for the paediatric population. However our results are good for a start and we are convinced that a retroperitoneal laparoscopic approach in children is less invasive than an open or intraperitoneal laparoscopic approach. This technique should soon become a routine approach for kidney, urinary tract and other organs located in the retroperitoneal space.

References

1. Anderson KR, Clayman RV (1995) Laparoscopic nephrectomy. In: Arregui ME, Fitzgibbons RJ Jr, Katkhouda N, McKernan JB, Reich H (eds) Principles of laparoscopic surgery. Springer, Berlin Heidelberg New York, pp 693–701
2. Chandhoke RS et al (1993) Pediatric retroperitoneal laparoscopic nephrectomy (abstract). J Endourol 138 [Suppl 7]:12
3. Clayman RV et al (1991) Laparoscopic nephrectomy: initial case report. J Urol 146:278–282
4. Clayman RV et al (1994) Laparoscopic nephrectomy: transperitoneal versus retroperitoneal (abstract 459). J Urol 151:342-A
5. Darzi A (1996) Retroperitoneoscopy. Medical Media, Oxford, p 151
6. Das S, Keiser JJ, Taschima M (1993) Laparoscopic nephro-ureterectomy for end stage reflux nephropathy in a child. Surg Laparosc Endosc 3:462–465
7. Doublet JD et al (1996) Retroperitoneal nephrectomy: comparison of laparoscopy with open surgery. World J Surg 20:713–716
8. Ehrlich RM, Gershman A, Fuchs G (1994) Laparoscopic renal surgery in children. J Urol 151:735–739
9. Elder JS, Hladky D, Selzman AA (1995) Outpatient nephrectomy for nonfunctioning kidneys. J Urol 154:712–715
10. Eraky I, El Kappany HA, Ghoneim MA (1995) Laparoscopic nephrectomy: Mansoura experience with 106 cases. Br J Urol 75:271
11. Figenshau RS et al (1994) Laparoscopic nephrectomy in the child: Initial case report. J Urol 151:740–741
12. Gaur DD (1992) Laparoscopic operative retroperitoneoscopy: use of a new device. J Urol 148:1137–1139
13. Gaur DD (1995) Retroperitoneal surgery of the kidney, ureter and adrenal gland. Endosc Surg 3:3–8
14. Gaur DD, Agarwal DR, Purohit KC (1993) Retroperitoneal laparoscopic nephrectomy: initial case report. J Urol 149:103–105
15. Gill IS, Delworth MG, Munch LC (1994) Laparoscopic retroperitoneal partial nephrectomy. J Urol 152:1539–1542
16. Guilloneau B et al (1996) Laparoscopic versus lumboscopic nephrectomy. Eur Urol 29:288–291
17. Himpems J (1996) Techniques, equipment and exposure for endoscopic retroperitoneal surgery. Semin Laparosc Surg 3(2):109–116
18. Jordan GH, Bloom DA (1994) Laparo-endoscopic genito-urinary surgery in children. In: Gomella LF, Kosminski M, Wingield HN (eds) In laparoscopic urologic surgery. Raven, New York, pp 223–246
19. Jordan GH, Winslow BH (1993) Laparoscopic upper pole partial nephrectomy with ureterectomy. J Urol 150:940–943
20. Kerbl K et al (1993) Retroperitoneal laparoscopic nephrectomy. Laboratory and clinical experience. J Endourol 7:23–26
21. Koyle MA, Woo JJ, Kavoussi LR (1993) Laparoscopic nephrectomy in the first year of life. J Pediatr Surg 28:693–695
22. MacFadyen BV (1996) Retroperitoneal surgery. Semin Laparosc Surg 3(2):59–60
23. Mandressi A et al (1995) Retroperitoneoscopy. Ann Urol 29:91–96
24. Moore RG et al (1995) Post-operative adhesion formation after urological laparoscopy in the pediatric population. J Urol 153:792–795
25. Parra RO et al (1995) Comparison between flank versus laparoscopic nephrectomy for benign renal disease. J Urol 153:153–1171

26. Rassweiler JJ et al (1994) Retroperitoneal laparoscopic nephrectomy and other procedures in the upper retroperitoneum using a balloon dissection technique. Eur Urol 25:229–236
27. Roberts JA (1976) Retroperitoneal endoscopy. J Med Primatol 5:124–127
28. Susuki K et al (1993) Laparoscopic nephrectomy for atrophic kidney associated with ectopic ureter in a child. Eur Urol 23:463–465
29. Tan HL (1995) Minimally invasive surgery in pediatric. Dial Pediatr Urol 18:1–8
30. Wickham JEA, Miller RA (1979) The surgical treatment of renal lithiasis. In: Wickham JEA (ed) Urinary calculus disease. Churchill Livingstone, Edinburgh, pp 145–198
31. Winfield HN et al (1995) Laparoscopic partial nephrectomy: initial experience and comparison to the open surgical approach. J Urol 153:1409–1414
32. Wolf JS et al (1995) The extraperitoneal approach and subcutaneous emphysema are associated with greater absorption of carbon dioxide during laparoscopic renal surgery. J Urol 154:959–963

CHAPTER 44

The Nonpalpable Testis

F. Ferro

Introduction

By the late 1970's, after the first case had been published (Cortesi et al. 1976), laparoscopy became first-choice examination for the impalpable testis (Diamond and Caldamone 1992; Moore et al. 1994). The first pediatric series was actually that of Scott in 1982, but only recently laparoscopy has been broadening its indications. In 1991 Bloom performed the first stage of the Fowler-Stephens procedure and, in the same year Jordan et al. (1992) carried out a single stage orchidopexy laparoscopically. In 1994 Caldamone and Amaral reported their experience about the second stage Fowler-Stephens orchidopexy with laparoscopic approach. Finally in the series of Docimo et al. (1995) evidence was given that laparoscopic orchidopexy for the high palpable undescended testes is possible, safe, effective, and with minimal morbidity.

Cryptorchidism is the most frequent anomaly of the male genital system and therefore one of the more frequent surgical conditions in the pediatric patient. Testicular maldescent has an incidence of approximately 0.8% at 1 year of age in otherwise normal term infants. The shorter the gestational age, the higher the rate of cryptorchidism; and in approximately 20% of cryptorchids the testis is nonpalpable. Although testicular maldescent is not a uniform disorder but rather a spectrum of clinical situations in which it may not be possible to define the exact etiology, pathogenesis, prognosis and appropriate treatment in the single case, there is quite uniform consent to relocate the cryptorchid testis in the scrotum before the onset of parenchymal damage, which is evident by 1 year of age under electronic microscope, and by 18 months by means of regular light microscope (Minimberg et al. 1982). Early orchidopexy seems to reduce the risk of future infertility and maybe also that of neoplastic transformation. In any case the testis would be in a more accessible site for postoperative follow-up.

Surgical orchidopexy repairs the associated groin hernia, prevents a possible torsion of the spermatic cord, and finally offers a cosmetic improvement of the genital area. Furthermore, early orchidopexy seems to have a higher rate of success, probably due to the shorter distance from the inguinal canal to the dependent scrotum. It has been generally believed that success after orchidopexy is related to the preoperative testicular position. On the base of numerous revised series it has been noted that the difference between the success rate for intra-abdominal and peeping testes (76.1%) and for canalicular testes (89.8%) appears highly significant (Docimo 1995).

The condition of nonpalpable testis may be due to difficulties in the physical examination (uncomfortable child, cold hands or environment), or to hypotrophy of a canalicular testis, excess fat over the groin, while rarely an unusual ectopia (cross-testicular or perineal ectopia) may lead to a misdiagnosis of impalpable testis.

Apart from the aforementioned instances, a nonpalpable testis falls into one of five categories:
- Absent gonad because of agenesis (rare) or as a consequence of intrauterine torsion in the abdomen or in the inguinal canal (the so-called *vanishing testis*).
- Gonad present but dysgenetic.
- Normal testis present in the abdomen, close to the internal ring and free to be mobilized into the inguinal canal (*peeping testis*).
- Low abdominal testis with long or short mesorchium.
- High intra-abdominal testis. Preoperative knowledge of the testis' position permits to chose the best operative strategy. This is especially true in cases of intra-abdominal gonads, where extensive groin and retroperitoneal exploration would be time-consuming and possibly fruitless.

Preoperative Workup

The diagnostic workup for impalpable testes differs for unilateral and bilateral cases. In bilateral ones, the human chorionic gonadotropin stimulation test has been advocated as a method of determining whether testicular tissue is present. In boys with a 46 XY karyotype and a male phenotype, the presence of substantially elevated gonadotropins and failure of serum testosterone to rise after stimulation strongly suggest that both testes are absent. This test may be negative in case of severe bilateral gonadal dysgenesis (Bartone et al. 1984), and Perovic and Janic (1994) reported on cases of negative tests in whom they found normal testes. Consequently, exploration should not be omitted and any dysgenetic tissue should be removed, because the risk of neoplastic transformation is higher in such cases.

Different means of investigation are still in use to preoperatively locate the impalpable testis. Ultrasonography has the advantage of being noninvasive and can be helpful in locating inguinal testes in fat boys. Its usefulness is otherwise nil having a sensitivity of only 13% in abdominal testicles (Weiss et al. 1986). Computerized tomography has a false negative rate of 44% in the pediatric population and the radioactivity exposure is of concern (Landa et al. 1987; Raijer et al. 1983). Magnetic resonance imaging offers several advantages in that it is noninvasive, nonionizing, capable of obtaining multiplanar images and has a potential for tissue characterization. However, MRI has long scanning times and needs sedation for optimal study in children under 5 years of age; furthermore, many authors experienced false negatives and false positive results (Tennenbaum et al. 1994). Spermatic venography is difficult in children under 4 years old, and anesthesia or heavy sedation is required (Weiss and Glickman 1982). In any case neither technique can ultimately prove that the testis is absent.

The primary surgical approach has been recommended to solve both the diagnostic and therapeutic aspects of the nonpalpable testis at the same time, as standard orchidopexy is possible in the vast majority of cases of intra-abdominal or canalicular testes (Ferro et al. 1992; Hazebroek and Molenaar 1992). Moreover, it offers the advantage of implanting an artificial testis through the same inguinal incision in case of vanishing or absent testis (Ferro et al. 1991). This approach, however, leads to a number of unnecessary extensive surgical procedures and should be revised in consideration of the new interventional possibilities offered by laparoscopy (Vaysse 1994). It is anyway necessary to be familiar with the techniques of *difficult orchidopexy*, with the alternatives such as the staged orchidopexy, with and without the Corkery modification (Ferro et al. 1990), the Fowler-Stephens technique and its anatomical background (Kogan et al. 1989; Poppas et al. 1996; Ransley et al. 1984), and with the microsurgical autotransplantation (Bukowsky et al. 1995). In fact, it may become necessary to employ such surgical alternatives either because of mistaken laparoscopic impression, or because laparoscopy must be interrupted for technical reasons or for unexpected complications.

Preoperative Preparation

Informed consent must include the following items: the possibility of converting from laparoscopic procedure to laparotomy during surgery, possible complications directly related to the technique, possible transfusion (cross-match), the possibility of having to perform orchiectomy or staged orchidopexy. The insertion of a testicular prosthesis and contralateral scrotal orchidopexy must also be discussed with the parents.

Most authors suggest to introduce a small pediatric feeding tube in the bladder and emptying the stomach. We don't introduce a bladder catheter routinely unless the bladder is palpable. Only in 2 out of 100 have cases we had to catheterize the bladder during laparoscopy, while in another case we were able to identify the vas deferens of one side after rotating the child to the contralateral side, thus moving the bladder out of the way. If the bladder is empty at the beginning of laparoscopy, it will probably remain so throughout the procedure, because of the reduction in diuresis due to the pneumoperitoneum.

Technique

Set-Up

- Diagnostic laparoscopy
  - Insufflator
  - Video system
  - (Veress needle)
  - 2- or 5-mm laparoscope
  - 3- or 5-mm reusable umbilical trocar (or Hasson trocar)
  - Electrocautery plate on patient
- Operative laparoscopy
  - Insufflator
  - Video system
  - (Veress needle)
  - Irrigator-aspirator
  - 5- or 10-mm laparoscope
  - 5- or 10-mm trocar (eventually a Hasson's trocar)
  - Two 3- or 5-mm trocars for working instruments
  - 5- or 10-mm endoscopic clip applier
  - 3- or 5-mm curved short dissector
  - 3- or 5-mm mini short scissors
  - 3- or 5-mm atraumatic grasper or endo-Allis
  - Cautery cord
  - Foot pedal cautery
  - Electrocautery plate on patient

Laparotomy equipment should be available at any time if conversion to open surgery is necessary.

Position of the Patient, Crew and Cannulae

The exploration of the abdominal cavity may be started with the patient supine. The surgeon stays opposite to the site to be explored. The monitor is located opposite to the surgeon. The assistant stays at the left side of the surgeon and the scrub nurse at the right side. In the majority of cases both internal inguinal rings may be observed in this position, and the diagnostic laparoscopy may be carried out entirely in this position. Failure to visualize the spermatic vessels and/or the vas deferens requires to put the patient in a 20°–30° Trendelenburg position and eventually to rotate him to the contralateral side. These modifications of position are necessary to carry out interventional laparoscopy.

As the average age of the patients is rather young, we suggest to use the open technique for the insertion of the first trocar. The approach is supraumbilical, with a curved 270° incision that enables to prepare a good portion of the supraumbilical linea alba, and to proceed into the peritoneum 2–3 cm rostrally to the subumbilical access. A purse-string suture (2/0 polyglycolic) is then applied around the trocar sheath (unless it is a Hasson's trocar) and is put into traction using a tourniquet made out of a small piece of feeding tube. At the end of the procedure the purse-string suture is tied closing the abdominal defect promptly and safely. Using this technique we have had no immediate or late umbilical hernia complications. Such umbilical access may be useful to remove the gonad as well, either because it is dysgenetic or because the patient has passed puberty. Even in the presence of an umbilical hernia, which some authors consider to be a contraindication, we advocate the use of the Hasson technique, with repair of the hernia at the end of the laparoscopy.

Depending on the age of the patient a pneumoperitoneum pressure between 8 and 12 mmHg is used.

Laparoscopic Diagnosis

Male Laparoscopic Pelvic Anatomy

Differences exist between the female laparoscopic pelvic anatomy, explored by gynecologists for several years, while the male laparoscopic pelvic anatomy is of more recent acquisition (Fig. 1) this must be learned in its normal anatomic landmarks and in its pathological aspects. Several vestigial structures, particularly those related to the umbilicus, are important in the endoscopic examination of the pelvis. The umbilical arteries persist in the deep pelvis as the internal iliac and proximal superior vesical artery, whereas the more anterior aspects remain as the medial umbilical ligament on each side. This is a very important landmark, perhaps the most visually obvious structure in the pelvis, permitting quick identification of the internal ring, which lies laterally; it is the key to an accurate diagnosis in patients with nonpalpable testis. Normal laparoscopic anatomy of the inter-

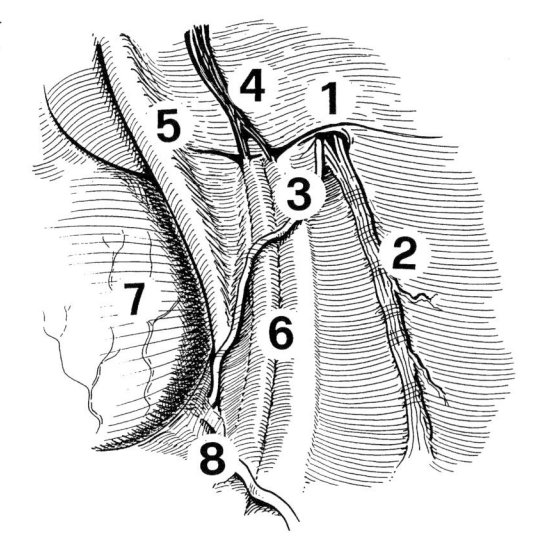

Fig. 1. Normal male pelvic anatomy. *1*, Internal inguinal ring; *2*, testicular vessels; *3*, vas; *4*, deep epigastric vessels; *5*, medial umbilical ligament; *6*, iliac vessels; *7*, bladder; *8*, ureter

nal ring consists of a substantial leash of spermatic vessels, without attenuation in caliber, proceeding into a closed ring, lateral to the vas deferens.

Laparoscopically the spermatic vessels and the vas are configured as an inverted V. Another fairly consistent finding in boys is the transverse vesical fold that blends into the anterior margin of the ring or fans out and disappears just above it. The ureter passes from a point medial to the distal spermatic vessels, deviating from them toward the midline across the iliac vessels to pass underneath the vas deferens. Sometimes, the most distal part of the ureter is hidden in fat and it therefore very important to have a confident sense of its position in order to avoid any injury to it. In cases of insufficient activity of müllerian inhibiting factor, one may encounter uterine or salpingeal structures, and, in cases of more complex disorders of the sexual differentiation, also ovaries or dysgenetic gonads, may be present (Bloom et al. 1994).

Findings in the Nonpalpable Testis

Cord structures entering the internal ring and appearing to be of normal size, i.e., equal to the one on the contralateral side, with or without a patent processus vaginalis.

Many authors believe that the presence of a hernial sac implies that the testicle is located at the level of the internal ring or more distally. If the sac is open, the testis may be pushed from the inguinal canal into the abdomen with a gentle pressure over the groin area, because of the usually long mesorchium. Otherwise, the testicle may be seen directly by pushing the lens into the inguinal canal.

In the case of atrophic testis (vanishing or vanished testis) the internal ring is generally closed and the spermatic vessels can appear smaller in caliber, are sometimes hardly visible or completely interrupted far from the internal inguinal ring, whereas the vas normally passes through it.

This finding must not to be confused with the abdominal vanishing testis or with blind ending vas.

In younger children the spermatic vessels may appear of normal size even if the testicle has undergone complete atrophy. This event is explained by the short period of time elapsed from the occurrence of testicular atrophy and laparoscopic exploration (Perovic and Janic 1994). In older children the vessels become hypotrophic in cases of vanishing testis. One of the questions in cases where the vas and vessels are seen entering the inguinal ring, is whether inguinal exploration is also necessary in slim children whose testes remain impalpable after anesthesia. In their series Weiss and Seashore (1987) reported the complete absence of viable testicular tissue in specimens excised from 7 patients who underwent inguinal exploration. Nogueira Castilho (1990) also did not find any testicular tissue in 8 spermatic cord structures removed at exploration, although he reported varying degrees of germinal hypoplasia or aplasia in 14 testes that were also removed. Plotzker et al. (1992) found microscopic islands of tubular epithelium within the small nubbins of tissue residing within the inguinal canal in 3 patients.

Since there are no documented cases of tumors arising from such nubbins, we feel that the significance of this finding is merely speculative. In our experience the problem is overcome by the request by the parents to implant a testicular prosthesis at the time of exploration or later if the child is too small. In such cases the excision of the eventual remnant is undertaken at the time of the implant. Another important issue is whether to pex the contralateral testis when a child is found to have a vanishing testis. Both the epidemiology of spermatic cord torsion in a solitary testis and the anatomical features of the testis contralateral to an atrophic one are not prone to a higher risk of torsion of a solitary testis with respect to any other scrotal testis. Nevertheless, we agree with Rozansky and Bloom (1995) who say *when a child is found to have only one testis, that gonad assumes a value beyond measure,* as the loss of a solitary testis is a catastrophic event. Therefore it is our practice to perform a prophylactic contralateral orchidopexy.

The laparoscopic identification of a blind-ending vas and spermatic vessels should be sufficient to establish the diagnosis of abdominal vanishing testis, which does not require further exploration.

Sometimes, the vessels are seen only after mobilization of the colon, they may end at some distance from the vas and may be very thin. The finding of an irregular terminal vas deferens, resembling an abdominal nubbing, toward which some vascular structures seen to approach, requires a very close evaluation. In fact these structures may be just a folding of the same vas and vessels which turn upwards to reach a high intra-abdominal testis, usually without mesorchium.

Laparoscopic visualization of the spermatic vessels alone, without the vas is a condition that is seldom referred to in the largest series and that we personally have never found.

The vas may be hidden behind the bladder if the latter is partially full. In one of our cases we identified the vas after inserting a feeding tube in the bladder during laparoscopy, as we do not routinely catheterize the bladder before starting the case. Levitt et al. (1978), after an extensive review, summarized that the finding of unilateral impalpable testis and vessels alone is present in 5% of cases.

The identification of only the vas blind ending in the abdomen or entering the internal ring without spermatic vessels is given different meanings depending on the investigators. Testicular absence, according to many reports, can be established only when blind ending vessels are found but not when a vas alone is present. These arguments are based on isolated reports of patients with complete separation between the testis and epididymis, in whom the vas and the epididymis were found in the scrotum or in the inguinal canal and the testis was found in the abdomen, or in the rare instance of an agenesis of the ductal system and an abdominal testis located close to the lower pole of the kidney. Others argue that a blind ending vas has the same diagnostic value of the blind ending vessels (Holcomb et al. 1994). Theoretically, testicular absence may be due to agenesis or perinatal torsion. The concept that testicular absence may be correctly diagnosed only when blind ending vessels are found does not take into consideration the rare (but documented) primary agenesis, in which the vessels have failed to develop along with the testis. Furthermore, there may be the case of antenatal torsion with complete reabsorption not only of the testicle, but also of the ductal structures and the vessels. This would account for the uncommon finding of testicular absence along with the absence of müllerian duct remnants. Guiney et al. (1989) reported failure to identify any structure that could possibly suggest the previous presence of a testicle. In two cases of a blind ending vas alone, when implanting the testicular prosthesis a nubbin was found in the scrotum, histologically resembling a vanishing testis (fibrosis, calcification).

Low abdominal and peeping testis

The finding of a testicle which lies between the abdomen and the internal inguinal ring (*peeping testis*), or in proximity with the internal ring, or behind the bladder is one of the instances when the testis is present. In the first case the gonad may be mobilized back and forth from the inguinal canal into the abdomen and vice-versa by means of gentle pressure on the groin or touching it with the camera. If there are doubts on the length of the vascular pedicle, a second trocar is inserted contralaterally to the abdominal testis and a grasper is used to mobilize the testis medially and/or rostrally, or to push the gonad in the inguinal canal if there is an open hernia sac. Despite the validity of these maneuvers, there may be cases in which the decision to perform a standard orchidopexy with high retroperitoneal dissection will appear too optimistic, due to the real brevity of the cord. However, the opposite is also true: section of the spermatic vessels to carry out a Fowler-Stephens repair have been performed in cases that probably would have not required anything else but a standard operation (Ferro et al. 1996). This diagnostic aspect is loosing importance nowadays as the tendency becomes that of an entirely laparoscopic single stage orchidopexy.

High intraabdominal testis

The finding of high intra-abdominal testis is less frequent than the low abdominal one. Usually the high abdominal gonad has an altered elongated anatomy, without mesorchium and thus little or not mobile at all, with an hypoplastic epididymis. The evaluation of these gonads requires the insertion of additional trocars, which is subsequently necessary to clip the spermatic vessels, as first step of a staged Fowler-Stephens repair, or to perform a laparoscopic orchiectomy.

Laparoscopic Therapy

Gonadectomy

The finding of a dysgenetic abdominal gonad, that of a very small testis, or unilateral cryptorchidism in the postpubertal age are considered indications for orchiectomy, which can be accomplished laparoscopically with two accessory ports, one 3- and one 5-mm if a 5-mm clip applier is available, or otherwise one of 5 mm and one 10–12 mm. Holcomb et al. (1994) recommend to insert the endoscopic clip applier in the suprapubic area and another port in the ipsilateral lower abdominal quadrant. Dissecting forceps are employed through the 5-mm abdominal port and used to dissect and expose the vas deferens and the testicular vessels. Endoclips are placed through the suprapubic port and vas and vessels are closed and divided. The testis is then removed through the suprapubic cannula. If the testis is too large to get into the cannula, the latter can be withdrawn and the testis exteriorized through the incision (Bogaert et al. 1993). Orchiectomy may be undertaken with two accessory ports inserted as described for laparoscopic orchidopexy, and, in small and poorly vascularized testes, the clip applier is not necessary. The vas and vessels may be fulgurated by means of bipolar cautery. The gonad may be taken out through the Hasson incision after passing the camera into an accessory port.

Two-Stage Fowler-Stephens Repair

The two-stage Fowler-Stephens repair was the first laparoscopic procedure popularized for high abdominal testes with a laparoscopic first stage followed by an open second stage or with a later laparoscopic second stage at another anesthetic session (Andze et al. 1990; Bloom 1991; Bogaert et al. 1993; Esposito and Garipoli 1997; Wilson-Storey and MacKinnon 1992). Step 2 is delayed for 6–8 months. The spermatic vessels can be cauterized and divided with either a uni- or bipolar cautery, using a single 5-mm accessory port inserted under laparoscopic control in the lower abdominal quadrant contralateral to the abdominal gonad (Bogaert et al. 1993). The use of a clip-applier requires two accessory ports, to prepare the vessels and to apply the clips to the spermatic vessels leash as far from the testis as possible (Bloom 1991).

One-Stage Laparoscopic Orchidopexy

When an abdominal low or peeping testis is localized, orchidopexy can be safely accomplished by means of laparoscopy alone, with minimal morbidity, while postoperative pain or discomfort may largely improve with respect to the traditional approach (Bogaert et al. 1993; Elder 1989; Froeling et al. 1994; Jordan et al. 1992; Jordan and Winslow 1994; Lindgren et al. 1998; Poppas et al. 1996). Favorable experience with laparoscopic orchidopexy techniques for intra-abdominal testes suggested a possible role for this technique in the high palpable testis, especially in the older child (Docimo 1995; Docimo et al. 1995). Some authors consider laparoscopy as a good diagnostic tool but many of them opt for an open surgical approach according to Jones as soon as an intra-abdominal testis is found (Gheiler et al. 1997). The technique of laparoscopic orchidopexy for testes located high in the inguinal canal does not differ from that described for abdominal or peeping testes, with the exception of a possible lesser dissection required to isolate the vessels and bring down the testis without traction (Docimo et al. 1995).

The 10-mm lens offers a better vision. The small size of the abdominal cavity in infants affects the placement of the trocars. If these are not high enough, instruments not exclusively dedicated to infants will be too close to the area of dissection to be used efficiently. Two accessory 5-mm trocars are inserted along the midclavicular line, approximately at the umbilical level. A suprapubic trocar is seldom necessary. When using of a suprapubic port, one must keep in mind that the infant bladder is mostly an intrabdominal organ and can be accidentally injured by the insertion of the trocar, even if the bladder has been drained by a transurethral catheter. The patient is positioned in 30° of Trendelenburg and rotated away from the operative side. Pneumoperitoneum is established and kept at 10–12 mmHg. The colon is pushed medially to gain access to the spermatic vessels. Before incising the peritoneum around and rostrally to the internal ring, it is important to note if the vas extends into the inguinal canal describing a loop along the gubernaculum. Such condition exposes to the risk of accidental transection of the vas when the gubernaculum is divided. The latter should be carried out as distally as possible in order to use the tissue around the gonad to manipulate the testis into the scrotum after the dissection time has been completed.

Special care must be taken in the hemostasis in order to keep the operative field clean and to avoid postoperative inguino-scrotal hematomas. The incision on the peritoneum is extended rostrally on the two sides of the spermatic vessels and vas (Fig. 2a,b), preserving a strip of peritoneum overlying the vas and the vascular connection at the vertix of the triangle formed with the spermatics. In case orchidopexy proves impossible without dividing the spermatic vessels, as described by Fowler and Stephens, sparing of the anastomotic arcades between the spermatic and deferential arteries results in a stronger blood flow to the gonad, thus reducing the risk of postoperative atrophy. Blunt dissection of the vas and vessels is extended as necessary. At this time one must identify the exact location of the new inguinal canal. There are three possibilities:

- Lateral to the epigastric vessels at the site of the original inguinal canal, in case of a good length of spermatic vessels (testes in the inguinal canal or peeping)

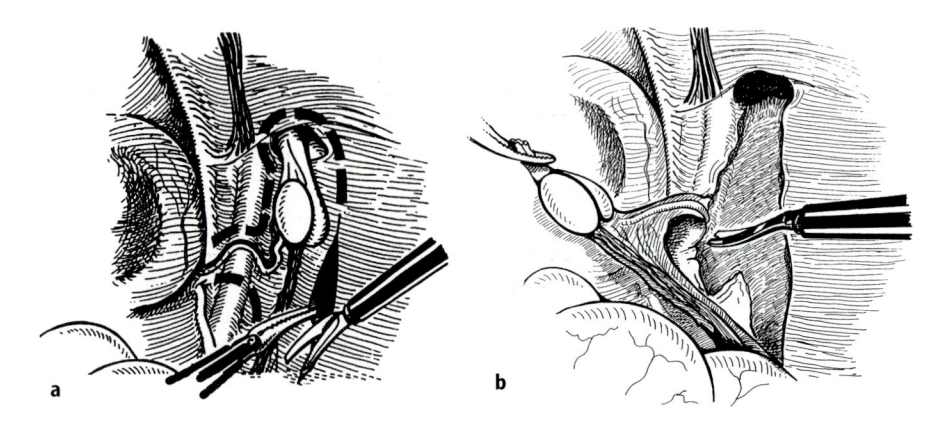

Fig. 2a,b. Dissection of the inpalpable testis. **a** The peritoneum is incised on both sides of the spermatic vessels and vas. **b** During mobilisation of the testis a strip of peritoneum overlying the vas and the vascular connections at the vertix of the triangle formed with the spermatic vessels is preserved

44 The Nonpalpable Testis

- Lateral to the umbilical ligament and medial to the epigastric vessels, performing the so-called *Prentiss maneuver*
- Medial to the umbilical ligament, between this and the bladder (Fig. 3).

The latter path is quite shorter but exposes to iatrogenic injuries of the bladder, and should be confined to cases with very short vessels or vas (Jordan and Winslow 1994).

The instrument is then followed in its path along the inguinal canal by palpating it over the pubis up to the hemiscrotum, where a dartos pouch is prepared. Once the dartoic fascia has been passed a 5-mm trocar sheath is placed over the instrument and pushed into the abdomen (Fig. 4). For large gonads it may be necessary to dilate the newly created pathway. The testis is then pulled into then scrotum with a grasper taking care not to rotate the vascular pedicle. Residual brevity of the vessels requires additional mobilization of these, and eventually of

Fig. 3. There are three possible routes for the pull through of the mobilized testis: *1* lateral to the deep inferior epigatric vessels, along the original inguinal canal, in case of a good length of spermatic vessels; *2*, between the medial umbilical ligament and the deep inferior epigatric vessels (Prentiss maneuver); *3*, between the bladder and the medial umbilical ligament, in cases of very short spermatic vessels or vas

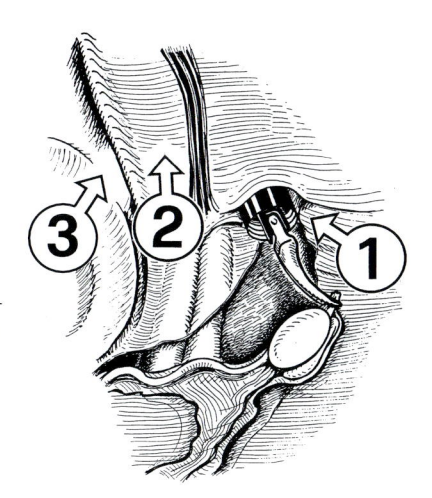

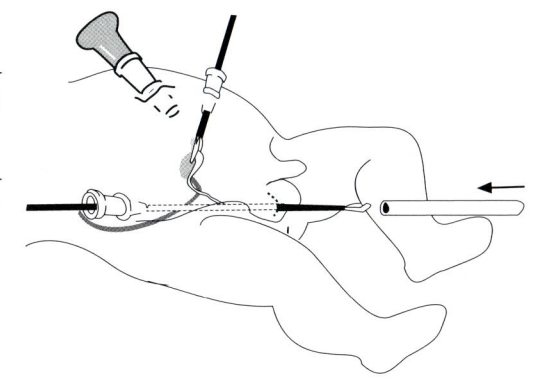

Fig. 4. Pull-through of the testis. An instrument is passed from the abdomen through the inguinal canal into the hemiscrotum, where a dartos pouch is created. Once the dartoic fascia is passed, a 5-mm trocar sheath is placed over the instrument and pushed into the abdomen. It may be necessary to dilate the newly created pathway

the vas deferens. Orchidopexy is then completed in the usual manner by passing polyglycolic sutures between the testis and septum and between the gubernaculum and the end of the scrotum. The parietal peritoneum overlying the area of dissection and the patent processus vaginalis are closed with vascular endoclips.

The apparently lesser vascular trauma appears to be related to the fact that in laparoscopic orchidopexy the spermatic vessels are isolated together with a parietal strip of peritoneum and the vas deferens, while in standard orchidopexy the posterior peritoneum remains intact and the vessels are separated from the peritoneum which results in greater trauma. In light of this, one should consider extending laparoscopic orchidopexy to the high palpable testis which requires a dissection of the vessels as high as possible.

Personal Experience

My personal experience is summarized in Tables 1 and 2. As a result of this experience an algorithm has emerged which is given in Table 3.

Table 1. Laparoscopic findings in nonpalpable testis (121 patients, 131 testes)

	n	%
Testis present	67	51
In the inguinal canal	11[a]	8.5
Peeping testis	10	7.5
In the abdomen	46[b]	35.0
Testis absent	64	49
Abdominal vanishing testis	17	13.0
Inguinal and scrotal vanishing testis	47	36.0

[a]One interstitial ectopia, two preperitoneal ectopia.
[b]One ovary in a case of true hermaphroditism with contralateral ovotestis.

Table 2. Surgical treatment of abdominal testes (n=41)

	n	%
Standard orchidopexy	30	73.0
Two-stage Fowler-Stephens orchidopexy	11[a]	27.0

[a]40.0% in the first 15 cases, 19% in the second 26 cases.

Closing Remarks

We emphasize that the laparoscopic finding of a blind ending vas and vessels does not necessarily imply that a intrauterine intra-abdominal torsion has occurred; as a matter of fact in three of our cases small "nubbins" with histological

Table 3. Laparoscopy in nonpalpable testis

Intra-abdominal gonad or peeping testis	
Normal testis	
Unilateral after puberty	Laparoscopic gonadectomy
	Prosthesis
	Contralateral orchidopexy
Uni- or bilateral before puberty	Standard open orchidopexy
	Laparoscopic orchidopexy
	Laparoscopic assisted orchidopexy
	Staged Fowler Stephens orchidopexy
	Microsurgical autotransplantation
Dysgenetic gonad	Laparoscopic gonadectomy
	Prosthesis
	Contralateral orchidopexy
No vas or vessels visualized	Prosthesis
	Contralateral orchidopexy
Vas and vessels blind ending in the abdomen	Prosthesis
	Contralateral orchidopexy
Vas and vessels entering the inguinal canal	
Closed internal ring	
Hypoplastic vessels	Prosthesis
	Contralateral orchidopexy
Normal vessels ⎫	Inguinal open exploration
Open internal ring ⎭	Inguinal or ectopic testis
	Standard orchidopexy
	Negative exploration/hypoplastic testis
	Prosthesis
	Contralateral orchidopexy

features of vanishing testis were found in the scrotum at the time of implantation of a testicular prosthesis; moreover the reason for the disappearance of gonadal structures right at theperitoneal level remains elusive.

Much attention should be paid to normal looking vessels entering a closed internal inguinal ring. As this finding may be associated with a dysmorphic gonad in preperitoneal or intestinal ectopia. Such a flattened gonad may be missed on palpation even in the anesthetized muscle relaxed patient.

As may other authors, we have the impression that the vast majority of intra-abdominal testes may be amenable to a one stage orchidopexy either in a classic open or laparoscopic way. It seems that too many first-stage Fowler-Stephens orchidopexies are performed at the present.

References

Andze GO et al (1990) La place de la laparoscopie thérapeutique dans le traitement chirurgical des testicules intra-abdominaux chez l'enfant. Chir Pediatr 31:299–302

Bartone FF et al (1984) Pitfalls in using human chorionic gonadotropin stimulation test to diagnose anorchia. J Urol 132:563–567

Bloom DA (1991) Two-step orchiopexy with pelviscopic clip ligation of spermatic vessels. J Urol 145:1030–1033

Bloom DA, Guiney EJ, Ritchey ML (1994) Normal and abnormal pelviscopic anatomy at the internal inguinal ring in boys and the vasal triangle. Urology 44:905–908

Bogaert GA, Kogan BA, Mevorach RA (1993) Therapeutic laparoscopy for intra-abdominal testes. Urology 42:182–188

Bukowsky TP et al (1995) Testicular autotransplantation: a 17-year review of an affective approach to the management of the intra-abdominal testis. J Urol 154:558–561

Caldamone AA, Amaral JF (1994) Laparoscopic stage 2 Fowler-Stephens orchiopexy. J Urol 152:1253

Cortesi N et al (1976) Diagnosis of bilateral abdominal cryptorchidism by laparoscopy. Endoscopy 8:33

Diamond DA, Caldamone AA (1992) The value of laparoscopy for 106 impalpable testes relative to clinical presentation. J Urol 148:632–634

Docimo SG (1995) The results of surgical therapy for cryptorchidism: a literature review and analysis. J Urol 154:1148–1152

Docimo SG et al (1995) Laparoscopic orchiopexy for the high palpable undescended testis: preliminary experience. J Urol 154:1513–1515

Gheiler EL, Barthold JS, Gonzalez R (1997) Benefits of laparascopy and the Jones technique for the nonpalpable testis. J Urol 158:1948–1951

Elder JS (1989) Laparoscopy and Fowler-Stephens orchiopexy in the management of the impalpable testis. Urol Clin North Am 16:399–411

Esposito C, Garipoli V (1997) The value of 2-step laparoscopic Fowler-Stephens orchiopexy for intra-abdominal testes. J Urol 158:1952–1954

Ferro F, Caterino S, Lais A (1991) Testicular prosthesis in children: a simplified insertion technique. Eur Urol 19:230–232

Ferro F, Lais A, Gonzales-Serva L (1996) Benefits and aftertoughts of laparoscopy for the nonpalpable testis. J Urol 156:795–798

Ferro F et al (1990) Staged orchidopexy: simplifying the second stage. Pediatr Surg Int 5:10–12

Ferro F et al (1992) Impact of primary surgical approach in the management of the impalpable testis. Eur Urol 22:142–146

Froeling FMJA et al (1994) The nonpalpable testis and the changing role of laparoscopy. Urology 43:222–226

Guiney EJ, Corbally M, Malone PS (1989) The management of the palpable testis. Br J Urol 63:313–316

Hazebroeck FWJ, Molenaar JC (1992) The management of the impalpable testis by surgery alone. J Urol 148:629–631

Holcomb GW et al (1994) Laparoscopy for the nonpalpable testis. Am Surg 60:143–147

Kogan SJ et al (1989) Orchiopexy of the high undescended testis by division of the spermatic vessels: a critical review of 38 selected transections. J Urol 141:1416–1419

Jordan GH, Robey EL, Winslow BH (1992) Laparoendoscopic surgical management of the abdominal/transinguinal undescended testicle. J Endourol 6:159–163

Jordan GH, Winslow BH (1994) Laparoscopic single stage and staged orchiopexy. J Urol 152:1249–1252

Landa HM et al (1987) Magnetic resonance imaging of the cryptorchid testis. Eur J Pediatr 146:16–17

Levitt SB et al (1978) The impalpable testis: a rational approach to management. J Urol 120:515

Lindgren BW et al (1998) Laparoscopic orchiopexy: procedure of choice for the nonpalpable testis? 169:2132–2135

Minimberg DT, Rodger JC, Bedford JM (1982) Ultrastructural evidence of the onset of testicular pathological conditions in the cryptorchid human testis within the first year of life. J Urol 128:782

Moore RG et al (1994) Laparoscopic evaluation of the nonpalpable testis: a prospective assessment of accuracy. J Urol 151:728–731

Nogueira Castilho L (1990) Laparoscopy for the nonpalpable testis: how to interpret the endoscopic findings. J Urol 144:1215–1218

Perovic S, Janic N (1994) Laparoscopy in the diagnosis of non-palpable testes. Br J Urol 73:310–131

Plotzker ED et al (1992) Laparoscopy for nonpalpable testes in childhood: Is inguinal exploration also necessary when vas and vessels exit the inguinal ring? J Urol 148:635–638

Poppas DP, Lemack GE, Minimberg DT (1996) Laparoscopic orchiopexy: clinical experience and description of technique. J Urol 155:708–711

Rajfer J et al (1983) The use of computerized tomography scanning to localize the impalpable testis. J Urol 129:972–974

Ransley PG et al (1984) Preliminary ligation of the gonadal vessels prior to orchidopexy for the intra-abdominal testicle. A staged Fowler-Stephens procedure. World J Urol 2:266–268

Rozansky TA, Bloom DA (1995) The undescended testis. Theory and management. Urol Clin North Am 22:107–109

Scott JES (1982) Laparoscopy as an aid in the diagnosis and management of the impalpable testis. J Pediatr Surg 17:14–16

Tennenbaum SY et al (1994) Preoperative laparoscopic localization of the nonpalpable testis: a critical analysis of a 10-year experience. J Urol 151:732–734

Vaysse P (1994) Laparoscopy and impalpable testis – a prospective multicentric study (232 cases). Groupe d'Etude en Coeliochirurgie Infantile. Eur J Pediatr Surg 4:329–332

Weiss RM, Carter AR, Rosenfield AT (1986) High-resolution real-time ultrasonography in the localization of the undescended testis. J Urol 135:936–938

Weiss RM, Glickman MG (1982) Venography of the undescended testis. Urol Clin North Am 9:387

Weiss RM, Seashore JM (1987) Laparoscopy in the management in the non palpable testis. J Urol 138:382–384

Wilson-Storey D, MacKinnon AE (1992) The laparoscopy and the undescended testis. J Pediatr Surg 27:89–92

CHAPTER 45

Laparoscopic Varicocele

G.A. MacKinlay

Introduction

Varicosities of the pampiniform plexus usually occur on the left side (90%). Rarely they are bilateral (9%) and very rarely (1%) on the right side (in which case situs inversus may be present; Wilms 1988). A varicocele is present in around 15% of the male population over the age of 15 (Steeno et al. 1976; Oster 1971; Yarborough et a. 1989). Idiopathic varicocele may occur as young as 10 years but if seen in children under 5 years it may be secondary to ingrowth of a Wilms tumour into the left renal vein or occasionally by compression of the left testicular vein by a hydronephrotic kidney. Surprisingly it is not seen in infants with renal vein thrombosis.

The testis has three sources of blood supply, the testicular artery from the aorta, the artery to the vas (the deferential branch of the vesical) and the cremasteric branch of the inferior epigastric artery. Any two can be divided without loss of the testis.

The testicular veins are formed from around 12 scrotal veins from the posterior testicular surface and epididymis, which form the pampiniform plexus. This is a chief component of the spermatic cord and ascends anterior to the vas deferens. Three or four veins traverse the inguinal canal coalescing into two or three veins, which ascend anterior to psoas major and the ureter behind the peritoneum on either side of the testicular artery. These veins join to form the testicular vein; the right opens into the inferior vena cava at an acute angle just inferior to the level of the renal veins but that on the left opens into the left renal vein at a right angle.

Various theories have been promulgated as to the aetiology of a varicocele. Ahlberg et al. (1966) and Kuypers et al. (1992) have reported the absence of valves in the left testicular vein as an aetiological factor. The upright posture in man leads to a high hydrostatic pressure predisposing to varicocele formation. Others have suggested that compression of the left renal vein occurs between the aorta and the superior mesenteric artery as occurs in compression of the duodenum in "cast syndrome". Certainly in my experience varicoceles are more common in tall thin boys who have recently undergone a "growth spurt". Differential growth may favour retrograde flow from the renal vein into the left testicular vein. Some believe that the sigmoid colon compresses the left renal vein. Another ingenuous suggestion has been that adrenaline (epinephrine) from the left suprarenal draining into the left renal vein may constrict the orifice of the left testicular vein!

Whatever the aetiology, the presence of a varicocele may be an incidental finding at a school medical examination (a common source of referral in my practice) or it may cause testicular discomfort or pain. The boy himself may notice the "bag of worms" in his scrotum, a finding that may cause grave anxiety that he has a tumour. The presence of a varicocele may lead to testicular atrophy or perhaps failure of growth of the testis on the affected side and has been shown to lead to subfertility in adults. A varicocele is present in 30%–40% of infertile men.

Some reports classify varicoceles according to their size using the grading system described by Dubin and Amelar in 1970. They classified them into small, moderate and large, now graded as I, II and III. Grade I is small and palpated with difficulty or detected by Valsalva's manoeuvre. Grade II is moderate in size and detected on physical examination. Grade III is large and clearly visible at a distance on inspection alone. Although Dubin and Amelar reported that in their experience the size of the varicocele was not significant it is noted in adolescents that the potential for testicular volume loss increases with the grade of the varicocele. Steeno et al. noted that testicular changes in volume and consistency were present in 34.4% of those with a grade II varicocele and 81.2% with grade III although grade I showed no change. Lyon et al. (1982) reported that in 77% of 30 adolescent boys with a palpable left varicocele there was volume loss of the left testis. Kass and Belman (1987) reported reversal of testicular growth failure in 16 of 20 patients post-varicocele ligation.

Indications

Whereas in the past the treatment of varicocele in adolescents was controversial, more and more authors are of the opinion that grade II and III varicoceles should be treated in adolescence.

Laparoscopic clip ligation of the testicular vessels can be safely carried out in adolescents with minimal morbidity.

Preoperative Workup

Although the risk is small it is advisable that all patients have a preoperative ultrasound scan of the renal tract to exclude a tumour of the kidney. Patients and their parents must be informed of the pros and cons of surgery and the minimal risks of laparoscopic surgery in experienced hands. They must be informed that there is a small risk of testicular atrophy post-operatively although this must be balanced against the risk of infertility.

As this procedure is a day-case one there is very little preoperative preparation required other than the standard for day-case surgery.

Preoperative Preparation

Patient Positioning/Skin Preparation/Draping. The patient is placed supine on the operating table under general anaesthesia (Fig. 1). The abdomen is prepared with antiseptic and surgical drapes applied to expose the abdomen from the epigastrium to the pubis and from the right iliac fossa to the left anterior axillary line.

Position of Surgeons and Staff. The surgeon stands on the patient's right side and his assistant (the cameraman) opposite him (Fig. 1). The scrub nurse stands to the left of the assistant with her instrument trolley towards the foot end of the table

Position of Monitor and Cables. Only one monitor is required for this simple short procedure. It is placed at the foot of the table, facing the head end, so that

Fig. 1. Position of the patient, crew, and equipment

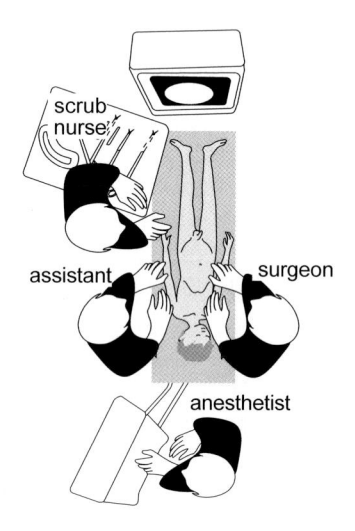

Fig. 2. Position of the trocars

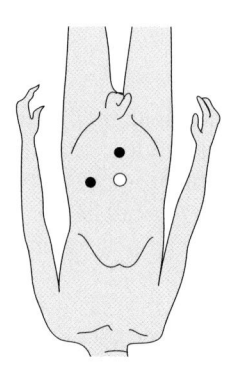

it can easily be viewed by the surgeon and his assistant and scrub nurse (Fig. 1). The laparoscopic insufflator and camera are mounted on the same trolley as the monitor and the camera cable and insufflation line are laid along the assistant's side of the table to avoid interference with the surgical field.

Positioning of Trocars. Each port site is first infiltrated with 0.25% marcaine with adrenaline, partly for postoperative pain relief but also to minimise any bleeding from the port site. The infiltration is from skin to peritoneum. First a 5-mm primary port is placed at the umbilicus, under direct vision (Fig. 2). A swab, held firmly against the skin infraumbilically, enables the lower fold of the umbilicus to be everted. Here a 5-mm incision is made using a scalpel with a number 11 blade. A towel clip is used to elevate the umbilicus. Two artery forceps grasp either side of the linea alba and direct vision incision of the peritoneum allows safe introduction of the primary port. If the incision is very small there is no need for a pursestring or other suture to anchor the port. The peritoneal cavity is insufflated with CO_2 at 0.3–1 l/min until the intra-abdominal pressure is 8–10 mmHg. It is maintained at this level with a flow rate of less than 1 l/min. During insufflation a 5-mm laparoscope (preferably 30° viewing) is inserted. Two further ports are then introduced visualising the insertion through the laparoscope. One is placed in the left iliac fossa above and medial to the anterior superior iliac spine. The other is placed slightly lower and to the right of the midline. The left one can be 5 mm or less to accommodate fine grasping forceps. The right one must be 5 mm to accommodate the dissecting shears and subsequently a 5-mm clip applicator.

Specific Instrumentation. Only three instruments are required for this procedure: (a) Dissecting scissors, (b) Fine grasping forceps for the peritoneum, (c) A 5-mm clip applicator with at least four clips.

Technique

The ports are inserted as above. The internal inguinal ring is identified. A head down position (Trendelenburg tilt) of the patient facilitates this and occasionally if the sigmoid colon obscures the view, the left side of the table may be slightly elevated. I have never had to mobilise the colon to expose the vessels. The testicular vessels can be seen clearly through the peritoneum above the inguinal ring and the vas with its vessels is seen to join them at the level of the ring (Fig. 3).

Using dissecting shears the peritoneum is incised over the testicular vessels a few centimetres above the internal ring. Care must be taken not to damage the underlying veins and an adequate window must be opened to clearly expose the vessels. Using the scissors the vessels are elevated from the posterior pelvic wall and grasped with the grasping forceps. Once a clear space has been developed behind the vessels the scissors are replaced by a 5-mm clip applicator. Two clips are applied above and two below the grasper prior to changing back to the scissors and dividing the vessels (Fig. 3b). Once they are divided the area behind the

Fig. 3. The actual clipping and transection of the spermatic vessels

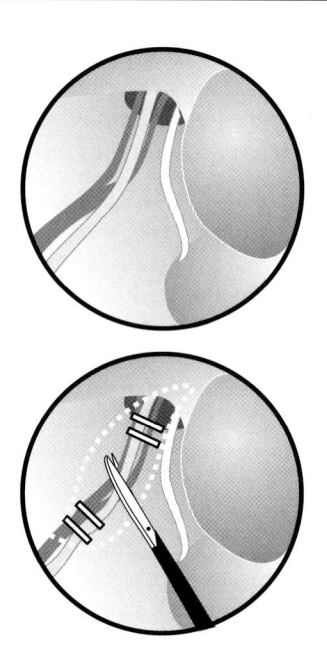

vessels is carefully inspected to ensure that no collaterals have been missed. In the past I endeavoured to preserve the testicular artery but recurrence of the varicocele in one case led to subsequent mass clip ligation of the vessels and 100% success in more than 20 consecutive cases. The ports are all removed under direct vision, the abdomen deflated and the wounds closed with subcutaneous 3/0 vicryl and 4/0 subcuticular dexon to the umbilical wound and subcuticular dexon alone to the other two. The procedure takes 10–20 min.

Some advocate ligation of collateral vessels such as those associated with the vas deferens. Once the main testicular vessels have been ligated the blood must drain from the testis somehow and to occlude all drainage pathways seems inappropriate. It is inappropriate to perform a procedure laparoscopically that would not be considered in open surgery. To ligate these vessels may lead to venous infarction and testicular loss.

Postoperative Care

The patient may be discharged home within a few hours or remain in overnight. They may eat and drink as soon as they feel able and paracetamol provides sufficient postoperative analgesia. With local anaesthetic wound infiltration often no further analgesia is required. No postoperative complications have been encountered. Outpatient review is carried out at 6 weeks.

Personal Experience

By the 6-week review the varicocele has resolved completely in 80% of cases. In 18 of the first 20 of my own personal series there was no residual varicocele. In the remainder the vessels may remain apparent but further progression does not occur and this is similar to the experience of adult surgeons using a conventional operative approach. These tend to be the cases that are grade III at the outset and they remain, as the veins were over distended at the outset and cannot regress completely.

Laparoscopic clip ligation of the testicular vessels is eminently suitable for day-case surgery, and the boy can return to school 1–2 days later.

Discussion

Many operative procedures have been devised to treat varicoceles. They are based on 3 surgical approaches to ligation of the vessels; scrotal, inguinal and retroperitoneal. The scrotal approach is the least favoured as the multiple veins of the pampiniform plexus are difficult to ligate in entirety and post-operative haematoma formation is common. The inguinal approach first described by Ivanissevich, in which all the venous channels are carefully ligated in the groin, has been the standard procedure for many years but has a significant failure rate in most series [Kass and Marcol (1992) reported a failure rate of 16%]. Alejandro Palomo from Guatemala in 1949 advocated a mass ligation of the retroperitoneal vessels, including the artery. He reported on 38 patients cured of their varicoceles without atrophy of the testicle. Kass and Marcol reported that with this technique a post-operative varicocele persisted in 7% of cases when the artery was preserved and in none of 18 cases where a mass ligation of the vessels included the artery. Testicular atrophy was not observed either. Microvascular venous bypass has also been used with variable success.

Interventional radiologists favour selective transvenous embolisation of the left testicular vein. There are, however, dangers of inadvertent venous perforation and late migration of the venous occlusion device and the technique is confined to centres with a radiologist skilled in such techniques. The failure rate is similar to that of surgery.

Kass and Marcol reported their experience using three different operative techniques for varicocele ligation in adolescents. The failure rate was 16% (9 of 53 patients) in whom a modified Ivanissevich (1960) inguinal approach was used, 11% (2 of 17 patients) with a high retroperitoneal technique but preserving the testicular artery and 0% (of 32 patients) using the Palomo high mass ligation technique. Testicular atrophy did not occur in any patient.

The above discussion illustrates that Palomo's technique is probably still the best and the operation is simplified by a laparoscopic approach. The first report of laparoscopic varicocelectomy is in 1992 by Hagood et al. who reported on the procedure in 10 patients aged 16–54 years, four of whom underwent bilateral ligation. Follow-up showed resolution of the varicocele in all patients and disappearance of pain in one patient treated for that symptom. No morbidity was encountered and all patients resumed normal activity in 2 days.

References

Ahlberg NE, Bartley O, Chidekel N (1966) Right and left gonadal veins: an anatomic and statistical study. Acta Radiol 4:593–601
Dubin L, Amelar RD (1970) Varicocele size and results of varicocelectomy in selected subfertile men with varicocele. Fertil Steril 21:606–609
Hagood PG et al (1992) Laparoscopic varicocelectomy: preliminary report of a new technique. J Urol 147:73–76
Ivanissevich O (1960) Left varicocele due to reflux: experience with 4,470 Operative cases in 42 years. J Int Coll Surg 34:742–755
Kass EJ, Belman AB (1987) Reversal of testicular growth failure by varicocele ligation. J Urol 137:475–476
Kass EJ, Marcol B (1992) Results of varicocele surgery in adolescents: a comparison of techniques. J Urol 148:694–696
Khupers P, Kang N, Ellis N (1992) Valveless testicular veins: a possible etiological factor in varicocele. Clin Anat 5:113–118
Lyon RP, Marshall S, Scott MP (1982) Varicocele in childhood and adolescence. Implications in adulthood fertility? Urology 19:641–643
Oster J (1971) Varicocele in children and adolescents. An investigation of the incidence among Danish school children. Scand J Urol Nephrol 5:27–32
Palomo A (1949) Radical cure of varicocele by a new technique: preliminary report. J Urol 61:604–607
Steeno O et al (1976) Prevention of fertility disorders by detection and treatment of varicocele at school and college age. Andrologia 8(1):47–53
Wilms G (1988) Solitary or predominantly right sided varicocele, a possible sign for situs inversus. Urol Radiol 9:243–246
Yarborough MA, Burns JR, Keller FS (1989) Incidence and clinical significance of subclinical varicoceles. J Urol 141:1372–1374

CHAPTER 46

Adnexal Pathology

H. Steyaert, Y. Heloury, V. Plattner, J-S. Valla

Introduction

Laparoscopy is a well-established diagnostic and therapeutic modality for adult gynecology. It was the first application of laparoscopy. In children the procedure can be used to extend our diagnostic capabilities as well as to facilitate minimal invasive therapeutic measures using laparoscopic tools or, if necessary, minimal inguinal incisions.

Diagnostic advantages of laparoscopy in girls has become increasingly apparent. Video laparoscopy allows the surgeon to thoroughly examine the lower and the upper abdomen to determine the exact etiology of a peritoneal irritation. Many reports and series confirm that therapeutic procedures give the same results by a laparoscopic approach after the necessary learning curve. What is more, video laparoscopy enhances probably the operation because it improves visualization.

Indications

The kind of lesions which can benefit from diagnostic and therapeutic use of the technique are dependent upon age. However, the same pathology, for example an ovarian cyst, may be present at different ages. So the indications are classified by organ.

Adnexal Pathology

Laparoscopy can be indicated in several circumstances.

Acute Pelvic Pain

Abruptly appearing pelvic pain can correspond with a torsion either of a healthy or a pathological adnexa. Ultrasonography remains the initial examination but any diagnostic doubt justifies an exploratory laparoscopy. Adnexal torsion is most of the time caused by an ovarian cyst and intracystic hemorrhage [11].

Torsion caused by a solid ovarian mass is not exceptional in children. Tumors are most of the time benign but malignant tumors are not exceptional [23].

Torsion of a normal adnexa occurs more frequently than is generally appreciated. Subsequent asynchronous torsion is possible and makes the management difficult [7].

Subacute Pelvic Pain

Adnexal pathology is the first differential diagnosis with appendicitis in girls. Laparoscopy is useful in cases in which the diagnosis remains unclear.

Very frequent is the detection of torsion of paraoophoric remnants. Some may be bigger than ovarian cysts.

Torsion of a normal fallopian tube without ovary is rare. A preoperative diagnosis is infrequently made [27].

In adolescents salpingitis is an other cause of subacute pelvic pain. Laparoscopy is an essential part of the diagnostic procedure and also an interestingly therapeutic procedure in severe cases [12].

Peritoneal adhesions after pelvic or appendicular operations may also have some advantages of a laparoscopic approach. This pathology is indeed one of the most important causes of future hypofertility in women.

Pelvic Mass

Clinical findings of pelvic diseases in children are different from the adult. The pelvic organs lie higher because the pelvis has not fully developed; therefore, abdominal or bimanual palpation may disclose a mass. If it is a solid mass, it can be a malignant tumor (yolk sac tumor, immature teratoma). Tumoral markers (e.g., HCG and CEA) must be analyzed. As in adults it would constitute a relative contraindication for laparoscopy. This procedure may, however, be of interest to determine the histological nature of an ovarian tumor [11].

A pure cystic tumor most often corresponds to a functional cyst. When to operate a functional cyst? First of all when the child presents with an acute abdomen or when ultrasonographic examination reveals signs of complication. In other circumstances "large" cysts are treated conservatively by ultrasonographic survey and hormonal therapy. If resolution does not occur laparoscopy and cystectomy is proposed [26].

Organic cysts are encountered before puberty (dermoid cysts). Surgical excision may be conducted or assisted by a laparoscopic approach.

In case of incidental ultrasonographic diagnosis:

Ultrasonography is the most used imaging technique in case of an abdominal complaint. It may show the presence of an ovarian cyst with some liquid in the Douglas in peripubertal girls. Differential diagnosis between tumors and uncomplicated cysts is easy. Differential diagnosis between tumors and cysts in case of torsion is very difficult. Laparoscopy may be helpful.

Prenatal diagnosis of a cystic mass in a female is encountered more and more frequently. Controversy still exists between conservative and early surgical management. The laparoscopic approach my be of interest to overcome this [25].

Uterovaginal Pathologies

Intersex

Indications for laparoscopy are well codified in neonates. It may be a diagnostic laparoscopy in case of suspicion of true hermaphrodism; or in case of male pseudohermaphroditism with persistent diagnostic difficulty. Later it can play an important therapeutic role in gonadal excision in cases of risk of gonadoblastoma or dysgerminoma (see also "Laparoscopy and Intersex," this volume). Laparoscopy is also useful when the surgeon discovers a female adnexa during exploration of an inguinal hernia or an impalpable testis in boys.

Uterovaginal Malformations

Laparoscopy can be indicated in cases of vaginal atresia or in utero-vaginal duplication to specify the magnitude of the malformation and determine the pelvic consequences of menstrual retention.

Endometriosis

Chronic pelvic pain in girls is rarely correlated with endometriosis. Detection of the importance of the disease and coagulation therapy is possible by a laparoscopic approach [6].

Other

Ovarian Transposition

The transposition of ovaries before radiotherapy is easy by laparoscopy. The transposition site depends on the area to be irradiated [11].

Ectopic Pregnancy

Pediatric surgeons interested in pubertal pathology must be aware about the possibility of pregnancy in young girls. One in 66 pregnancies is an ectopic pregnancy. The success of laparoscopic management of this pathology has been well documented. Various laparoscopic techniques can be used [19].

Technique

Installation and General Considerations

The patient is placed in a supine position. If the child does not empty his bladder immediately prior to surgery, catheterization is performed. The surgeon is positioned opposite the adnexa to be operated with the assistant by his side (along the legs). The monitor is positioned at the feet of the child. When the preoperative diagnosis is certain and the expected operative time long, then the position of the patient and crew may be changed as follows: The surgeon stays at the head of the patient and the anesthesiologist on the left. The assistant helps on the right side and the monitor is placed between the open legs. Handling of the operating tools is made much more comfortable in this position.

Three laparoscopic puncture sites including the umbilicus are used. Open laparoscopy is systematically used. The size of trocars depends on the age of the child (3, 5, 8, or 10 mm). The lower quadrant trocar sleeves are placed just above the pubic hairline and lateral to the deep epigastric vessels. These vessels are located by direct laparoscopic inspection of the anterior abdominal wall. In some cases were the pathological side is identified preoperatively the 2 operating trocars may be inserted on the same opposite side, one supra-pubic, one para-umbilical.

This type of surgery needs of course a Trendelenburg position. Left or right rotation is also of great interest.

Aquadissection is particularly useful in some gynecological pathologies (e.g., tubo-ovarian abcess, and ovarian cyst). It creates cleavages planes in the least resistant spaces, making further division easy and safe using blunt dissection, scissors or electrosurgery [20]. Irrigation and suction is of main importance in adnexal procedures. It helps to obtain a perfect hemostasis. Voluminous cysts can be suctioned in this way or by supra-pubic peroperative puncture. At the end of the procedure, we currently leave intraperitoneal Ringer's lactate solution in the peritoneal cavity to prevent adhesions which can be a cause of infertility in women.

Cystectomy

During exploration the wall of the cyst is checked. Cysts with a translucent wall are usually functional. Most organic cysts have thick walls. Any excrescence is suspicious for malignancy.

The intraparietal cystectomy begins by the incision of the tunica albuginea of the ovary. The cyst is removed using hydrodissection and divergent traction with 2 forceps, one holding the albuginea, the other the cyst. The remaining ovarian parenchyme is left open and the cyst is ideally placed in a bag for extraction. Biological glue may be used to perfect hemostasis. In case of a large dermoid cyst, puncture under protection of the peritoneal cavity may be necessary. The risk of chronic granulomatous reaction is real [16]. To avoid this complication cystectomy may be performed after exteriorization of the mass by a suprapubic or a low inguinal incision.

Ovarian cystectomy is not a common laparoscopic procedure in children and conversion must be ever in mind.

Acute Adnexal Torsion

In all cases detorsion must be tried. Indeed ovarian recovery is frequent because vascularization is of double origin (ovarian, uterine) and presents many connections. Evacuating puncture may help the "untwisting" in voluminous cysts. Liquid samples are systematically taken for biological analysis (e.g., HCG).

Oophorectomy and Adnexectomy

Before starting with an oophorectomy or salpingo-oophorectomy, the surgeon must imperatively visualize the course of the ureter. The ovary is released from the pelvic sidewall and bowel adhesions. A necrotic adnexa is excised only after previous detorsion and a long time of observation for potential recuperation. The section of the lumbo-ovarian and utero-ovarian pedicles are performed after bipolar coagulation or by using clips and linear staplers [5]. The fallopian tube is sectioned at the edge of the uterus. The adnexa is placed in an endoscopic bag and extracted by a trocar site enlargement. When possible the fallopian tube is preserved.

Tubo-ovarian Abscess

A diagnostic laparoscopy is the first step in the treatment of salpingitis. Extent of the tubo-ovarian involvement is thoroughly noted. Some cases are acute with pus in the peritoneal cavity. Some are old with interuretero-adnexal abscess and pelvic adhesions.

If there is a diagnostic doubt, the palpator is used to press on the fallopian tube and to look for pus appearance. Bacteriological samples are taken [12].

Exploration must also visualize the hepatic region. False membranes and diaphragmatic or anterior wall adhesions are pathognomonic of the Fitz-Hugh-Curtis syndrome.

Simultaneously definitive treatment is undertaken. Purulent fluid is aspirated. Necrotic inflammatory excudative tissue is excised and peritoneal lavage is started. An antiseptic solution and/or antibiotics are instilled at the end of the procedure.

Endometriosis

Red lesions are the most common in adolescents. Peritoneal lesions are most frequently seen. Ovaries are also an important site of implantation at this age. Laparoscopy is of main importance to detect subtle lesions because laparoscopy provides important magnification [6]. Electrocoagulation is preferred to excisional techniques in adolescents. It gives good pain relief without the risk of infertility consecutive to radical dissection. Temporarily suspension of the ovaries may be indicated during extensive electrocoagulation of pelvic lesions. Extension of the thermal injury to the ureter must be kept in mind. Laparoscopy is imperatively followed by ovulation suppression.

Oophoropexy

The main indication for oophoropexy is to protect ovaries from irradiation [24]. The technique differs depending on the irradiation technique. For external irradiation, the ovaries are transposed in the parieto-colic area after section of the utero-ovarian pedicle. Ovaries are fixed by stitches and marked with two titanium clips. In case of curietherapy for vaginal tumors (yolk sac tumor, rhabdomyosarcoma), ovaries are fixed in the abdominal cavity to the retroperitoneum. When irradiation is completed, relaparoscopy is programmed. The thread is cut allowing the return of the ovaries to normal position.

Oophoropexy should also be considered in torsion of a normal adnexa (for the twisted ovary in case of salvation but also for the opposite ovary in case of oophorectomy). Various methods of fixation are described. The ovary may be fixed to the uterine serosa with absorbable suture. Fixation to the broad ligament is also possible [10]. We prefer fixation of the upper part of the ovary to the peritoneum in front of the iliac vessels. Thus, ovaries lies close to the fallopian pavilion. This position decreases probably the potential hypofertility due to the technique. The use of nonabsorbable suture is recommended in securing the ovary.

Particularities in Babies

In babies suspension by a purse string suture around the umbilical trocar sleeve is of great interest. So the intra-abdominal pressure can be limited by using this simple technique. Trocar introduction is also specific. After introduction of the first trocar by open periumbilical technique, the operating trocars are introduced transparietally in the umbilical sleeve. Visual control through the sleeve is permanent. This technique avoids the danger of great vessel or bowel damage. The 3-mm trocars are fixed to the skin with the help of a ring manufactured at half the length of the sleeve. Small accessory instruments can be inserted directly through the abdominal wall. In neonates it may be of interest to modify the installation. With the patient across the table, the surgeon is in the most comfortable position at the head of the child to operate in the pelvis. The anesthesiologist remains in his normal place. A long connector between the endothracheal tube and the respirator is necessary.

Complications

Specific complications due to gynecological laparoscopic procedures are rare. Monopolar hook handling must be limited in a little pelvic space. Surgeon has always to be attentive to the ureter. Conversion is easy and quickly performed if necessary. Scars are small even after conversion.

Personal Experience

We report 89 cases.

Neonatal Period (*n*=7)

We operated 7 neonates by laparoscopy after prenatal diagnosis of an ovarian cyst. All were complicated at ultrasonographic examination. We performed 4 adnexectomies and 2 oophorectomies. Only one cystectomy seemed feasible. One of our cases presented with a neonatal bowel occlusion due to adhesions from a free ovarian cyst. There was no complication and no conversion in this small neonatal series.

Childhood (*n*=82)

Fourteen girls have undergone a laparoscopic procedure for adnexal torsion. We performed 4 adnexectomies, 3 oophorectomies and 1 salpingectomy for isolated fallopian tube torsion. Six adnexae were untwisted and salvaged. The beginning symptom was acute abdominal pain in 13 cases and the presence of a mass in 1. Torsion was due to an ovarian mass in 8 cases and to a normal adnexa in 6. Three of the masses were solid tumors: 2 teratomas and 1 dysgerminoma. The other were complicated functional cysts.

Untwisted ovarian cysts were preventively operated on in 27 cases by evacuating puncture and biopsy (10 cases) or by cystectomy (11 cases) in case of cystic hemorrhage.

In the same period we operated 30 twisted paraoophoric remnants. One of them contained 180 cc liquid. We diagnosed four times a salpingitis and once an endometriosis. Four ovaries were fixed (2 before radiotherapy and 2 after torsion of a normal controlateral adnexa). In two cases of unilateral occlusion of duplicated müllerian ducts complicated with hydrometrocolpos, a laparoscopically assisted hemihysterectomy was performed.

Mean hospital stay was 3 days (range 1–16). There were six conversions and one complication, namely fibrinolysis after untwisting an adnexa. Secondary laparotomy was mandatory in order to remove the adnexa. We did not see other complications.

Discussion

The laparoscopic approach of gynecological disease in children seems ideal. It allows thorough visualization of the anatomy of the pelvis and of the rest of the peritoneal cavity, securing the diagnosis, and allowing for adaptation of treatment. This minimal access surgery avoids as in the other procedures the painful access wounds of conventional incisions and minimizes trauma inside the body cavity. Realimentation is started promptly. The patient is generally discharged at 24 or 48 h depending on symptoms. A learning curve must be considered for operative procedures. Discovery of a malignant tumor is rare in children and may be difficult to manage.

Neonatal Ovarian Cysts

Near all cases of neonatal torsions are caused by a follicle cyst appearing in the third trimester of the pregnancy [22]. In our series of 7 cases, only one cystectomy was possible. To avoid such bad results, some authors advocate an evacuating puncture just before delivery in case of a cyst larger than 40 mm (14–21). This kind of management is not practicable by everybody and, perhaps, is not in proportion to the disease. Recurrence seems frequent [18]. Misdiagnosis is possible: four cases in our experience (intestinal duplication, cystic lymphangioma, biliary cyst, hydrometrocolpos on uterine duplication). On the other hand, other authors have very conservative views [1]. Because of the decrease in hormonal stimulation that occurs after birth, cysts should spontaneously regress; so they recommend surgical treatment only for neonates' cysts containing debris or septae, or in case of simple cysts that do not decrease in size. However, radiological signs of complication are, most of the time, late.

Others base their management on infant's gestational age and hormonal serum levels [28]. Postnatal percutaneous puncture is also proposed in simple cysts that are larger than 30, 40 or 50 mm [21]. Definition of "large" cyst remains debatable [13–28]. These punctures may be complicated (transvesical puncture, or puncture of one of the many other organs present in the area); moreover recurrence is frequent (more than 10%), and other diagnostic possibilities are not eliminated. Based on our poor results and a review of the literature we modified our management of neonatal intra-abdominal cysts [23]. After birth this pathology must be considered as an emergency. Ultrasound is performed on the first day of life. If there are obvious echographic signs of a complication, the ovary is certainly lost, and surgical removal by a laparoscopic approach is proposed without emergency. If there are no echographic signs of complication, the laparoscopic approach is proposed as soon as possible. The procedure starts by a peritoneal exploration and, once an exact diagnosis is established, is carried on as surgical intervention [25]. Collaboration of specialized anesthesiologists is, of course, mandatory. Some clinically complicated cases are meanwhile emergencies: organ compression or intestinal occlusion; laparoscopic approach in these cases is more debatable but possible.

Premenarcheal Adnexal Torsion

Most of the adnexal cysts and torsions are on the right side (80% in our series).

Differential diagnosis between uncomplicated and complicated adnexae seems difficult [26]. Signs are frequently sparse and various: liquid-liquid level, intratubal hemorrhage, thinner pathological tube, pathological adnexa inseparable from the uterus, impression of multilocular cortical follicles (three cases in our series) of unilaterally enlarged ovary [9]. Surgery, especially by a laparoscopic approach, seems to be the best method in an attempt to increase the salvaged adnexae number [4]. It seems clear now in all cases that the surgeon endeavors to preserve as much as possible if ovarian parenchyma can still be identified [2]. Some authors plea for detorsion in most of the cases with a laparoscopic control 6 weeks later [3-17]. They suggest that there is no danger in untwisting the twisted adnexa. They describe frequent ovarian recovery. Thromboembolic complications, however, have been reported. Laparoscopy has the same advantages as in neonates, for example, correction of the clinical diagnosis and application of the ideal treatment, reduced hospital stay, and minimal scars [11-23]. Oophoropexy of the controlateral ovary is not necessary.

Torsion of a Normal Adnexa

Torsion of a normal adnexa in children is rare [7]. This pathology may, however, be serious. One of our cases presented an asynchronous torsion with definitive loss of her genital potential. Torsion may occur at any age but most likely between 8 and 14 years old. Torsion of the right adnexa is more frequent (66%). It is a surgical emergency [15]. Laparoscopy is the first proposed procedure to make exact diagnosis and to treat the adnexa by detorsion and/or by oophorectomy or adnexectomy. At the question of whether to perform an oophoropexy there are currently no clear answers [10]. However, given our results and reports of the literature about subsequent asynchronous ovarian torsion, we believe that oophoropexy should be considered.

Paraoophoric Remnants and Fallopian Tube Torsion

Subacute pelvic or infra-abdominal pain is often related to torsion of juxtatubal remnants. Since the expansion of explorative laparoscopy there are increasing descriptions of this remnants [11-23]. Treatment by removal is easy. Isolated torsion of a normal fallopian tube is extremely rare [27]. Laparoscopy is, here again, most of the time diagnostic and therapeutic. Untwisting is the treatment of choice wherever possible.

Salpingitis

Laparoscopic exploration is of main importance in this pathology. It confirms the diagnosis, gives clues regarding the etiology, permits bacteriological sampling, gives an indication about prognosis and is the first part of the treatment. Some authors recommend this procedure in any suspicion of salpingitis [12]. Laparoscopy is certainly indicated in serious infections for adnexal abscesses when medical treatment is ineffective; but also when preoperative diagnosis is uncertain.

Pelvic Tumors

Ovarian cysts are more frequently functional but organic cysts are not exceptional. Prevention of ovarian torsion by puncture or exeresis of "large" cysts is mandatory. The problem is the definition of the term "large," that is debatable as for prenatal diagnosis. We think that cysts larger than 40 mm must be treated by percutaneous puncture or by a laparoscopic approach.

There are two etiologies in organic cysts: dermoid cyst (teratoma) or cystadenoma. The second is rare in the pediatric age group. Laparoscopic excision of the cyst is the ideal treatment. In case of teratoma the controlateral ovary must be controlled. 10% of the cases are bilateral. A laparoscopic-assisted ovarian evisceration technique may be helpful because it enables palpation of ovarian tissue and permits, if necessary, excision without undue loss of ovarian tissue [8].

Malignant tumors represents 3% of all the malignant tumors in children. The most frequent are Yolk sac tumors, choriocarcinoma and immature teratoma. Malignant tumors are regularly discovered during laparoscopy for ovarian torsion. Adnexectomy is the initial treatment. May this be carried out laparoscopically? The implantation of tumor in trocar tracts used during laparoscopy is an undeniable possibility that must be considered. There is no clear answer to that problem. Protocols for the use of laparoscopy in the management of ovarian malignant tumors in children must be devised.

Endometriosis

Laparoscopic treatment of endometriosis in adolescents seems superior to laparotomy because of improved visualization and dissection [6]. Vision is indeed essential to treat all lesions and obtain pain relief. There is still a lack of long-term studies. Performance of electrocoagulation in comparison with more difficult and aggressive excision therapy must be evaluated. However, electrocoagulation is probably the less invasive solution for young girls and preserves at best fertility.

Ectopic Pregnancy

Conservative treatment of an ectopic pregnancy by the laparoscopic approach is proved to be effective because it's sure and preserves further fertility [19]. Laparoscopic visualization permits accurate assessment of pregnancy status and location, treatment of tubo-ovarian adhesions, complete hemostasis and evacuation of all blood clots. The laparoscopic procedure is possible in more than 80% of the cases. Trained surgeons are mandatory.

Conclusion

Bruhat wrote in his book about operative laparoscopy in gynecology that the development of laparoscopic procedures obeyed to some fundamental principles: elegance, efficacy and economy [3].

As in adults, laparoscopic gynecological procedures in children and babies are elegant.

Tissue aggression is decreased and incisions are cosmetically minimal. Sutures are reduced because magnification permits microsurgery and because minimally invasive surgery helps spontaneous tissue restoration.

Efficacity is the same as in open surgery but the diagnostic power of laparoscopy improves that greatly. By a laparoscopic approach the surgeon knows always exactly where to go in this somewhat diversified pathologies.

Minimal invasive surgery results also in decreased pain, shorter hospital stay and significant reduction in recuperation time.

Minimal aggression to the treated organs is, last but not least, an ideal guarantee for decreased long-term morbidity and preservation of fertility of future women.

References

1. Bagolan P et al (1992) Prenatal diagnosis and clinical outcome of ovarian cysts. J Pediatr Surg 27(7):879–881
2. Bayer A, Wiskind A (1994) Adnexal torsion: can the adnexa be saved? Am J Obstet Gynecol 17:1506–1511
3. Bruhat R et al (1989) Operative coelioscopy. McGraw-Hill, New-York
4. Cohen Z et al (1996) The laparoscopic approach to uterine adnexal torsion in childhood. J Pediatr Surg 31(11):1557–1559
5. Davidoff AM et al (1996) Laparoscopic oophorectomy in children. J Laparoendosc Surg 6(1):115–119
6. Davis G (1995) The laparoscopic management of endometriosis for the relief of pain. In: Arregui ME, Fitzgibbons RJ, Katkhouda N, McKernan JB, Reich H (eds) Principles of laparoscopic surgery. Springer, Berlin Heidelberg New York, pp 538–544
7. Davis AJ, Feiss NR (1990) Subsequent asynchronous torsion of normal adnexa in children. J Pediatr Surg 6:687–689
8. Dokler ML, Mollitt DZ (1997) A laparoscopic technique for pediatric ovarian evaluation and salvage. Ped Endosurg Inn Tech 1(1):55–57
9. Graif M, Itychak Y (1988) Sonographic evaluation of ovarian torsion in childhood and adolescence. AJR 150:647–649
10. Grunewald B, Keating J, Brown S (1993) Asynchronous ovarian torsion. The case for prophylactic oophoropexy. Postgrad Med J 69(810):318–319
11. Héloury Y et al (1993) Laparoscopy in adnexal pathology in the child: a study of 28 cases. Eur J Pediatr Surg 3:75–78

12. Henrion R, Aubriot FX (1992) Salpingitis and sexual related illness in adolescent. In: Salomon Y, Thibaud E, Rappaport R (eds) Gynécologie médicochirurgicale de l'enfant et de l'adolescente. Doin, Paris, pp 165–174
13. Ikeda K, Suito S, Nakano H (1988) Management of ovarian cyst detected antenatally. J Pediatr Surg 23(5):432–435
14. Meagher SE et al (1993) Fetal ovarian cyst: diagnosis and therapeutic role for intrauterine aspiration. Fetal Diagn Ther 8:195–199
15. Jan D, Lortat-Jacob S (1992) Normal adnexa torsion. In: Salomon Y, Thibaud E, Rappaport R (eds) Gynécologie médicochirurgicale de l'enfant et de l'adolescente. Doin, Paris pp 123–129
16. Nezhat C, Winer WK, Nezhat F (1989) Laparoscopic removal of dermoid cysts. Obstet Gynecol 13:278–280
17. Oelsnr G et al (1993) Long term follow up of the twisted ischemic adnexa managed by detorsion. Fertility Steril 60(6):976–979
18. Philippe HJ, Nisand I, Paupe A (1994) Therapeutique foetale. Maloine, Paris
19. Reich H, Kader N (1995) Ectopic pregnancy. In: Arregui Me, Fitzgibbons RJ, Katkhouda N, McKernan JB, Reich H (eds) Principles of laparoscopic surgery. Springer, Berlin Heidelberg New York, pp 578–594
20. Reich H, Parker WH (1995) Laparoscopic ovarian surgery. In: Arregui Me, Fitzgibbons RJ, Katkhouda N, McKernan JB, Reich H (eds) Principles of laparoscopic surgery. Springer, Berlin Heidelberg New York, pp 566–577
21. Sapin E et al (1994) Management of ovarian cyst detected by prenatal ultrasounds. Eur J Pediatr 4:137–140
22. Scully RE et al (1995) Case records of the Massachusetts General Hospital, case 6-1995. N Engl J Med 332:522–527
23. Steyaert H, Meynol F, Valla JS (1998) Torsion of the adnexa in children a current problem. Value of laparoscopy. Pediatr Surg Int 13:384–387
24. Thibaud E et al (1992) Preservation of ovarian function by ovarian transposition performed before pelvic irradiation during childhood. J Pediatr 121:880–884
25. Van der Zee D et al (1995) Laparoscopic approach to surgical management of ovarian cysts in the newborn. J Pediatr Surg 30 (1):42–43
26. Warner BW, Kuhn JC, Barr LL (1992) Conservative management of large ovarian cysts in children: the value of serial pelvic ultrasonography. Surgery 112(4):749–755
27. Weir CD, Brown S (1990) Torsion of the normal fallopian tube in a premenarcheal girl: a case report. J Pediatr Surg 25(6):685–686
28. Zachariou Z et al (1989) Three year's experience with large ovarian cysts diagnosed in utero. J Pediatr Surg 24(5):478–482

Laparoscopy and Intersex

Y. Heloury, V. Plattner

Introduction

The use of laparoscopy in intersex patients is currently being evaluated (Yu et al. 1995). Either alone or in association with conventional surgery, the use of laparoscopy should permit a better orientation in more difficult cases, or a less invasive surgical approach for certain pelvic excisions.

Indications

Surgery is undertaken to correct the discordance between the chosen phenotype and the ambiguity, and to remove the dysgenetic gonad and/or the gonad at risk of malignancy (Kazin 1985; Kulkarni et al. 1990).

Female Pseudohermaphroditism. Most surgical corrections can be performed by perineal approach; laparoscopy has very few indications in female pseudohermophroditism. It's use in the dissection of the colic patch for rare indications of neo-vagina construction could be proposed. This avoids a laparotomy, a cosmetic detriment which is not insignificant in female patients.

True Hermaphroditism. The female orientation seems preferable with spontaneous puberty and menstruations if the müllerian ducts are complete. We must try to keep the parenchyma in agreement with the sex assignment, especially if the child has been raised as a girl (Nihoul-Fékété et al. 1984). The most frequent encountered gonadic structure is the ovotestis in 33.4% (Nihoul-Fékété et al. 1984); the gonadic removal must be meticulous; optical amplification can help in recognizing the demarcation between the ovary (irregular white surface, firm consistency) and the testicle (smoother, shiner, softer and yellow at the section). The rare ovarian-testicle dispositions (25%) represents the indication of choice to perform gonadal removal using laparoscopy.

Male Pseudohermaproditism. In case of female orientation, the ablation of the gonads is performed at the same time as the genitoplasty (during the first weeks of life). Laparoscopy gives also precise anatomical knowledge of the internal genital organs (presence of an uterus or an hemi-uterus) which is not always possible preoperatively by ultrasonography, genitography or endoscopy of the urogenital sinus. This knowledge of the internal genital organs can be one of the elements for sexual orientation. In these cases, laparoscopy may be necessary during the first few days of life before making the definitive sex declaration. In addition, this helps to inform the parents of the consequences of the intersex (possibility of menstruation, hope of medically assisted fertility). In cases of male orientation, laparoscopy allows ablation of the internal genital organs which don't need to be conserved (uterus and/or vagina) and eventually an intra-abdominal rudimentary gonad.

Pure Gonadal Dysgenesis. The diagnosis is made during puberty for a primary amenorrhea. Due to the presence of chromosome Y, the risk of a malignant gonadal tumor, such a dysgerminoma is high (Olsen et al. 1988; Shalev et al. 1992; Wilson et al. 1992). Indication for removal of a dysgenetic gonad is indubitable. Bilateral gonadectomy is a simple procedure by laparoscopy. If the diagnosis is made early (familial history), laparoscopy can be proposed as soon as the diagnosis is confirmed.

Male Pseudohermaphroditism Due to Müllerian Inhibiting Factor Deficiency. Diagnosis is often made during surgery for impalpable testis, leading to the discovery of an uterus. Currently, laparoscopic exploration of impalpable testis is accepted, with the possibility of lowering the testis in one or two steps. In müllerian inhibiting factor (MIF) deficiency the intra-abdominal position of the testis seems to be related to the presence of müllerian structures. They are difficult to bring to the scrotum. The necessity to remove the müllerian structures is still debatable but seems better to facilitate the complete testicular lowering (Josso et al. 1983). Treatment can be performed by laparoscopy in spite of some difficulties to dissect the vas deferens through the uterine wall.

Technique

Preparation of the child and technique are identical to those described in the preceding chapter (see Steyaert et al., "Adnexal Pathology"). As laparoscopy is performed in many cases in the first weeks of life, short instruments and small size trocars (3 or 5 mm) are used. In doubtful cases laparoscopy is used during the same session as the genitoscopy.

Results

From 1991 to 1995 nine pediatric surgical services, members of the French study group in pediatric laparoscopic surgery (GECI) participated in a retrospective multicentric study which gathered 18 cases of laparoscopy for intersex. The 18 patients included 4 Turner-like syndromes, 5 pure gonadal dysgenesis, and 3 male pseudohermaphroditism due to MIF deficiency. The mean age of the children was 8.3 years old, ranging from 1 month to 17 years.

Turner-like syndromes: laparoscopy was indicated for bilateral gonadectomy in 4 cases. Histology confirmed the presence of gonadal streaks, without tumor.

Pure gonadal dysgenesis: five observations of pure gonadal dysgenesis were clarified. Laparoscopy was indicated for primary amenorrhea in 4 cases, and for a family history in a 2-year-old girl. Laparoscopy was performed for bilateral gonadectomy, the pathological examination confirming pure gonadal dysgenesis in every case, without associated tumor.

Dysgenetic male pseudohermaphroditism: in two cases a male orientation was chosen. In both cases laparoscopy was indicated for nonpalpable testis, and discovered intra-abdominal dysgenetic gonads, associated with an uterus in one case. A bilateral gonadectomy in one case and a first step Fowler-Stephens operation in another case was performed. In the patient with male pseudohermaphroditism with female assignment, laparoscopy was carried out to verify the condition of the internal genital organs.

Mixed gonadal dysgenesis: in both patients with male orientation, laparoscopy was indicated for unilateral gonadectomy of an intra-abdominal dysgenetic gonad. Histological examination of the gonad did not show any associated tumoral lesion. In the case with female orientation, laparoscopic bilateral gonadectomy was combined with clitoridoplasty. Laparoscopy allowed more precise verification of the state of the internal genital organs (left hemi-uterus). The pathological examination showed the presence of a gonadoblastoma in the left gonad.

Male pseudohermaphroditism due to MIF deficiency: three patients were diagnosed during laparoscopy for bilateral nonpalpable testis. Laparoscopy detected an uterus and allowed the diagnosis to be made. None of the müllerian elements were excised.

Conclusion

In intersex patients laparoscopy represents an excellent diagnostic aid and optimal method for the removal of structures which are contrary to the assigned sex or of gonads with a high risk of malignancy.

References

1. Josso N et al (1983) Persistance of Müllerian ducts in male pseudohermaphroditism, and its relationship to cryptorchidism. Clin Endoc 19:247–258
2. Kazim E (1985) Intra-abdominal seminomas in persistent Müllerian duct syndrome. Urology 26:290–292
3. Kulkarni JN, Kamat MR, Borges AM (1990) Bilateral synchronous tumors in testes in unrecognized mixed gonadal dysgenesis: a case report and review of literature. J Urol 143:362–364
4. Nihoul-Fékété C et al (1984) Preservation of gonadal function in true hermaphroditism. J Pediatr Surg 19:50–55

5. Olsen MM et al (1988) Gonadoblastoma in infancy: indications for early gonadectomy in 46 XY gonadal dysgenesis. J Pediatr Surg 23:270–271
6. Shalev E et al (1992) Laparoscopic gonadectomy in 46 XY female patient. Fertil Steril 57:459–460
7. Wilson EE, Vuitch F, Carr BC (1992) Laparoscopic removal of dysgenetic gonads containing a gonadoblastoma in a patient with Swyer syndrome. Obstet Gynecol 79:842–844
8. Yu TJ et al (1995) Use of laparoscopy in intersex patients. J Urol 154:1193–1196

Part V
Orthopedics and Neurosurgery

Thoracoscopic Anterior Spinal Diskectomy and Fusion

G.W. Holcomb III

Introduction

In 1910 Jacobeus first described the technique of thoracoscopy for dissection of intrapleural adhesions in patients with pulmonary tuberculosis [1]. In the following 60 years, this technique was employed sporadically as a diagnostic tool in patients with diffuse pulmonary disease but never gained great popularity because of the relatively poor optical systems available. With development of the Hopkins fiberoptic lens system, optical visualization was substantially improved. In 1976 Rodgers reported his experience in nine children. One of the advantages described was the use of intravenous anesthesia which eliminated many of the hazards of endotracheal inhalational anesthesia in those patients [2]. Rodgers subsequently reported his experience with thoracoscopy for children with intrathoracic neoplasms, for diagnosis of interstitial pneumonitis and for management of spontaneous pneumothoraces [3–6]. In the past 5 years, a number of authors have described the thoracoscopic approach in children for a variety of indications including parenchymal biopsy, ligation of patent ductus arteriosus, management of chronic effusions and empyema, sympathectomy for palmer hyperhidrosis, biopsy and excision of mediastinal masses and, recently, pneumonectomy for tumor [7–16].

The use of thoracoscopy in the surgical management of patients with spinal conditions was initially reported in adults by Regan and colleagues in 1995 [17]. This study described 12 adults undergoing video-assisted thoracoscopy (VATS) primarily for diskectomy and fusion. At the 1996 meeting of the Section on Surgery of the American Academy of Pediatrics in Boston, we reported our initial experience utilizing thoracoscopy for anterior spinal diskectomy, release, and fusion in eight children [18].

Advantages to the thoracoscopic approach for spinal conditions include a decreased operative time, the potential for reduced postoperative discomfort and pain, muscle sparing trauma with subsequent weakness, improved access to the entire length of the thoracic vertebral column and cosmesis. Landreneau and colleagues reported reduced postoperative pain, a shortened hospital stay, and an improved early shoulder girdle function in 106 adults undergoing VATS for peripheral lung lesions compared with patients undergoing thoracotomy [19]. This experience confirms the supposition that the thoracoscopic approach should result in less morbidity and early return of muscle function than a similar operation using open thoracotomy. The traditional approach for access to the anterior spine has been a posterolateral thoracotomy. This operation carries the same known incisional morbidity of any intrathoracic operation including respiratory difficulties and postoperative pain. In addition, there is a significant incidence of persisting chronic pain following open thoracotomy [20].

This chapter describes the thoracoscopic approach to anterior spinal diskectomy and fusion and summarizes the author's experience with this technique.

Preoperative Preparation

From the perspective of the pediatric surgeon, these patients are originally seen and evaluated by pediatric orthopedic colleagues. Indications for the thoracoscopic approach are the same as for the open operation. Presently, the only absolute contraindications to the thoracoscopic technique would be an uncontrollable bleeding condition. However, this condition should rarely arise. Relative contraindications include the inability to establish an adequate working space within the thoracic cavity. This problem might occur in patients who have undergone previous thoracic operations with the development of numerous intrapleural adhesions obliterating the pleural space which could not be satisfactorily lysed using the endoscopic technique.

Another relative contraindication is the inability to deflate the ipsilateral lung satisfactorily. At present, the smallest double-lumen tube available has a diameter of 6.0 F. Therefore this technique can be utilized in children older than 8–9 years who usually have a sufficient size trachea to accommodate a 6.0-F endotracheal tube. However, for younger children, it may be necessary to utilize alternative techniques to deflate the ipsilateral lung. If the apex of the thoracic curve is to the left, it is quite likely that intubation of the right mainstem bronchus with subsequent collapse of the left lung would be satisfactory. However, intubation of the left mainstem bronchus for access to the right thoracic cavity is usually less satisfactory. In this situation, placement of a bronchial blocker in the right mainstem bronchus may be necessary.

A Fogarty catheter may be used for this purpose to occlude ventilation to the right lung either with left mainstem bronchial intubation with an uncuffed tube or tracheal intubation (Fig. 1). A useful technique to accomplish ipsilateral bronchial occlusion in younger children is to place the Fogarty catheter into the trachea under direct laryngoscopy. The endotracheal tube is inserted beside the catheter followed by flexible bronchoscopy through the endotracheal tube to visualize location of the catheter in the appropriate mainstem bronchus. With this technique, it is important to auscultate the lungs after turning the patient into the lateral decubitus position to insure the bronchial blocker has not become dislodged. An optional technique to effect ipsilateral lung deflation is insufflation of the thoracic cavity with up to 5 mmHg. of carbon dioxide. The possibility

Fig. 1. For thoracoscopic diskectomy it is necessary to deflate the ipsilateral lung. One technique is to intubate the right mainstem bronchus for left lung collapse (*left*). However, it is usually difficult to intubate the left mainstem bronchus. Therefore an alternative technique is to occlude the right mainstem bronchus with a catheter passed along the endotracheal tube to effect right lung collapse (*right*)

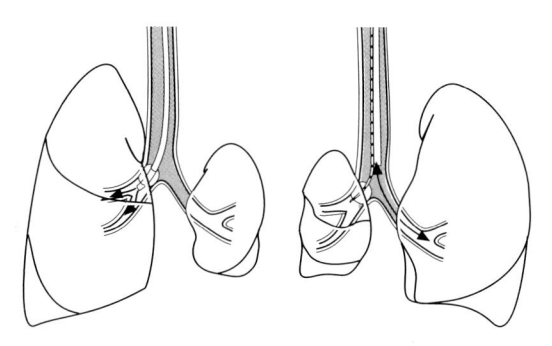

of creating a tension pneumothorax using this technique may develop but this complication seldom occurs at such low pressures.

A final relative contraindication, at present, is the need for extension of the operation into the lumbar vertebral column. Although a number of reports have described laparoscopic lumbar diskectomy in adults [21–23], takedown of the diaphragm and thoracolaparoscopic exposure of the thoracic and lumbar spine simultaneously has not been described in either adults or children.

It is important to have a preoperative discussion with the orthopedic surgeon regarding the nature of the indicated procedure, the number of diskectomies required and any potential problems which might be encountered in each specific patient. A thorough preoperative conference with the family is also imperative to describe the nature and risks of the operation, and the possibility of conversion to the open operation if necessary. Surprisingly, the operation may be less satisfactory in a very thin asthenic patient with a severe scoliotic curve. In such patients, the ipsilateral thoracic cavity is quite small and the distance from the thoracic vertebral column to the chest wall may measure only a few centimeters. This situation creates technical difficulties because the collapsed lung may still impair visualization.

Operative Technique

As previously mentioned this is an elective procedure and the patients usually are admitted to the hospital the day of the operation. The operative preparation is the same as for the open anterior approach for the correction of the spinal anomaly. The anesthetic preparation, however, differs in that collapse of the ipsilateral lung is necessary for exposure to the anterior vertebral column. Techniques used for this purpose have previously been discussed (Fig. 1). Endotracheal anesthesia using a double-lumen endotracheal tube or blockade of the ipsilateral mainstem bronchus with endotracheal intubation is performed with the patient in the supine position. In addition, two peripheral intravenous catheters, a urinary catheter and an arterial catheter are inserted. The patient is then

Fig. 2. As the target for thoracoscopic diskectomy is the posterior mediastinum and vertebral column, it is helpful to position the patient relatively face down, which allows the lung to fall away from the posterior aspect of the chest cavity and improve visualization

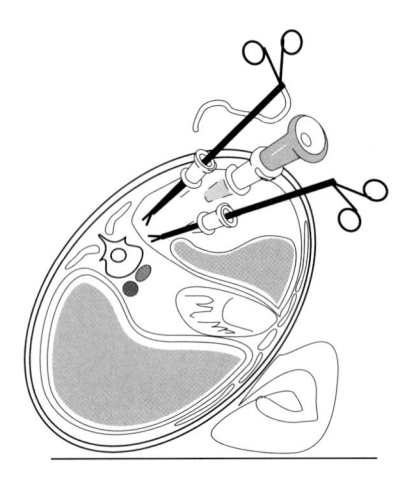

turned to the lateral decubitus position in preparation for the thoracoscopic operation. As the target of the operation is the posterior mediastinum and vertebral column, it is helpful to rotate the patient more face down, which allows the lung to fall away from the posterior aspect of the chest cavity and improve visualization (Fig. 2).

The patient is then prepped and draped similarly for the open operation. As a general rule, three to four short incisions are required depending on the number of intervertebral disks which need to be excised. Usually at least three incisions are necessary for three or four disks, but four incisions are likely required for excision of five or six disks. These incisions are placed in a vertical direction along the patient's lateral chest wall in the anterior or middle axillary line and need to be individualized according to the patient's body habitus and length of the vertebral column (Fig. 3). The incisions are 7 mm in the length as the cannulas used (Flexipath, Ethicon Endosurgery, Cincinnati, Ohio) have a diameter of 7 mm. The advantage of these cannulas is that the sleeve is malleable and can be cut to the appropriate length so that the cannula does not extend into the thoracic cavity sufficiently to impair the operation. It is best to cut the sleeve at a length slightly longer then the thickness of the chest wall. Standard rongeurs, currettes and osteotomes can readily be used for most cases.

The first incision is made in the midaxillary line at a 90° angle from the apex of the thoracic deformity. It is important to realize that if the apex of the curve is at the eighth thoracic vertebral body, the interspace that is at a 90° angle in the midaxillary line may be at the T-6 or T-7 level. Therefore, it is necessary to utilize the interspace which is approximately 90° from the apex of the curve. In general, it is important to maintain this 90° working angle as it provides the optimal approach for diskectomy so that the surgeon is not working at a difficult angle into the intervertebral disk. In such a circumstance, the vertebral body on each side of the disk may impair complete diskectomy. When placing this initial cannula, it must be remembered that the lung may not have been completely deflated by

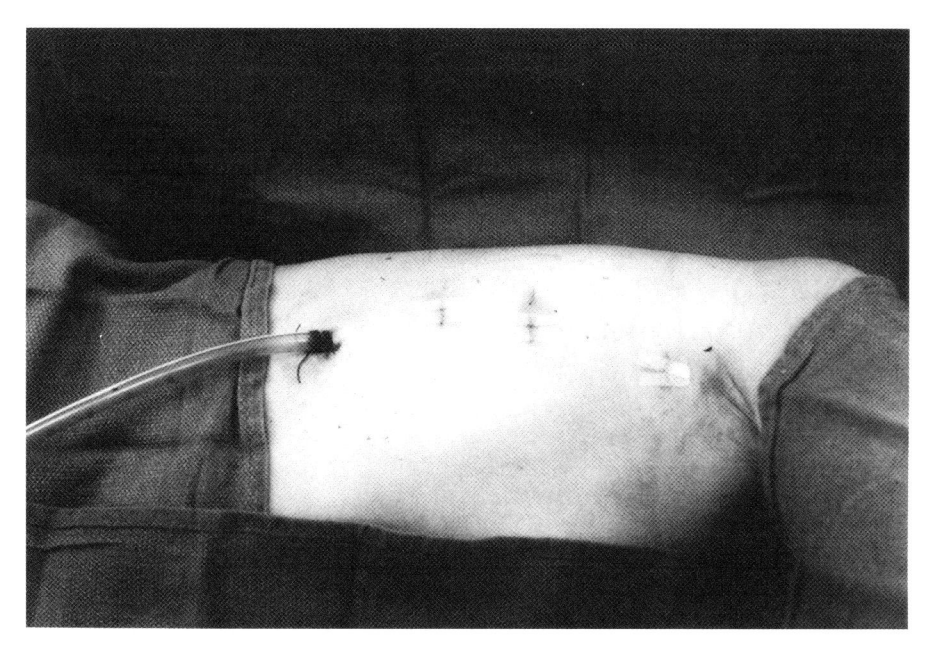

48 Thoracoscopic Anterior Spinal Diskectomy and Fusion

Fig. 3. In this patient, who underwent five diskectomies, the incisions are oriented vertically along the patient's right chest wall. Notice the spacing between the incisions to accomplish the diskectomies (T_{5-6}–T_{9-10}). Also notice that the chest tube has been inserted through the most inferior incision

the anesthesiology team. Therefore, the first cannula should be inserted cautiously to avoid injury to an inflated lung. Following placement of the first cannula, a 5-mm 0° telescope is inserted through the cannula and diagnostic thoracoscopy performed. If the lung has not been completely deflated, it is possible to manually apply external pressure on the lung using the camera to assist with deflation. (If the lung cannot be completely deflated, it may be necessary to place a retractor through one of the accessory cannulas for retraction during the operation.) During the diagnostic thoracoscopy, special attention should be focused on the vertebral column to identify the correct anatomy. If this first incision was not placed directly across from the disc at the apex of the scoliotic curve, this incision may be used for the diskectomy either above or below the apex. Another incision should be made at 90° to the apex. At this point, it is possible to plan placement of the other three incisions and, if necessary, identify a fourth site. If the first incision is placed correctly, the other two incisions are located either one or two interspaces above and below the apex so as to be able to perform diskectomies above and below the apex of the vertebral curve. When deciding if the other incisions should be placed one or two interspaces above or below, try to imagine a 90° working angle for optimal diskectomy between that incision and the involved disk space.

Having oriented three incisions vertically in the interspaces in the midaxillary line along the lateral chest wall, a Steinman pin is inserted through one of the cannulas and into one of the intervertebral disks. A lateral chest radiograph is then taken to confirm the correct anatomy so that the first diskectomy is performed in the proper disk space allowing the other diskectomies to be accomplished appropriately. Following the radiograph, the Steinmann pin is removed and diskectomy initiated. The telescope is inserted through one of the ports, the second port is used for insertion of a suction/irrigation instrument and the third port is used to perform the diskectomy. Each diskectomy is accomplished in a similar fashion. The pleura overlying the disk is incised (Fig. 4a). The vessels lie over the vertebral bodies and the disks are in the middle between these vessels which usually do not require ligation. Following pleural incision overlying the

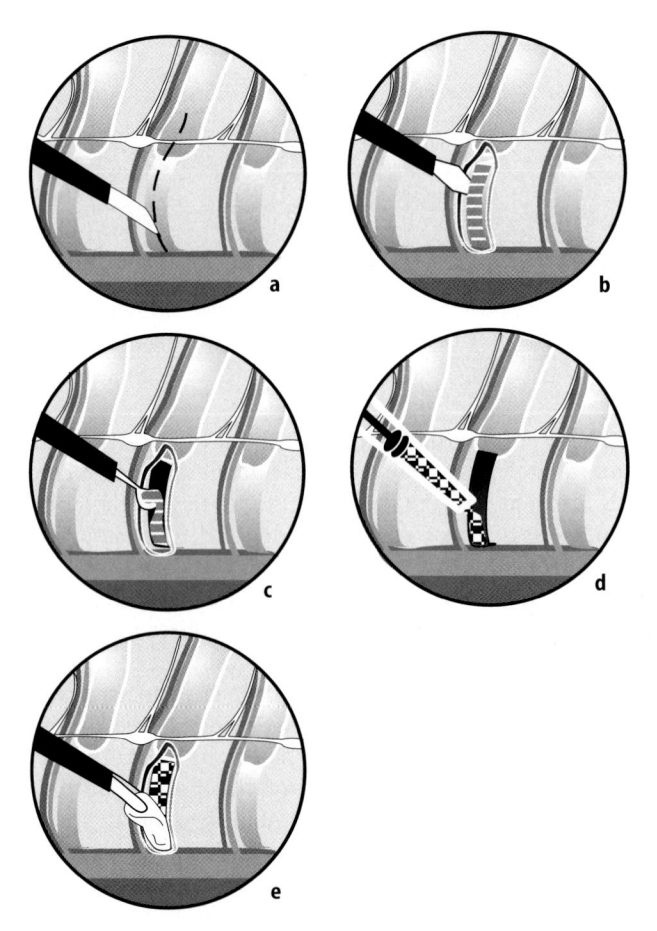

Fig. 4. **a** The initial step in performing the diskectomy is incision of the pleura overlying the disk using the electrocautery. It is usually not necessary to divide the vertebral vessels as the disk lies in the middle between these vessels. **b** An osteotome is used to perform the diskectomy. **c** A curette is shown cleaning the vertebral body end plates. **d** Following removal of the disk material, cancellous bone is placed within the excised disk space for fusion. **e** Following placement of the cancellous bone graft, gel foam is used to cover the cancellous bone to aid in hemostasis

disk, the annulus of the disc is excised and a rongeur is utilized to extract the disc material. The end plates of the vertebral bodies are cleaned with a curette.

On occasion, an osteotome with mallet facilitates the diskectomy (Fig. 4b,c). Visualization is important during this time to insure that dissection does not extend outside the disk space and into the adjacent vertebral body. Some of the instruments have depth markings on the shafts and a depth of 2 cm is the ideal limit during the diskectomy. Bleeding is not usually a problem although there may be some visible oozing. However, this usually stops following diskectomy. Once the diskectomy has been performed, the disk space is packed with either allograft cancellous bone or autogenous graft harvested from the adjacent rib and covered with Gelfoam (Fig. 4d,e). Cancellous bone is utilized primarily by the author because it is more time efficient than harvesting the adjacent rib and provides comparable results.

Once the first diskectomy has been accomplished, the remaining diskectomies are performed in a similar fashion. It is necessary, however, to rotate the instruments such that the working port remains opposite the disk to be excised. It may be necessary to change from a zero to a 30° telescope during these diskectomies so that optimal visualization is achieved. As previously mentioned, if more than three diskectomies are required, a fourth, and occasionally, a fifth incision may be needed. The same principle for placing these incisions is utilized as previously described. A fourth incision can also be made earlier if required for retraction although the suction/irrigator works as a retractor when not being utilized for suction or irrigation. Heparinized saline is used for irrigation to prevent clot formation in the thoracic cavity.

After all diskectomies are completed, the thoracic cavity is irrigated and all debris removed. Hemostasis is confirmed and attention turned toward closure. Depending on the child's size, a 24- or 28-F. chest tube is inserted through the most inferior incision under direct visualization (Fig. 3) and the most distal hole in the tube is positioned just inside the thoracic cavity. The anterior fascia of the muscles of the remaining incisions are closed with 3.0 absorbable suture and the skin closed with 5.0 absorbable suture. Steri-strips and dressing are then applied. (When removing the chest tube, it is important to remember that a tunnel through the soft tissues of the chest wall has not been created and care must be taken not to allow air entry into the thoracic cavity upon pulling the tube.) At this time, the patient is turned supine and a single-lumen endotracheal tube inserted. The patient is then turned prone for the posterior instrumentation and fusion which is accomplished solely by the orthopedic surgeons.

Personal Experience

The first thoracoscopic anterior diskectomy at Children's Hospital- Vanderbilt University Medical Center was performed in November 1995. In the following 13 months, a total of 12 patients have undergone the operation (Table 1). Most of the children had idiopathic adolescent scoliosis as the indication for the operation. The number of diskectomies per patient has ranged from 2 to 5, with a

Table 1. Results of thoracoscopic diskectomy (*n*=12) (1995–1996)

Pat. no.	Age (years)	Sex	Disease	Site of diskectomies (total no.)	Operative time (min)	Estimated blood loss (cc)	Posterior instrumentation and fusion	Complications
1	13	F	Congenital scoliosis, hemivertebra (T_5)	T_{4-5}–T_{6-7} (3)	180	145	Yes	None
2	5	F	Congenital scoliosis, hemivertebra (T_8)	T_{7-8}–T_{8-9} (2)	90	75	Yes	None
3	16	M	Thoracic kyphosis	T_{6-7}–T_{10-11} (5)	205	150	Yes, staged 1 week	None
4	20	F	Idiopathic scoliosis, adolescent	T_{5-6}–T_{9-10} (5)	150	175	Yes	None
5	10	F	Neuromuscular scoliosis, spina bifida	T_{6-7}–T_{10-11} (5)	225	125	Yes	None
6	11	F	Idiopathic scoliosis, adolescent	T_{6-7}–T_{10-11} (5)	210	200	Yes, staged 1 week	None
7	17	M	Neuromuscular scoliosis, syringomyelia	T_{7-8}–T_{10-11} (4)	195	725	Yes, staged 1 week	Intraoperative bleeding, controlled (Intercostal vessel)
8	25	F	Idiopathic scoliosis, adolescent	T_{6-7}–T_{10-11} (5)	140	30	Yes	None
9	9	M	Idiopathic scoliosis	T_{5-6}–T_{9-10} (5)	125	150	Yes	None
10	12	F	Idiopathic scoliosis, adolescent	T_{6-7}–T_{9-10} (4)	105	145	Yes	None
11	13	F	Scoliosis, Marfan's syndrome	T_{5-6}–T_{9-10} (5)	105	200	Yes	None
12	11	F	Idiopathic scoliosis, adolescent	T_{6-7}–T_{9-10} (4)	100	120	Yes	None

mean of 4. A learning curve exists for this combined operation between pediatric orthopedic surgeons and pediatric thoracic surgeons. In the first seven patients, the time required to complete the operation averaged 179 min (mean of 43 min per diskectomy). In the last five patients the mean time required for the operation has been 115 min (mean of 25 min per diskectomy). Nine patients underwent posterior spinal instrumentation and fusion immediately following the anterior thoracoscopic procedure under the same anesthesia. Three patients were staged with the posterior fusion being performed 1 week following the anterior thoracoscopic operation. Only one peri- or postoperative complication has occurred. In the seventh patient, a significant amount of bleeding occurred following injury to an intercostal vessel. However, this was quickly controlled and did not require conversion to an open operation.

In addition to what is perceived to be less discomfort and an easier recovery for the patient, the reduced operative times for the thoracoscopic approach compared with the open operation means that the entire combined procedure (anterior and posterior) is accomplished in less time as well. The anterior thoracoscopic and posterior open fusion operations are now being completed in approximately 6 h compared with eight or nine for the open anterior and posterior fusions which is advantageous for our pediatric patients. In our experience, the thoracoscopic approach for anterior diskectomy, release and fusion followed by the traditional open posterior instrumentation and fusion is now the preferred approach for children requiring both anterior and posterior correction of their thoracic spinal condition.

References

1. von Jacobaeus HC (1910) Über die Möglichkeit die Zystoskopie bei Untersuchung seröser Höhlungen anzuwenden. Munchener Med Wochenschr 40:2090–2092
2. Rodgers BM, Talbert JL (1976) Thoracoscopy for diagnosis of intrathoracic lesions in children. J Pediatr Surg 11:703–708
3. Rodgers BM, Moazam F, Talbert JL (1979) Thoracoscopy: early diagnosis of interstitial pneumonitis in the immunologically suppressed child. Chest 75:126–130
4. Rodgers BM et al (1981) Thoracoscopy for intrathoracic tumors. Ann Thorac Surg 31:414–420
5. Ryckman FC, Rodgers BM (1982) Thoracoscopy for intrathoracic neoplasia in children. J Pediatr Surg 17:521–524
6. Tribble CG, Selden RF, Rodgers BM (1986) Talc poudrage in the treatment of spontaneous pneumothoraces in patients with cystic fibrosis. Ann Surg 204:677–680
7. Burke RP (1994) Video assisted thoracoscopic surgery for patent ductus arteriosus. Pediatrics 93:823–825
8. Laborde F et al (1993) A new video-assisted thoracoscopic surgical technique for interruption of patent ductus arteriosus in infants and children. J Thorac Cardiovasc Surg 105(2):278–280
9. Kern JA, Rodgers BM (1993) Thoracoscopy in the management of empyema in children. J Pediatr Surg 28:1128–1132
10. Daniel TM et al (1993) Thoracoscopic surgery for diseases of the lung and pleura. Ann Surg 217:566–575

11. Kao MC et al (1994) Palmer hyperhidrosis in children: treatment with video endoscopic laser sympathectomy. J Pediatr Surg 29(3):387–391
12. Dillon PW, Cilley RE, Krummel TM (1993) Video-assisted thoracoscopic excision of intrathoracic masses in children: report of two cases. Surg Lap Endo 3:433–436
13. Craig SR, Hamzah M, Walker WS (1996) Video-assisted thoracoscopic pneumonectomy for bronchial carcinoid tumor in a 14-year-old girl. J Pediatr Surg 31:1724–1726
14. Rodgers BM (1993) Thoracoscopic procedures in children. Semin Pediatr Surg 2:182–189
15. Holcomb GW III et al (1995) Minimally invasive surgery in children with cancer. Cancer 76:121–128
16. Rodgers BM (1994) Thoracoscopy. In: Holcomb GW III (ed) Pediatric endoscopic surgery. Appleton and Lange, Norwalk
17. Regan JJ, Mack MJ, Picetti GD III (1995) A technical report on video-assisted thoracoscopy in thoracic spinal surgery. Spine 20:831–837
18. Holcomb GW III, Mencio GA, Green NE (1997) Video assisted thoracoscopic diskectomy and fusion. J Pediatr Surg 32:1120–1122
19. Landreneau RJ et al (1993) Postoperative pain related morbidity: video assisted thoracoscopy vs. thoracotomy. Ann Thorac Surg 56:1285–1289
20. Hazelrigg SR et al (1991) The effect of muscle-sparing versus standard posterolateral thoracotomy on pulmonary function, muscle strength, and postoperative pain. J Thorac Cardiovasc Surg 101:394–401
21. Mahvi DM, Zdeblick TA (1996) A prospective study of laparoscopic spinal fusion: technique and operative complications. Ann Surg 224(1):85–90
22. Slotman GJ, Stein SC (1996) Laparoscopic L5-S1 diskectomy: a cost-effective minimally invasive general surgery – neurosurgery team alternative to laminectomy. Am Surg 62:64–68
23. Slotman GJ, Stein SC (1995) Laparoscopic laser lumbar diskectomy. Surg Endosc 9:826–829

Indications, Techniques and Results of Pediatric Neuroendoscopy

J.A. Grotenhuis, W.P. Vandertop

Introduction

In 1910, Dr. V. L'Espinasse used a cystoscope to remove the choroid plexus in two patients to treat their hydrocephalus. This is considered the beginning of neuroendoscopy (Davis 1939). In 1922, Walter Dandy first coined the term "ventriculoscope" when he used a cystoscope to avulse the choroid plexus in the lateral ventricles of two children with hydrocephalus. One year later, in 1923, Mixter reported the first, and successful, endoscopic third ventriculostomy in a patient with obstructive hydrocephalus. The endoscopes were rigid and quite large, and the procedures had high morbidity and mortality rates because of the technical limitations of that time. After the introduction of implantable CSF-shunts for the treatment of hydrocephalus, endoscopes were virtually abandoned.

The widespread use of the operative microscope in neurosurgery pushed the development of neuroendoscopic techniques into the background, although there were some promising attempts to visualize the spinal canal (Burman 1931; Stern 1936; Pool 1942; Fukushima and Schramm 1975; Olinger and Ohlhaber 1974; Ooi et al. 1973), the cerebellopontine angle (Fukushima 1978; Prott 1974; Oppel and Mulch 1979) and the cisterna magna, the C1–2 space and Meckel's cave (Crue 1977; Fukushima et al. 1978).

The refinements in recent years of endoscopic instrumentation have revitalized neuroendoscopy, and many more applications of endoscopes in research and clinical neurosurgery have been elaborated since (Bauer and Hellwig 1994; Caemaert et al. 1994; Cohen 1993a,b, 1994; Grotenhuis and Tacl 1993; Grotenhuis et al. 1994, 1995, 1996, 1998; Hüwel et al. 1993; Knosp 1993; Liston et al. 1987; Manwaring and Crone 1992; Oka et al. 1993). Neuroendoscopy has now gained a widespread acceptance, particularly among neurosurgeons who deal with the pediatric population.

Because the use of neuroendoscopes and instruments is inherently different from classical microneurosurgical techniques, careful planning and preparation are very important to avoid complications and poor outcomes.

Indications

The indications for neuroendoscopy include 1) treatment of obstructive hydrocephalus by fenestrating the floor of the third ventricle or dilatating or stenting an obstructed aqueduct, 2) direct positioning of a proximal shunt catheter, 3) fenestration of intraventricular membranes, 4) opening of the septum pellucidum in unilateral obstruction of the foramen of Monro, 5) evacuation of intraventricular hematomas and abscesses, 6) biopsy or excision of intraventricular tumors, 7) fenestration of intra- and paraventricular arachnoid cysts, and marsupialization of neuro-epithelial cysts.

In addition to these indications, the endoscope is also used increasingly as an adjunct to open microneurosurgical procedures to look around corners to visualize otherwise hidden structures, for example, during craniotomy for craniopharyngioma or tumors of the fourth ventricle.

Preoperative Workup

Magnetic resonance (MR) imaging is the diagnostic modality of choice as it gives exact anatomical details in three planes which greatly enhances preoperative planning. Sometimes, for example, for multiloculated hydrocephalus, a CT with intraventricular contrast is better for demonstrating the communicating and noncommunicating parts of the ventricular system.

For precise placement of the burr hole and calculation of the appropriate, often angled trajectory and guidance of the neuroendoscopes towards the target, the neuroendoscope can be used in conjunction with frame-based or frameless stereotaxy.

Preoperative Preparation

Neuroendoscopes

Two types of endoscopes are commonly employed for neuroendoscopy: rigid endoscopes, which can be either lenscopes or fiberscopes, and flexible endoscopes which are based on fiberoptic technology. The lenscope provides the best image clarity, resolution and illumination. Its straight design makes it easy to introduce and also allows easy orientation and hence makes it the best type of endoscope to start with and to master basic neuroendoscopic skills. However, the disadvantage of rigid lenscopes is the comparatively large diameter of the endoscope.

Nowadays, a variety of rigid neuroendoscopes is available, such as the 6-mm cerebral endoscope from Wolf, designed by Caemaert, with four channels, one for the 5° optic, one for the 2.2-mm working channel and two channels for suction and irrigation; the 6-mm Gaab neuroendoscope, with an angled eyepiece and a straight operating sheath and the MINOP system with trocars and an 2.7-

mm angled neuroendoscope which can also be used for endoscope-assisted microneurosurgery. The rigid fiberscope, such as the Workscope, is as easy in handling as the lenscopes. Its weight is much less than that of lenscopes but its particular advantage is the small size of the optical fibers, which permits a much larger instrument channel relative to the total endoscope diameter. The image quality however, is inferior to that of a lenscope, although incorporation of 30,000 fibers has improved much of the image quality.

The main advantage of the flexible fiberscope is the deflection and hence "steering" capability of the working tip, enabling both looking and working "around the corner." Because the shaft of the endoscope is flexible, the endoscopic image rotates during deflection of the tip and this pairs a more challenging anatomical orientation with an inferior image quality. In addition, as its working channel is quite small the flexible instruments for these endoscopes are so small that they are difficult to manipulate precisely because they exhibit delay or rotation on actuation.

Flexible and steerable neuroendoscopes are available with an outer diameter of 4-mm, and with fiberoptics providing a 5- to 50- mm depth of field, a 90° field of view (in water 64°), a steerable tip that can be rotated 100°/160°, one working channel of 1 mm and a flexible working length of 38 cm with 10-cm markings.

A fiberscope mainly used for placement of the proximal shunt catheter, is the stylet or the 1.2-mm Neuroview neuroendoscope, which is a semirigid fiberscope that can be introduced into the ventricular catheter during a shunting procedure. It also has a flushing channel and it can be used for other procedures such as diagnostic ventriculoscopy, and some neurosurgeons also use it for third ventriculostomy. About the same size is the Neuroguide, but is has no flushing channel. The Neuroguide is only used in shunting procedures.

Light Source

Nowadays, the incandescent lamp is no longer used but rather an external light source which is directed towards a fiber cable. It should be a cold light source, preferably a xenon light of daylight intensity. An auto-iris which automatically adjusts the brightness maintains an optimum image while moving the endoscope.

Camera and Videosystem

As the video camera, with appropriate optical coupler, is mounted on the eyepiece of the endoscope, it should be as small and as light as possible. With most fiberscopes there is no eyepiece, so the camera is directly plugged into the image cable. With the charged-couple device (CCD) technology, there are now cameras available as small as a match-box. The image is transmitted to a video monitor which is an important part of the equipment because all pictures from the endoscope are projected there. It should have a high resolution and color balance. Furthermore, it should not be too small so that it can be placed at a sufficient distance to maintain sterility of the operating field. A video recorder can be practical for documentation of the procedure, which is useful for evaluation and teaching purposes.

Irrigation Device

Irrigation is important during neuroendoscopy as visualization rapidly diminishes without it. If the amount of perfusate is small, ordinary physiological saline solution is suitable, but its prolonged use can lead to a wash-out of ventricular electrolytes, which is potentially dangerous. Therefore, the use of Ringer's solution is preferable. In any neuroendoscopic procedure, it is of the utmost importance that the irrigation fluid can escape in order to prevent a sudden rise of intraventricular pressure or even tentorial herniation with acute cardiac arrest.

The simplest way of irrigating is manual flushing with a syringe by an assistant. However, it is difficult to control the exact amount of perfusate and its pressure. A simple infusion system set at a rate of 2–3 ml/min can be sufficient, but the solution cools off very quickly due to the distance between the infusion and the entrance in the endoscope. This is eliminated by the Hotline Fluid Warmer HL-90INT (HFW), designed for safe inline warming of blood and intravenous fluids as they are administered to patients at low flow rates. An 8' Disposable Set allows fluid to be delivered to the patient at near body temperature at flow rates up to 3000 ml/h (50 ml/min). Furthermore, the HFW employs an unique Gas Eliminator which vents the micro-bubbles of gas which are always released from fluids as they are warmed up, preventing these bubbles from hampering the view through the endoscope.

A more sophisticated system is the Malis Irrigation Module, controlled with a foot pedal. It allows gentle pulsatile irrigation, which can be of greater use than continuous irrigation because the pulsating movements can assist in dissecting membranes and any bleeding source can be detected and controlled easier.

Fixation of the Endoscope

It is difficult to keep an endoscope still for any length of time. An assistant can do for very short procedures but a mechanical stabilizer is more reliable and with the endoscope fixed, bimanual manipulation with instruments becomes possible. Almost any self-retaining retraction system used in daily neurosurgery can be modified to hold the endoscope. A stereotactic frame and holder is also very useful but time consuming and hardly practicable for very small children.

Instruments for Neuroendoscopy

Endoscopes used for therapeutic procedures should have a working channel through which instruments can be inserted. Instrumentation during neuroendoscopy is a major part of a training program. It is important to remember that the instrument enters the viewing field from the side and not through the center. This can be difficult whenever a target in the center of the viewing field is focused on too closely because the instrument passes it by. The second difficulty is to choose the right working distance for the instrument. When the tip of the endoscope is too far away from the target and the working area of the instrument, it is difficult to see how the instrument is acting, but when the endoscope is too close, the instrument fills up a great part of the viewing field which obstructs the visual control of the instrument tip and the target area. For example, with the 4-mm flexible endoscope, the tip of the instrument should extend about 10 mm beyond the imaging tip of the endoscope.

Ventricular Cannula

The ventricles can be reached directly with a rigid lenscope without a previous ventricular puncture, if the endoscope is blunt-nosed or bullet-shaped. With the flexible endoscope it is necessary to use a guide to access the ventricle. It must have a slightly larger inner diameter than the outer diameter of the flexible endoscope, for example, for a 4-mm flexible endoscope a 14-F cannula should be used while a 10-F cannula is appropriate for a 2.8-mm endoscope, so it can permit smooth movement of the endoscope. It is essential to allow free passage of irrigation fluid outside the endoscope but within the cannula.

For endoscope-assisted shunt procedures a special peel-away sheath is helpful. With its blunt-nosed stylet it is used for ventricular puncture and then used as a conduit to guide the endoscope from the entry point to the target. For prolonged procedures it is more convenient to use a rigid ventricular cannula, based upon the same principles as the Dandy or Cushing ventricular needle. Such a cannula can be fixed in a self-retaining arm. Several types of metal ventricular cannulas according to the kind of endoscope can be used. Usually we coagulate the arachnoid and open the superficial cortex according to the diameter of the cannula, then puncture the ventricle with a Dandy or Cushing needle, followed by insertion of the cannula.

Grasping and Biopsy Forceps

The forceps should be large enough to take representative samples for histology, but the smaller the endoscope, the smaller the working channel and the corresponding instrument. With the forceps of the 4-mm flexible neuroendoscope it is still possible, though difficult, to take a representative biopsy. The toothed grasping forceps is very useful for seizing small foreign bodies, a loose ventricular catheter, parts of a cyst wall or an arachnoid membrane. The flexible forceps for fiberscopes do not open gradually but they more or less snap open suddenly with a short delay and often they rotate on actuation, which results in a reduced manual control.

Scissors

Scissors are only available for rigid endoscopes and can be very helpful in dissecting membranes or cyst walls. The action is straightforward, such as the use of microscissors in open microneurosurgical procedures.

Laser Equipment

Lasers were introduced as surgical tools in the 1960s. At first a ruby crystal was used, later, the Helium Neon gas laser was created, followed by the carbon dioxide gas laser, the Argon laser and the neodymium-doped yttrium aluminum garnet (Nd:YAG) laser. One of the newest lasers, introduced in 1981, is the potassium titanyl phosphate (KTP/532) laser. The experience with lasers in neurosurgery is mainly focused on tumor resection.

The conversion of photons from laser light into heat, and the tissue's reaction to this heat, produces the ultimate biological effect. The penetration and absorption of laser energy into and by tissue varies from organ to organ and according to the kind of laser energy applied. It would be beyond the scope of this chapter to go into more detail about the different types of lasers used in neurosurgery. An excellent review article on the use of lasers in specific neurosurgical applications has been published recently, which every neurosurgeon who wishes to start laser-assisted surgery is encouraged to consult (Krishnamurthy and Powers 1994).

For neuroendoscopy, the CO_2 laser is not suitable because it is highly absorbed by water (Grotenhuis 1995). Furthermore, the CO2 laser can be used only with rigid endoscopes because development of flexible fibers and fiber tips is in its infancy. The continuous wave (cw) Nd:YAG, argon, KTP and Diode lasers have proven to be very effective for resecting highly vascularized tissues and can be transported efficiently through fibers.

To date, the Nd:YAG laser (1064 nm) has been used most frequently, in both contact and noncontact modes, for coagulation of the choroid plexus, blood vessels and for tumor resection (Yamakawa 1995). Noncontact Nd:YAG laser light is not really suitable because the laser light is readily absorbed by cerebrospinal fluid (CSF) leading to large scattering and possible thermal damage to surrounding tissue. The contact-tipped Nd:YAG laser partly overcomes this problem, as 10%–20% of the laser energy is absorbed at the tip, but many surgeons still do not feel comfortable using high-energy laser endoprobes in close proximity to vital structures such as the basilar artery (e.g., in third ventriculostomy; Jones et al. 1995).

From studies on the basic ablation mechanism of cw lasers using contact probes, it is known that carbonization of tissue followed by efficient heat absorption and vaporization of that tissue is the main mechanism of ablation (Verdaasdonk et al. 1995b). Using regular uncoated fiber tips, laser light is converted into heat by absorption in tissue only. The white (nonpigmented) ependymal tissues and arachnoid membranes during neuroendoscopy poorly absorb visual and near-infrared laser light. The light is scattered and absorbed in a large volume of tissue and therefore, a large amount of energy is needed for the tissue to carbonize (10–20 W for many seconds). Experimental data have now indeed confirmed that noncoated, direct-contact fiber tips should not be used near critical structures, because once carbonization is followed by vaporization, the dispersion of heat using uncoated fiber tips transgresses far beyond the intended depth with possible damage to deeper structures (Vandertop et al. 1998; Willems et al., submitted).

To overcome the above mentioned dangers, we have developed a special laser catheter with an atraumatic ball-tip which was pretreated with a layer of carbon particles. This layer absorbs approximately 90% of the laser light which is very effectively converted into heat (Verdaasdonk et al. 1995a). This enables us to drastically limit the amount of laser light used and the length of the exposure needed, thereby increasing safety, even around critical structures. As the carbon particles absorb a broad range of wavelengths very efficiently, any cw laser source which can be transmitted by optical fibers, is suitable for this application. Because only a few Watts of power is needed using our specially developed 'black' fiber tips, battery driven diode lasers in the size of a flashlight might even be used in the future.

Radiofrequency Dissector

This device is a most adaptable tool for neuroendoscopy. It is comparable with the monopolar ball electrode or the Bugbee wire used by urologists. The RF dissector and its improved version the ME2-electrode (Codman) developed for the use with flexible endoscopes, uses saline as an electrically conductive medium between the recessed electrode and the face of the ceramic tube that is brought down over the tip of a bare wire while this tip can be extended step by step a few millimeters beyond it. The depth of thermal penetration is controlled by the length of wire exposed beyond its tip. When the face of the ceramic catheter is brought on a membrane (e.g., the thinned floor of the third ventricle or an arachnoid cyst wall) keying of the electrode causes a vaporization to be induced which cuts a hole with exactly the dimensions of the ceramic tube. Prolonged dissection, however, is associated with the sticking of debris on the electrode tip, which can be a problem. An advantage over the Bugbee wire is that much lower wattage suffices to achieve equivalent dissection.

For dissecting a membrane, a dot-to-dot fashion can be used. Thinner membranes can be dissected by making a hole and then slowly moving the tip of the endoscope in a circular fashion so that the tip of the ceramic tube cuts a circular hole into the membrane. There is, however, one difficulty in working with the RF dissector. It is not possible to advance the wire through the end of the working channel when the tip is flexed more than 30°.

Bipolar Coagulation Electrode

A bipolar coagulation electrode is also available for neuroendoscopes, however, only for rigid endoscopes with large working channels, although the development of such a bipolar electrode for the use with flexible endoscopes is in progress. As in microneurosurgery it is an important tool for hemostasis and, contrary to the monopolar electrode, it prevents excessive heating of the CSF.

Puncturing Needle

A sharp puncturing needle can be useful to enter a cyst with a thick wall and then aspirate the cyst's content. A blunt needle can be helpful for taking a biopsy from a more firm tumor. At present, puncturing needles of different kinds are available for rigid endoscopes and also (but more limited) for flexible endoscopes.

Balloon Catheter

Balloon catheters can be useful for enlargement of holes in membranes up to a predetermined diameter. For third ventriculostomy, a 3- or 4-F Fogarty balloon catheter is used, or a so-called figure-8 balloon catheter.

For other indications, such as dilatation of the aqueduct, catheters with longer and sometimes larger balloons are necessary, including angioplasty balloon catheters such as are used for coronary angioplasty (e.g., the Monorail Piccolino, the Small Vessel Balloon Dilatation Catheter or the USCI Pronto Balloon Dilatation Catheter with Pro/Pel Coating, with a shaft size of only 2.9 F, a balloon length of 20 mm and a balloon diameter of 3.5 mm). Before using any balloon catheter it is necessary to read the instructions about the amount of fluid and pressure needed to inflate the balloon carefully. Be sure that the balloon catheter is long enough and that it fits into the working channel of the endoscope.

Hydrojet

This is not an instrument in its true sense, but irrigation through a small (1 mm or less) channel creates a very fine but forceful water column that can be used for dissection and defining tissue planes. Most of the time it is used to detect segments of free mobility which are the easiest and safest sites to fenestrate, for example, to find from inside a cyst the part of the cyst wall adjacent to the ventricle (this part shows its deformability while the wall adjacent to the white matter does not) or to find the optimal point for fenestration of the septum pellucidum.

Technique

Neuroendoscopic procedures require careful planning and preparation by the operating room staff. Presently, there are entire neuroendoscopic systems available, consisting of a control panel, a remote control for sterile field operation, video camera and optical coupler, xenon light source, infusion pump, super VHS recorder, color printer, video floppy disc recorder and a picture-in-picture character generator, which make the set-up more easy.

It is crucial to set up the neuroendoscopic equipment systematically in order to manage the diversity of instruments and their interconnections. Furthermore, the specific tasks of anyone in the team: the scrub nurse, the circulating nurse, the neurosurgeon and the assistant, should be clearly depicted. Experience shows that a drawing or even a photograph of the set-up helps more than any written description (Fig. 1).

It is important to be familiar with the normal endoscopic anatomy of the ventricular system and examine the large amount of landmarks within the different parts of the ventricles (Figs. 2, 3) before trying to perform an endoscopic procedure in a patient with a pathological condition of the ventricles. The following landmarks help in orientation:
- Within the lateral ventricles
  - Foramen of Monro
  - Choroid plexus
  - Septal and thalamostriate veins
  - The corpus callosum with its typical appearance caused by multiple small, transverse grooves

Fig. 1. Position of the patient, crew, and equipment. *L*, Light; *I*, irrigation; *S*, suction; *B*, bipolar electrocautery

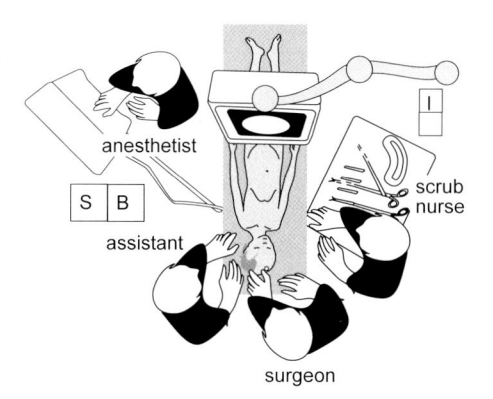

Fig. 2. Sagittal view of the brain showing trajectory of endoscope through frontal burrhole via the right lateral ventricle into third ventricle

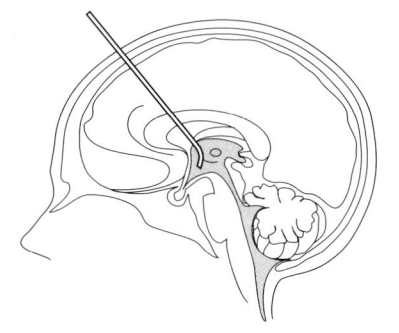

Fig. 3. View into the right lateral ventricle with enlarged foramen of Monro, through which the floor of the third ventricle can be seen from anterior (dorsum sellae) to posterior (aqueduct)

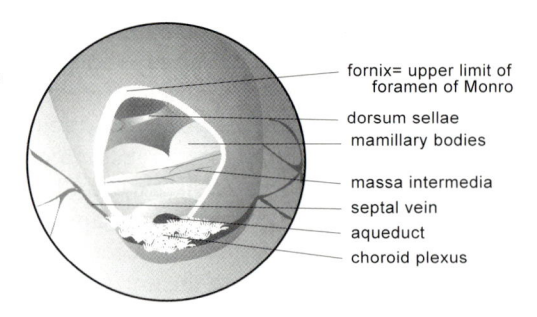

- Within the anterior third ventricle
  - Mamillary bodies
  - Tuber cinereum
  - Infundibular recess
  - Optic chiasm
  - Supraoptic recess and lamina terminalis
- Within the posterior third ventricle:
  - Entry of aqueduct
  - Posterior commissure
  - Pineal gland and suprapineal recess

To enter the ventricles, several techniques can be used. Stereotactic guided placement of the cannulating trocar, either frame-based or frameless, is the most reliable, but also a time consuming method. The outline of the human skull varies greatly, but nevertheless external bony landmarks such as the bregma, the meeting place of the coronal and sagittal sutures and, in the fetal skull the site of the anterior fontanelle, and the inion, which is the most salient point on the external occipital protuberance in the median plane, can be very helpful for orientation. Of course, careful study of the MR images should be always be performed.

Specific Endoscopic Techniques

In general, endoscopic procedures within the ventricular system are performed through one burr hole, also referred to as a monoportal procedure compared to a biportal procedure in which two different approaches are used. In some instances, such as procedures for ventricular tumors, this can be advantageous because it broadens the possibilities of manipulation and it gives the possibility to control the shaft of each endoscope by the other. One should keep in mind that using trajectories for, for example, two 4-mm endoscopes (together a cross-sectional area of 25 mm^2) is less invasive than one trajectory for a 6-mm endoscope (cross-sectional area of 28 mm^2).

Endoscopic Treatment of Hydrocephalus

The preferred treatment for symptomatic *communicating* hydrocephalus is ventriculoperitoneal shunting although sometimes lumboperitoneal shunting can suffice.

One key to long-term success of a shunt probably is the correct placement of the ventricular catheter. The use of an endoscope allows precise positioning of the proximal catheter away from the choroid plexus. We advise anyone to rehearse catheter placement as often as possible on a teaching-head because, although it sounds quite simple, there is a steep learning curve for successful performance of this procedure (as is for all endoscopic procedures). In what is called the direct method, a very small stylet-like endoscope is placed directly through the ventricular catheter so there is no need for additional passage of a cannula through the brain.

Obstructive hydrocephalus can be treated effectively with an endoscopic procedure which avoids the insertion of a shunt: endoscopic third ventriculocisternostomy, fenestration of obstructive cysts or balloon dilatation of aqueduct stenosis with or without stenting are now the primary treatment options for patients with an obstructive hydrocephalus.

Endoscopic third ventriculostomy has proven to be effective and safe if some precautions are taken. The procedure is performed in cases of obstructive hydrocephalus with patent subarachnoid spaces and a dilated third ventricle. Making a connection between the subarachnoid space (interpeduncular cistern) and the third ventricle through its floor can cure the hydrocephalus and eliminate the need for a shunt. Crucial for the success of this treatment is proper patient selection. Mandatory is a preoperative MRI, revealing large ventricles, ballooning of the third ventricle, thinning of its floor and a confirmation of the site of CSF obstruction. Cine-MRI, showing the lack of a CSF flow void signal in the aqueduct, is desirable.

The endoscope is introduced through a burr hole at or slightly in front of the coronal suture and about 2.5 cm paramedian, which mostly equals the midpupillary line. After entering the anterior horn one should identify the choroid plexus or a vein, which is followed towards the foramen of Monro where the choroid plexus enters the third ventricle and the septal vein and thalamostriate vein coalesce. The foramen should be large enough (which is usually the case in obstructive hydrocephalus) to allow entrance of the endoscope without touching the fornix. When using a peel-away sheath the best method is to retract the endoscope a little until the edges of the sheath become visible and thus the sheath with the endoscope can be safely put through the foramen of Monro into the third ventricle. Within the third ventricle, the mamillary bodies are rapidly recognized (although they can be less prominent in infants, but then they are recognizable by their vascular pattern). In front of the mamillary bodies the thinned out, translucent floor of the third ventricle and the basilar artery beneath it are often visible. Somewhat more frontally the hypervascularized area of the infundibular recess is a well-recognizable landmark. By staying exactly in the midline and within the anterior third of a line from the anterior border of the mamillary bodies to the infundibular recess, opening of the floor should be safe.

There are many techniques to perforate the floor of the third ventricle. As blunt perforation can be hazardous, especially when vital structures are obscured, several methods and instruments have been described and used (Sainte-Rose 1992). A gentle thrust of the endoscope itself is simplest, but not without danger (Jones et al. 1992). A puncturing needle can be adequate, allowing the introduction of a balloon catheter to dilate the orifice of a ventriculostomy. In addition to monopolar coagulation wires and radio-frequency dissectors, laser-assistance has also proven to be valuable. However, conventional laser-tips require large amounts of energy for ablation of the floor of the third ventricle with considerable risk to underlying, vital structures such as the basilar artery and its branches.

We have developed a special laser catheter with an atraumatic ball-tip, pretreated with a layer of carbon particles, which absorbs approximately 90% of the energy. As the heat is generated in this very thin layer of carbon coating, only a few Watts of energy are necessary for a fraction of a second in order to reach ablative temperatures instantly at the tip with virtually no heat effect on surrounding tissues or deeper structures. The precoated tip enables the surgeon to predict the depth of ablation and the extent of coagulation. The procedure is started with very low energies to ensure coagulation before perforation. After each pulse the lesion can be examined and the dosimetry can be adapted depending on the effect observed. At the moment of perforation, the light emitted from the fiber is minimal and highly scattered so no temperature increase can be created in distal structures. This combination of low energy and high absorption makes the application safe and controlled (Vandertop et al. 1998).

Arachnoid Cyst Fenestration

Intraventricular arachnoid cyst can lead to hydrocephalus. The goal of the neuroendoscopic procedure is to open the cyst and to establish communication between the cyst and ventricles and between the cyst and the basal cisterns, together with shrinkage of the cyst wall. The flow of cerebrospinal fluid within these cysts is low and given the ability of these cysts to heal (and thus causing recurrent obstruction) simple endoscopic puncture rarely gives a good long-term result. In these cases a wide fenestration (as large as possible but preferably more than 1 cm) is necessary.

The difficulty in these cases is the thickness and initial elasticity of the cyst wall, which makes it difficult to perforate. When the cyst wall is opened, the cyst collapses, and the remaining wall floats away from the instruments, which can make it difficult to make a second hole for free communication of CSF between cyst and basal cistern. The ME-2 electrode or the laser are very helpful in making the large opening that is necessary.

Ventricular Tumors

Hypothalamic tumors are frequently found in children. They usually fill up the whole third ventricle, obstructing CSF flow and causing hydrocephalus. Total removal, restoring normal CSF flow, is hardly possible, but sometimes substantial debulking of the tumor can be achieved endoscopically. When inserting a shunt, an endoscopic septum pellucidum fenestration should be performed, preventing the need for a bilateral shunt.

For posterior 3rd ventricle and pineal region tumors a direct surgical approach is preferred, especially in those tumors that seem to be well circumscribed on the MRI. Nevertheless, if there is an obstructive hydrocephalus (as is often the case), CSF can be sampled and the hydrocephalus can be relieved by an endoscopic third ventriculostomy. This allows also inspection of the tumor and, if it seems indicated, a biopsy can be performed. The tumor is approached directly with the endoscope, either with or without stereotactic guidance. The biopsy forceps is brought towards the mass and one can feel the consistency of the tumor. The forceps is opened and pushed into the tumor under continuous irrigation, which keeps the image clear by flushing away small amounts of venous blood from the biopsy site. Under direct visualization, the forceps is closed and with gentle traction, the biopsy specimen is removed from the tumor. Typically, the bleeding that follows the biopsy is minor and stops with irrigation. Once the biopsy specimen is grasped, the entire endoscope together with the biopsy forceps is removed. If one would try to remove the forceps back through the working channel this results in loss of the specimen.

At present, there is hardly any indication for an endoscopic biopsy of a 4th ventricle tumor. However, if an endoscopic third ventriculostomy is considered for relief of an obstructive hydrocephalus, the tumor can be inspected, and even a biopsy can be performed through the widened aqueduct. One should always consider the risk and the benefit of such a biopsy.

Endoscope-Assisted Microneurosurgery

For quite some years this specific applications was thought of as a more frontier type application of neuroendoscopy but now it is an emerging field. The basic principle is that endoscopes need not be introduced through a burr hole to be effective but they can be used during open procedures to look around blind corners that would otherwise be invisible to the operating microscope. They are helpful in directing the removal of suprasellar tumors such as craniopharyngiomas, posterior fossa tumors, and during surgery for tethered spinal cord.

Complications of Neuroendoscopy

Every surgical intervention harbors the risk of a complication. During neuroendoscopy, several complications can occur. For practical reasons it seems justified

to divide the complications in minor complications, generally without lasting sequelae for the patient and major complications, often causing (sometimes irreversible) neurological deficit or even death.
- Minor complications
  - Minor bleeding
  - Air entrapment causing nausea and vomiting
  - Fever, unrelated to infection, and other manifestations of increased heat loss
  - Late arousal from anesthesia
  - Depressed breathing
- Major complications
  - Major endoscopically uncontrollable bleeding
  - CSF fistula
  - Infection
  - Ventricular collapse with subdural hematoma
  - Injury of brain structures

Minor bleeding occurs during almost every neuroendoscopic procedure. It can be caused by cannulation of the ventricle, during intraventricular manipulation especially at the choroid plexus, during opening of a cyst wall or opening of the floor of the third ventricle and during tumor biopsy. Generally this type of bleeding ceases with continuous irrigation. Bleeding from the choroid plexus can be minor, but it can be very lasting and can finally lead to blurred vision that compels to end the procedure. Therefore, it can be advisable to coagulate the part of the choroid plexus that enters the foramen of Monro whenever performing a procedure within the third ventricle, because this prevents hindrance-causing bleeding from the plexus due to movement of the endoscope.

Entrapment of air is very difficult to avoid. Beside the fact that air bubbles can distort the view, it often leads to postoperative nausea and sometimes vomiting. This discomfort is fortunately not a lasting one and in the majority of cases stops within 24 h.

Fever during the first postoperative days, especially a moderate fever that appears immediately after the procedure, not related to infection (negative blood and CSF cultures) and other manifestations of increased heat loss such as cutaneous vasodilatation, sweating or even panting, can be seen after neuroendoscopic procedures within the third ventricle. It is probably related to a form of chemical, sterile "ventriculitis," or due to a rise of temperature in the anterior hypothalamus or even direct electrical stimulation during prolonged use of an energy source within the third ventricle.

Some believe that changes in the ionic composition of the CSF following prolonged irrigation with normal saline is responsible for late arousal. Changes in the ionic composition and in the temperature of the CSF undoubtedly underlies the occurrence of depressed breathing. An irrigation solution that is too cold acts on the chemosensitive areas of the medulla and depresses breathing, as does a high concentration of bicarbonate in the irrigation solution leading to change in pH of the CSF.

Endoscopically uncontrollable bleeding is the most dangerous and dreaded complication during neuroendoscopy. It is always caused by injury of a major vessel. A large septal vein or vessels of the choroid plexus or even a previously undetected crossing vein within the ventricle can cause a bleeding that cannot be stopped by irrigation and often not even by attempts of coagulation, which are difficult to accomplish because the view is instantly hindered by the bleeding. This type of bleeding may not inevitably lead to a neurological deficit. However, arterial bleeding, for example, from a biopsy site of a tumor or even worse from an artery in the interpeduncular fossa following third ventriculocisternostomy, is disastrous. The devastating effect of this type of bleeding can hardly be reversed by switching to an open approach, because the site of bleeding is difficult to reach.

A CSF fistula can be a very lasting and annoying problem, especially with infants. The risk of a CSF fistula or pseudomeningocele at the entry site of the endoscope is more likely to occur with larger endoscopes. A CSF fistula interferes with primary healing of the wound and subsequent infection is a major risk. We try to avoid CSF fistulas by using smaller endoscopes in infants, by closure of the dura with a piece of periosteum, the use of fibrin glue and by filling up the burr hole with collagen or Gelfoam and bone-dust.

Infection can occur as a consequence of CSF leakage, but also as contamination during a prolonged procedure. A regimen of perioperative antibiotics should eliminate this source of infection. Fever in the postoperative phase should urge prompt clinical investigation for infection, including sampling of CSF, because ventriculitis is still hazardous with long-lasting sequelae for the patient.

Collapse of the ventricles, often with bilateral subdural hematoma, can occur in patients with an extremely enlarged ventricular system and a thin brain mantle, and is found more often in infants and children than in adults. This complication can be avoided in most cases by careful execution of the neuroendoscopic procedure, first by avoiding rapid release of a large amount of CSF following the cannulation of the ventricle and introduction of the endoscope, and secondly by starting the irrigation immediately after the tip of the endoscope has reached the ventricular system (but not earlier!).

Injury to brain structures depends on the site of entrance of the endoscope and the type of procedure, but generally all brain structures that form the boundaries of the ventricular system can be injured. It should be possible to avoid all these injuries. Lesions of the thalamus or caudate nucleus or the posterior margin of the foramen of Monro, resulting in intracerebral or intraventricular bleeding, are caused by wrong cannulation of the ventricles (too deep or too lateral). Starting too early with irrigation before entering the ventricle results in forced brain edema. Damage to the nuclei of the oculomotor and trochlear nerves within the central grey occurs when using an inappropriate balloon dilatation catheter for aqueductoplasty. Cranial nerve damage of oculomotor or abducent nerve has been reported in 3rd ventriculostomies.

Personal Experience

In this section we present our clinical experience with neuroendoscopic procedures in children

Patients

From December 1991 to November 1997, 566 consecutive patients underwent 576 endoscopic procedures at the University Hospital Nijmegen and the University Hospital Utrecht/Wilhelmina Children's Hospital Utrecht, The Netherlands. All operations were performed by the authors in their respective hospitals. From this series, 152 patients were under the age of 16.

At the University Hospital Utrecht/Wilhelmina Children's Hospital Utrecht, 75 consecutive patients underwent 77 endoscopic procedures, using pretreated "black fiber" tips with a Nd:YAG contact laser and a new generation of diode lasers in a variety of neuroendoscopic procedures in children.

Only three procedures were merely diagnostic without the need for use of the laser and in one patient the floor of the third ventricle was fenestrated using only a guide wire and Fogarty balloon catheter. Laser-assisted procedures were all attended to by a clinical laser physicist.

There were 11 girls and 12 boys, their age ranging from 3 weeks to 15 years (mean 6.5 years). Signs and symptoms were usually attributable to a raised intracranial pressure caused by an obstruction of normal CSF flow.

At the University Hospital Nijmegen, 491 consecutive patients underwent 499 endoscopic procedures. 158 procedures were intra- or paraventricular endoscopic operation (third ventriculostomy, aqueductoplasty, aqueductal stenting, cyst fenestration, septostomy, shunt implantation and shunt revision, tumor biopsy), 11 procedures were spinal procedures (syringomyelia) and 330 procedures were endoscope-assisted operations. From this total number of patients, 129 were under the age of 16 (ranging from 2 days to 15 years with a mean of 4.8 years)

Endoscopic Equipment

At the University Hospital Utrecht/Wilhelmina Children's Hospital Utrecht, a selection of different flexible and steerable fiberscopes was used: the 4-mm Neuroendoscope, the 2.3-mm NeuroviewR endoscope, the 4.6-mm NeuroviewR endoscope and the 2.7-mm Clarus NeuroflexR. The for each endoscope designated fiberoptic cables and lighting equipment were used, in combination with a standard camera and TV-monitor. The Malis irrigation module was used for continuous irrigation with either a physiological saline solution or Ringer's solution. The laser equipment used was a standard 1064 nm Nd:YAG laser and a new generation 810-nm diode laser.

At the University Hospital Nijmegen, the same array of fiberscopes was used but also the 4.5- and 3.5-mm Clarus WorkSCOPE neuroendoscopes and rigid neuroendoscopes based on the rod lens system such as the Angled Neuroview and a custom-made neuroendoscope were used.

Results in the Pediatric Group

Third Ventriculostomy with Laser (n=17). The most frequent indication for a 3rd ventriculostomy was a shunt dysfunction in 5 patients and an aqueductal stenosis in 4 patients. The remaining patients had a tectal mass (4), a pineal/thalamic/cerebellar tumor (1/1/1), and a hydrocephalus associated with myelomeningocele (1). In 16 of the 17 patients a wide hole of 4–7 mm was made. Patency was confirmed in 16 patients with postoperative MRI for a ventriculostomy success rate of 94%. Twelve patients clearly improved clinically, for a patient outcome success rate of 70%. Preoperatively, 8 patients had a shunt. Postoperatively, 5 of these 8 patients remained shunt-dependent. The baby with a myelomeningocele developed progressive hydrocephalus despite an open ventriculostomy and was subsequently shunted. Four patients who were shunt-dependent preoperatively, became fully shunt-independent.

Third Ventriculostomy Without Laser (n=32). The most frequent indication is this group of children (their age ranging from 2 days to 15 years with a mean age of 5.4 years) was a primary aqueductal stenosis or secondary aqueductal stenosis due to tumor in the tectum or pineal region. The third ventriculostomy was performed either with the radio-frequency dissector or a balloon dilatation catheter or a combination of the two methods. In 28 of the 32 patients the third ventriculostomy was effective, both clinically and on postoperative MRI. In 4 children a second third ventriculostomy was performed and in two of them a second obstructing membrane was found and opened in the interpeduncular fossa and both children remained shunt-free afterwards. In the remaining two patients a widely open floor of the third ventricle was found without any further obstruction and both children had a subsequent shunt implantation. So the primary success rate of the procedure was 87.5% and the final success rate (including the two children that had two procedures) was 93.8%.

Cyst fenestration with Laser (n=6). The most frequent indication for cyst wall fenestration was a third ventricular arachnoid cyst or suprasellar cyst in 4 patients. The remaining patients had a right frontal cyst (1) and an anterior interhemispheric cyst (1). Marsupialization of the cyst contents to the lateral or third ventricles by partially resecting the cyst wall was obtained in all cases. In all cases a VP-shunt (4) or second shunt (2) could be avoided.

Cyst Fenestration Without Laser (n=22). In this group the typical cyst also was the suprasellar arachnoid cyst, followed by a cerebellar arachnoid cyst and the interhemispheric arachnoid cyst. In two children with a cerebellar arachnoid cyst fenestration the cyst recurred after 3 and 9 months respectively. A second fenestration was performed in both children and they remained symptom-free and shunt-free afterwards. In two older children with multiple shunt dysfunctions (the 15-year-old boy had three implanted shunt, the 10 year-old girl had a bilateral shunt) had endoscopic fenestration of their intraventricular cysts and endoscopic septostomy and they only needed one single shunt afterwards. In one child (10 months old) a subdural bleeding occurred during the cyst fenestration (April 1994), probably due to collapse of the cyst and a craniotomy had to be performed directly. The bleeding could be stopped and the fenestration remained open since.

Tumor Biopsy (n=13). In 13 children an endoscopic biopsy of an intraventricular tumor, mostly located within the third ventricle was performed. In one child (16 months old) the first biopsy did not reveal a histological diagnosis and so a second biopsy was performed which showed a malignant rhabdoid tumor. Although some bleeding from the biopsy site is inevitable during tumor biopsy in this series it was never a reason to stop the procedure nor was the minor bleeding of any major consequence for the patients, although most of them had nausea and vomiting in the first 24 h after the biopsy.

Endoscope-Assisted Procedures (n=33). The endoscope was used, with increasing frequency during the past 3 years, as an adjunct during open microneurosurgical procedures in children. While in the adult group the endoscope is most frequently used during surgery for vascular lesions, in the pediatric group it is most frequently used during surgery for tumors, for example, in the suprasellar region, such as craniopharyngioma ($n=8$) and optic/hypothalamic glioma ($n=2$), tumors of the posterior fossa, including medulloblastoma ($n=5$), ependymoma ($n=3$), cerebellar astrocytoma ($n=3$), PNET ($n=2$), choroid plexus carcinoma within the foramen of Luschka ($n=1$), pontocerebellar teratoma ($n=1$), clivus/foramen magnum meningioma ($n=1$) and other locations such as a choroid plexus papilloma of both lateral ventricles ($n=1$), a choroid plexus carcinoma of the trigonum ($n=1$) and pineal gland tumors ($n=2$). Another indication for the adjunctive use of an endoscope is during surgery for tethered spinal cord syndrome ($n=3$).

Complications

In the group of patients treated at the University Hospital Utrecht/Wilhelmina Children's Hospital Utrecht, there was no mortality, nor increased morbidity. Four patients did not benefit clinically from a technically successful endoscopic procedure and in one patient the ventriculostomy was too small for it to be successful (documented on a postoperative MRI) for an overall patient outcome success rate of 83%.

In the group of patients treated at the University Hospital Nijmegen there also was no mortality, but in 4 patients there was increased postoperative morbidity. There was one permanent oculomotor nerve palsy in a child after a second endoscopic third ventriculostomy and in an adult patient there was a quadrant hemianopia following endoscopic third ventriculostomy. There were two adult patients with a permanent short-term memory deficit after endoscopic removal of a colloid cyst of the third ventricle. There were two children with a CSF fistula requiring a second operation, one of these patients having a postoperative ventriculitis after the first operation and one having subdural effusion after a third ventriculostomy requiring operative drainage. Additionally, in two cases a bleeding during the endoscopic procedure could not be controlled effectively, and craniotomy had to be performed. However, these events remained without sequelae for the patients.

Conclusions

The revival of neuroendoscopy first started within the field of pediatric neurosurgery and the indications and techniques within this group of patients have now matured and neuroendoscopic operations can be considered as standard procedures. Neuroendoscopy offers great benefits to the patients as it is a minimally traumatic and yet maximally effective treatment not only for hydrocephalus but for a great variety of intracranial and intraventricular lesions.

References

Bauer BL, Hellwig D (1994) Minimally invasive neurosurgery - a survey. Acta Neurochir (Wien) [Suppl 61]:1–12
Burman MD (1931) Myeloscopy or the direct visualization of the spinal canal and its contents. J Bone Joint Surg 13:695
Caemaert J, Abdullah J, Calliauw L (1994) A multipurpose cerebral endoscope and reflection on technique and instrumentation in endoscopic neurosurgery. Acta neurochir (Wien) [Suppl 61]:49-53
Cohen AR (1993a) Endoscopic laser third ventriculostomy. N Engl J Med 328:552
Cohen AR (1993b) Endoscopic ventricular surgery. Pediatr Neurosurg 19:127–134
Cohen AR (1994) Ventriculoscopic surgery. Clin Neurosurg 41:546–562
Crue BL (1977) Needle scope attached to stereotactic frame for inspection of cisterna magna during radiofrequency trigeminal tractotomy. Appl Neurophysiol 39:58–64
Dandy WE (1922) Cerebral ventriculoscopy. Johns Hopkins Hosp Bull 33:189–190
Davis L (ed) (1939) Neurological surgery, 2nd edn. Lea and Febiger, Philadelphia, p 439
Fukushima T (1978) Endoscopy of Meckel's cave, cisterna magna, and cerebellopontine angle. Technical note. J Neurosurg 48:302–306
Fukushima T, Schramm J (1975) Klinischer Versuch der Endoskopie des Spinalkanals: Kurzmitteilung. Neurochirurgia 18:199–203
Fukushima T et al (1973) Ventriculofiberscope: a new technique for endoscopic diagnosis and operation. Technical note. J Neurosurg 38:251–256
Griffith HB (1986) Endoneurosurgery: endoscopic intracranial surgery. Adv Techn Stand Neurosurg 14:3–24
Grotenhuis JA (1995) Manual of endoscopic procedures in neurosurgery. Uitgeverij Machaon, Nijmegen
Grotenhuis JA (1996) Endoscope-assisted craniotomy. Techn Neurosurg 1:201–212
Grotenhuis JA (1998) The use of endoscopes during surgery in the suprasellar region. In: Hellwig D, Bauer BL (eds) Minimally invasive techniques for neurosurgery. Current status and future perspectives. Springer, Berlin Heidelberg New York, pp 107–110

Grotenhuis JA, Tacl S (1993) The use of flexible micro-endoscopes for visualization of blind corners during microneurosurgical procedures. Abstract book of the 1st international congress on minimal invasive techniques in neurosurgery, Wiesbaden, p 16

Grotenhuis JA, de Vries J, Tacl S (1994) Angioscopy-guided placement of balloon-expandable stents in the treatment of experimental carotid aneurysms. Minim Invasive Neurosurg 37:56–60

Hüwel NM, Perneczky A, Urban V (1993) Neuro-endoscopic techniques in operative treatment of syringomyelia. Acta Neurochir (Wien) 123:216

Jones RF, Stening WA, Brydon M (1990) Endoscopic third ventriculo-stomy. Neurosurgery 26:86–91

Jones RFC et al (1995) Neuroendoscopic third ventriculostomy. In: Cohen AR, Haines SJ (eds) Minimally invasive techniques in neurosurgery. Williams and Wilkins, Baltimore, pp 33–48

Knosp E (1993) Endoscopic assisted microneurosurgery. Abstract book of the 1st international congress on minimal invasive techniques in neurosurgery, Wiesbaden, p 22

Krishnamurthy S, Powers SK (1994) Lasers in neurosurgery. Lasers Surg Med 15:126–167

Liston SL et al (1987) Nasal endoscopes in hypophysectomy. J Neurosurg 66:155

Manwaring KH, Crone KR (eds) (1992) Neuroendoscopy, vol 1. Liebert, New York

Mixter WJ (1923) Ventriculoscopy and puncture of the floor of the third ventricle. Preliminary report of a case. Boston Med Surg J 188:277–278

Oka K et al (1993) Flexible endo-neurosurgical therapy for aqueductal stenosis. Neurosurgery 33:236–242

Olinger CP, Ohlhaber RL (1974) Eighteen-gauge microscopic-telescopic needle endoscope with electrode channel: potential clinical and research application. Surg Neurol 2:151–160

Ooi Y, Satoh Y, Morisaki N (1973) Myeloscopy, possibility of observing lumbar intrathecal space by use of an endoscope. Endoscopy 5:90–96

Oppel F, Mulch G (1979) Selective trigeminal root section via an endoscopic transpyramidal retrolabyrinthine approach. Acta Neurochir (Wien) [Suppl] 28:565–571

Pool JL (1942) Myeloscopy: intrathecal endoscopy. Surgery 11:169–182

Prott W (1974) Möglichkeiten einer Endoskopie des Kleinhirnbrückenwinkels auf transpyramidalem-retrolabyrinthärem Zugangsweg – Cisternoskopie. HNO 22:337–341

Sainte-Rose C (1992) Third ventriculostomy. In: Manwaring KH, Crone KR (eds) Neuroendoscopy, vol 1. Liebert, New York, pp 47–62

Stern EL (1936) The spinascope: a new instrument for visualizing the spinal canal and its contents. Med Rec 143:31–32

Vandertop WP, Verdaasdonk RM, van Swol CFP (1998) Laser-assisted neuroendoscopy using Nd:YAG and diode contact laser with pretreated fiber tips. J Neurosurg (in press)

Verdaasdonk RM, Vandertop WP (1995a) Endoscopic ventricular fenestration and choroid plexus coagulation using diode and ND:YAG contact laser ablation with pretreated fiber tips. Lasers Surg Med [Suppl] 7:26

Verdaasdonk RM, Borst C (1995b) Optics of fibers and fiber probes. In: Welch AJ, van Gemert MJC (eds) Optical-thermal response of laser irradiated tissue. Plenum, New York, pp 619–666

Vries JK (1980) Endoscopy as an adjunct for hydrocephalus. Surg Neurol 13:69–72

Willems PWA, Vandertop WP, Verdaasdonk RM, van Swol CFP, Jansen GJ et al (1998) Pretreated 'black' fibre tips can be applied safely in contact laser-assisted neuroendoscopy: experimental data. (submitted)

Yamakawa K (1995) Instrumentation for neuroendoscopy. In: Cohen AR, Haines SJ (eds) Minimally invasive techniques in neurosurgery. Williams and Wilkins, Baltimore, pp 6–13

Part VI
Oncology

CHAPTER 50

Endoscopic Surgery in Paediatric Oncology

H.A. Steinbrecher, A.S. Najmaldin

Introduction

There is now abundant literature describing the application of minimal invasive surgery MIS in adults with malignancy (Gouma et al. 1996; Cuschieri 1995; Dalgic et al. 1994) or suspected malignancy (Chu et al. 1994; Vander Velpen et al. 1994). Both thoracoscopic and laparoscopic techniques have been developed in adults for diagnosis (Cuschieri 1994; Kern et al. 1993), tumour staging (Fiocco and Krasna 1992; Anderson et al. 1996) and treatment (Bourtin et al. 1993). Increasing numbers of intestinal resections (Cuschieri et al. 1992; Cohen and Wekner 1993), operations for pancreatic carcinoma (Cuschieri 1994), radical nephrectomies (McDougall et al. 1996; Ono et al. 1997), adrenalectomies (Elashry et al. 1997; Takeda et al. 1997) and pelvic lymphadenectomies (Parra et al. 1992) are being performed in the adult oncological patient. However, the role of endoscopic surgery in oncology in particular that of organ resection has remained highly controversial. There are fears of inadequate access for complete resection (Guillou et al. 1993), the possibility of malignant seeding (Pezet et al. 1992; Leather et al. 1994) and concerns regarding the histological integrity of specimens taken for examination (Lobe et al. 1994).

The treatment protocols of most if not all Paediatric Oncological conditions now involve the multi-modality approach of chemotherapy, radiotherapy and surgery. Traditional imaging, Ultrasound guided or computed tomography guided biopsies and open procedures are still most commonly employed for childhood tumours. However, imaging and attempted image guided biopsy may fail to establish the diagnosis (Scherer et al. 1978; Watt et al. 1989). More and more laparoscopies and thoracoscopies are, therefore, being carried out instead of, or prior to open surgery. This is largely because of the difficulty in localisation or safe access, or the need for larger pieces of tissue to improve diagnostic yield (Jori and Peschle 1972; Pagliaro et al. 1983).

This chapter highlights the current opinion and experience with the use of endoscopic surgery in the management of oncological conditions in children. Further information, in particular that of indications and techniques of diagnostic and theraputic laparoscopy and thorascopy procedures as well as organ resection can be found in their respective chapters.

Indications

As in adult oncology surgery, the use of endoscopic surgery in children with tumours broadly covers the main areas of diagnosis, tumour staging, and treatment.

The diagnosis of solid tumours in children has traditionally relied on the relatively non-invasive imaging of the plain X-ray, contrast X-ray, the ultrasound scanning (USS), computed tomography (CT) and more recently magnetic resonance imaging (MRI). With chemotherapy and radiotherapy, as opposed to surgical resection previously, rapidly becoming primary therapies for the treatment of malignancy, the reliance on confirmatory tissue sampling for definitive diagnosis has often been reduced to biopsy only, be it in the form of true-cut biopsy, fine needle aspiration (FNA), or open biopsy. This non-invasive approach is not always the most accurate for diagnostic purposes. For example, in adults, small peritoneal deposits, small liver metastases or local in-growth in gastrointestinal tumours are said to be missed in 10%–40% of patients using noninvasive radiological methods (Watt et al. 1989). This is mainly due to the resolution qualities of the machines and the inability to clearly detect different tissue plains and lesions less than 5–10 mm in size. The development of laparoscopic visualisation and laparoscopic ultrasonography has markedly increased the preoperative predictability of tumour resectability (Cuesta et al. 1993).

In the child, not only does the tissue diagnosis determine the treatment regime, but often the tumour staging is vital to decide the intensity of treatment given. The commoner intra-abdominal tumours in children are neuroblastoma, nephroblastoma, ovarian "cysts", lymph node masses and liver tumours. As a result of a possible discrepancy in up to 30% of cases between diagnostic imaging and surgical findings for intra-abdominal malignancy (Haase et al. 1995), an adjunct to the traditional investigative methods has been the development of new diagnostic techniques such as contact ultrasound scanning (Fornari et al. 1989; Pietrabissa et al. 1993), target needle biopsy (Mackenzie et al. 1992), and fine needle cytology carried out under laparoscopic guidance (Jori and Peschle 1972). These can provide more information regarding localised invasion and tissue type prior to definitive treatment. Laparoscopy enables assessment of resectability vs inoperability and is the only reliable method of detecting peritoneal deposits (Cuschieri 1995).

When the diagnosis as to the cause of the acute abdomen is in doubt, laparoscopy has been shown to be a reliable method by which other causes such as acute appendicitis, perforated or ischaemic bowel or intestinal adhesives obstruction can be excluded (VanderVelpen et al. 1994). Children who are undergoing chemotherapy and are neutropenic may also present with an acute abdomen due to typhlitis, or due to any other cause, and laparoscopy may prove to be the only reliable method of diagnosis.

Thoracoscopy is commonly used in some centres to evaluate mediastinal or pleural masses. Diagnostic accuracy for thoracoscopic evaluation of mediastinal masses varies from 86% to 100% (Rogers et al. 1992; Ryckman and Rodgers 1982).

The staging of lymphoma relies on the detection of lymph node involvement throughout the body. Laparoscopy can easily identify lymph node masses in remote areas that are poorly visualised with other modalities, for example, Porta hepatis (Canavese et al. 1996). A study comparing CT and lymphography with laparotomy showed that staging laparotomy affected the stage of the disease for 37% of patients (Baker et al. 1990). Often it is the retroperitoneal and splenic involvement that is misdiagnosed with conventional imaging.

The use of endoscopic surgery in the definitive treatment of childhood tumours has been exceedingly limited to date to occasional tumour resection, usually of lung recurrences (Holcomb et al. 1995), elevation of ovaries out of radiotherapy fields (Tan et al. 1993) and laparoscopic ligation of feeding vessels to tumours, for example, sacro-coccygeal teratoma and median sacral artery (N.M.A. Bax, personal communication, 1997). Recurrent tumour excision is usually limited to thoracoscopic resection of lung metastases since these are most often found in the periphery (Coppage et al. 1982). Occasionally persistent malignant pleural effusions may require pleurodesis which can be carried out thoracoscopically (de Campos et al. 1997). The elevation of an ovary out of a radiotherapy field arose out of the observation that a major morbidity associated with pelvic irradiation is ovarian ablation. This is said to occur in 68% of children with ovaries within the radiation field, in 14% with ovaries at the edge of the radiation field and in no ovaries outside the radiation field (Stillman et al. 1981).

A number of isolated cases involving specific whole organ resections such as the kidney (Gill et al. 1994) and adrenal gland (Staren and Prinz 1996) have been reported, although a number of issues as to the applicability of laparoscopy in this situation are still left unanswered (as discussed later in this chapter).

Pre-operative Preparation

Common to all surgical procedures, the preoperative preparation for endoscopic surgery pivots around many areas. There must be a full assessment of the indications and potential benefits of endoscopic surgery over either conventional surgery or a non-surgical strategy. Full parental-child consent must be obtained. The operation should be planned adequately, especially with reference to the patient position, placement of ports, instruments required and potential sequelae. All patients should be informed of the possibility of having to convert a minimally invasive procedure to an open one.

In the case of diagnostic procedures, the possibility of proceeding to definitive treatment, be it endoscopic or open, under the same anaesthetic must be considered. It is vital that there be a good liaison with the pathologist in the case of fresh biopsy samples sent for frozen section, cytology or later analysis. Similarly, many surgeons are unfamiliar with the ultrasonographic features of lesions and so close cooperation with a radiologist is paramount when using an endoscopic intra-operative ultrasound probe.

Instrumentation

For most minimally invasive procedures on the oncology patient a small armamentarium of instruments is sufficient. Two or more 3.5- to 12-mm cannulae, depending on the patients' size, shape, surgeon's preference and the type of procedure to be carried out are essential. A 3.5- to 10- mm 0° or preferentially 30° telescope is used. An angled telescope provides versatility required during diagnostic or therapeutic procedures. Two or more atraumatic grasping forceps are needed to manipulate tissues. Therapeutic manoeuvres, such as adhesiolysis or tissue biopsy are carried out using a pair of dissecting scissors, preferably insulated for diathermy usage or a needle diathermy probe. For small biopsy samples biopsy needles or endoscopic forceps are required. For larger biopsies or whole tissue organ removal a nonpermeable retrieval bag is employed. An organ or tissue retractor is helpful for access and a number of different types are available. Specific instruments for various therapeutic procedures, for example, lung resection, oophorectomy, nephrectomy, adrenalectomy, splenectomy are available and described elsewhere in this book.

Techniques

General anaesthesia with muscle relaxation are essential. Laparoscopic procedures are aided by the placement of a nasogastric tube. An empty bladder, achieved either with or without a urinary catheter is helpful. Abdominal operations are usually carried out with the patient in a supine position. However, steep Trendelenburg, reverse Trendelenburg or a lateral tilt position are often used to improve access. Video recording of all procedures should be carried out if possible for review and discussion with those involved in the primary management of the child, including oncologists, pathologists and radiologists. For laparoscopic procedures we advocate that a modified Hassan's approach is used to place the primary 3.5- to 12-mm cannula (Humphrey and Najmaldin 1994). This is particularly so in patients who have ascites, intestinal dilation, organomegaly or large palpable masses. The primary cannula may be placed anywhere in the abdomen but should be away from the operating field (see Najmaldin and Grousseau, "Basic Techniques"). In general, however, a periumbilical primary cannula is adequate for most diagnostic and therapeutic procedures.

After a preliminary exploratory laparoscopy the size and site of one or more secondary "working" cannulae may be assessed, depending on the procedure to be carried out. Endoscopic ultrasonography is performed using a 7.5 MHz linear array ultrasound probe through a 10-mm cannula if and when required. Biopsies may be taken under direct laparoscopic vision with or without intra-operative ultrasonic guidance, using a needle or forceps, either percutaneously or through a cannula. The latter route may prevent the theoretical risk of wound tumour seeding. Alternatively samples of tissue and lymph nodes may be obtained using a formal resection procedure.

The transposition site of an ovary prior to radiotherapy depends on the area to be irradiated. In the event of total medullary irradiation, for example, for medulloblastoma, the ovary is transposed laparoscopically to the level of the anterior superior iliac spine. If inverted gamma radiation is to be given for Hodgkin's disease, the ovary is transposed on to the median line. For pelvic irradiation, the ovary is transposed into the right upper quadrant. Metallic clips are often placed to each ovary to allow radiation doses to be calculated and to verify ovary position during treatment using plain X-rays.

Resection of neoplastic tissue or organs such as the kidney, adrenal gland, ovary or spleen, may be carried out in a fashion similar to that described in the relevant other chapters of this book. Extreme care must be taken not to compromise the radical nature of the procedure, the margins of resection, or the nature of the specimens taken for histological examination. Furthermore, manipulation of the affected organ should be minimal and contamination of the surrounding spaces and cannula sites are to be avoided. The use of impermeable retrieval bags is mandatory for all appreciably sized specimens to be removed. To preserve these rules, large extracting abdominal wounds are sometime unavoidable.

For thoracoscopic procedures patients are placed either supine with arms extended laterally or in a complete lateral position. In the former position a lateral tilt of 30°–45° allows the lung to fall away with gravity after the pneumothorax is established. This is especially useful for patients with suspected anterior or posterior mediastinal lesions. More often than not, however, the patient must be safely and securely strapped to the operating table. For apical lesions a reverse Trendelenberg position is helpful and for basal lesions a standard Trendelenberg position is adopted (Rogers et al. 1992). Under general anaesthesia, either a double lumen tube intubation method or selective main stem bronchus intubation is used for major pulmonary and mediastinal procedures. A simple endotracheal tube with a pleural insufflation of 4–6 mmHg is adequate for most diagnostic maneuvers with or without biopsy on the pleural and lung surfaces. As in laparoscopies the site and size of the cannulae used are dependent on the nature of the procedure to be carried out. In general a small midaxillary line stab incision is made in the 4th or 5th intercostal space to allow open insertion of the primary 3.5- to 10-mm cannula. A maximum insufflation pressure of 6–8 mmHg is adequate for good visualisation. Further working cannulae for instruments are placed under thoracoscopic guidance appropriate to the site of any suspected lesion to allow biopsies or resections to be carried out. Full visualisation of all the parietal surface, the hilum and all the pleura is possible by gently manipulating the lung. Tissue biopsies are easily obtained using a needle or biopsy forceps, inserted either through a secondary port or percutaneously. A wedge of lung tissue may be removed using a ligature technique or a linear stapler. As for laparoscopic oncological procedures, the quality and integrity of tissue removed must be preserved by careful handling, adequate exposure and an appropriate incision for organ removal.

Outcome

To date there are still only a small number of reports in which a series of paediatric patients treated laparoscopically or thoracoscopically for malignancy are described. A retrospective review of all patients undergoing a laparoscopic or thoracoscopic procedure in Childrens Cancer Group Institutions in the United States over a 3-year period yielded 85 patients in 15 participating centres (Holcomb et al. 1995). Twenty-five had laparoscopies and 60 had thoracoscopies. Tissue biopsies taken in 67 cases gave a 99% diagnostic result. Of the 25 laparoscopies, 9 patients had evaluation of a new malignancy, 6 a staging procedure, 4 a second look procedure, 2 an assessment for hepatoblastoma resectability, 2 patients with cancer had evaluations for suspected infection, 1 resection of recurrence and 1 evaluation of metastatic disease. There were no complications in this group. Indications for thoracoscopy included evaluation for mediastinal mass, suspected metastatic disease, lung biopsy, wedge resections of lung metastases, and evaluation for recurrent tumours. There were 7 complications with 6 conversions to open procedures because of adhesions in 2, bleeding in 1 and poor visualisation of nodularity in 1. One patient developed hypercarbia on attempted single lung ventilation and therefore the procedure was converted to an open thoracotomy and 1 patient was converted because of the inability to get adequate biopsies for Hodgkin's lymphoma. One patient developed atelectasis post-operatively.

In another series of 5 children who had laparoscopies for lymphoma in the abdomen (Canavese et al. 1996), there were no complications. In 3 cases neoplastic masses were excluded, one had a liver metastases of a large cell anaplastic lymphoma, and one had a diagnosis of chronic myeloid leukaemia made.

The potential of thoracoscopy in diagnosing malignancy was first recognised by Jacobaeus in 1921 who identified 6 cases of intra-thoracic carcinoma by this technique (Jacobaeus and Key 1921). In an early original description of thoracoscopy for diagnosis of intra-thoracic lesions in children (Rogers and Talbert 1976), of nine patients aged 17 months–16 years, 1 had a thoracoscopy for mycoplasma pneumonia, and 6 patients developed diffuse pulmonary parenchymal infiltrates requiring biopsy for further treatment planning. These 6 patients were receiving chronic immunosuppressive treatment for either systemic malignancy, following renal transplantation, or for the treatment of collagen vascular disorders. Two further patients underwent thoracoscopy for suspected diagnosis of intra-thoracic malignancy (1 apical chest wall Ewing's sarcoma, 1 apical chest recurrent Hodgkin's). In all cases, sufficient tissue was obtained on biopsy for a definitive diagnosis to be made. There were 2 small pneumothoraces and 1 minor bleed post-operatively (a 13-year-old requiring 150 ml transfusion) in 3 of the nine patients.

A later series of 150 thoracoscopies included 25 thoracoscopies in 23 children aged 8 months–18 years for the diagnosis or staging of intra-thoracic tumours (Ryckman and Rodgers 1982). Eleven had a mediastinal mass, with 6 having undergone previous invasive procedures without achieving a definitive diagnosis.

Tumour was confirmed in 9 of these patients and 2 had inflammatory disease. Further areas of previously unsuspected tumour involvement were diagnosed by thoracoscopy in 5 of the 9 patients. Two children underwent thoracoscopy for pleural abnormalities and metastatic disease was identified in both. In this series, the overall diagnostic accuracy for mediastinal disease was 91%, for pleural disease 92%, and for parenchymal disease 100% (2 patients).

More recently Lung biopsies through the thoracoscope has been used successfully as a day-case procedure (Rogers et al. 1992). Our experience so far is limited to 3 thoracoscopic and 8 laparoscopic diagnostic procedures (age 2.5–13 years). Successful assessment and biopsy using multiple Tru-Cut needle stabs or wedge resection biopsies were carried out using one two secondary cannulae. One para-aortic lymph node biopsy had to be converted to an open technique due to access difficulties and bowel retraction. There were no technique related complications. An additional two patients had successful ovariopexies to avoid radiation damage. We have also successfully used laparoscopy in 4 patients with acute abdomens during chemotherapy to exclude adhesion intestinal obstruction, ischaemic bowel or perforation, and in 2 patients having chemotherapy and acute appendicitis for appendicectomy.

Discussion

There is now ample evidence that for a variety of major procedures both in adults and children a laparoscopic surgical approach can be carried out safely and cost-effectively (Waldhausen and Tapper 1997; Farah et al. 1997), with reduced hospital stay (Collins et al. 1995), reduced analgesia requirement (McMahon et al. 1994) and morbidity to patients (Curran and Raffensperger 1996). In most diagnostic circumstances, laparoscopy and thoracoscopy obviate the need for laparotomy and thoracotomy respectively. In a patient with malignancy additional factors make the minimally invasive technique attractive.

Inflammatory mediators are believed to modify the host response to surgical trauma (Waydhas et al. 1992). Inflammatory mediators are also involved in host response exposed to endotoxin (Welbourn and Young 1992). Since endotoxin has been found to be present in circulatory air, less exposure of viscera to the open air potentially reduces the postoperative immune response in already immune compromised patients (Watson et al. 1995; da Costa et al. 1996).

A lower incidence of adhesive obstruction and reduced post-operative pain also reduces the immune response, and laparoscopy in itself may have less of an effect on the immune response than open surgery (Trokel et al. 1994).

A number of specific features of endoscopic surgery in oncology remain to be addressed. On a practical level, with endoscopy the loss of tactile sense in identifying mobility or fixation of tumour, especially recurrent tumour is a disadvantage. The inability of the laparoscopic ultrasound probe to detect local and vascular invasion will undoubtedly be conquered in the near future by more sophisticated probes.

Another concern is the scattered reports in the literature of tumour seeding to port sites (Mathew et al. 1996; Sartorelli et al. 1996). This complication may be inherent due to the laparoscopic technique or because any wound may give rise to metastases in it. Conventional colectomy for colorectal carcinoma gives a 1% incidence of metastases to the wound (Hughes et al. 1983). Tumour metastases may be a function of the advanced stage of the tumour. Tumour spillage during mobilisation has been suggested as a cause of wound metastases (Mathew et al. 1996). Other theories include the effect of gas leak and pneumoperitoneal pressure causing tumour cells to lodge in the wounds (Cuschieri 1994). None the less, the exact incidence of wound metastases due to a laparoscopic procedure is not known but may not be more than for open procedures. Further studies are clearly needed to clarify the situation. Furthermore, some of the important potential disadvantages of endoscopic surgery such as those of tissues crushing, compromise of margins of resection and tumour extraction using bags and larger incisions (Cohen and Wekner 1993) need to be recognised and overcome.

Conclusion

The treatment of childhood malignancy is increasingly being supplemented by the use of endoscopic surgery. Both thoracoscopic and laparoscopic techniques are available to help in diagnosis, staging and treatment of various malignancies. Every effort must be made not to compromise safety and the value of adequate treatment. At present routine laparoscopy and thoracoscopy should be limited to diagnostic measures, assessment of tumours, biopsies and vascular access. As equipment becomes more refined, imaging technology improves, and our understanding of tumour behaviour and experience grows, endoscopic surgery will take its full place in the surgery of paediatric oncology patients.

References

Anderson DN, Campbell S, Park KGM (1996) Accuracy of laparoscopic ultrasonography in the staging of upper gastrointestinal malignancy. Br J Surg 83:1424–1428
Baker LL et al (1990) Staging of Hodgkin disease in children: comparison of CT and lymphography with laparotomy. Am J Radiol 154:1251–1255
Bourtin C et al (1993) Thoracoscopy in pleural malignant mesothelioma: a prospective study of 188 consecutive patients. Cancer 72:394–404
Canavese F et al (1996) The role of laparoscopy in pediatric cancer patients. It J Ped Surg Sci 10(1–2):39–41
Chu CM et al (1994) The role of laparoscopy in the evaluation of ascites of unknown origin. Gastrointest Endosc 40(3):285–289
Cohen SM, Wekner SD (1993) Laparoscopic colorectal resection for cancer: the Cleveland Clinic Florida experience. Surg Oncol 2 [Suppl 1]:35–42
Collins JB III et al (1995) Comparison of open and laparoscopic gastrostomy and fundoplication in 120 patients. J Ped Surg 30(7):1065–1071
Coppage L, Shaw C, Curtis AM (1982) Metastatic disease in the chest in patients with extra thoracic malignancy. J Thorac Imag 2:24–37

Cuesta MA et al (1993) Laparoscopic ultrasonography for hepatobiliary and pancreatic malignancy. Br J Surg 80:1571–1574
Curran TJ, Raffensperger JG (1996) Laparoscopic Swensons pull-through: a comparison with the open procedure. J Ped Surg 31(8):1155–1157
Cuschieri A (1994) Laparoscopic surgery of the pancreas. J R Coll Surg Edinb 39:178–184
Cuschieri A (1995) Laparoscopic management of cancer patients. J R Coll Surg Edinb 49:1–9
Cuschieri A, Shimi S, Banting S (1992) Endoscopic oesophagectomy through a right thoracoscopic approach. J R Coll Surg Edinb 37:7–11
Dalgic A et al (1994) Pretransplant investigations of primary liver tumours with minimal access surgery. Transplant Proc 26(6):3566–3567
da Costa ML et al (1996) Increased tumour establishment and growth after laparotomy vs laparoscopy. Arch Surg 131:1003
de Campos JRM et al (1997) Thoracoscopy in children and adolescents. Chest 111:494–497
Elashry SM et al (1997) Laparoscopic adrenalectomy for solitary metachronous contralateral adrenal metastasis from renal cell carcinoma. J Urol 157:1217–1222
Farah RA et al (1997) Comparison of laparoscopic and open splenectomy in children with haematological disorders. J Pediatr 131:41–46
Fiocco M, Krasna MJ (1992) Thoracoscopic lymph node dissection in the staging of esophageal carcinoma. J Laparendosc Surg 2:111–115
Fornari F et al (1989) Laparoscopic ultrasonography in the study of liver disease. Preliminary results. Surg Endosc 3:33–37
Gill IS, Delworth MG, Munch LC (1994) Laparoscopic retroperitoneal partial nephrectomy. J Urol 152 (5/1):1539–1542
Gouma DJ et al (1996) Laparoscopic ultrasonography for staging of gastrointestinal malignancy. Scand J Gastroenterol 31 [Suppl 218]:43–49
Guillou PJ, Darzi A, Monson JRT (1993) Experience with laparoscopic colorectal surgery for malignant disease. Surg Oncol 2 [Suppl 1]:43–49
Haase GM et al (1995) Surgical management and outcome of locoregional neuroblastoma; comparison of the Children's Cancer group and the International Staging System. J Ped Surg 30:289–295
Holcomb GW III et al (1995) Minimally invasive surgery in children with cancer. Cancer 76:121–128
Hughes ESR et al (1983) Tumour recurrence in the abdominal wall scar tissue after large bowel cancer surgery. Dis Colon Rectum 26:571–572
Humphrey GME, Najmaldin AS (1994) Modification of the Hasson technique in paediatric laparoscopy. Br J Surg 81:1319
Jacobaeus HC, Key E (1921) Some experiences of intra thoracic tumours, their diagnosis and their preoperative treatment. Acta Chir Scand 53:573–620
Jori PJ, Peschle C (1972) Combined peritoneoscopy and liver biopsy in the diagnosis of hepatic neoplasms. Gastroenterology 63:1016–1019
Kern JA et al (1993) Thoracoscopic diagnosis and treatment of mediastinal masses. Ann Thorac Surg 56:92–96
Leather AJM et al (1994) Detection of free malignant cells in the peritoneal cavity before and after resection of colorectal cancer. Dis Colon Rectum 37:814–819
Lobe TE et al (1994) The suitability of automatic tissue morcellation for the endoscopic removal of large specimens in pediatric surgery. J Ped Surg 29:232–234
Mackenzie DJ et al (1992) Laparoscopic diagnosis of Ewing's sarcoma metastatic to the liver. Case report and review of the literature. J Ped Surg 27(1):93–95
Mathew G et al (1996) Wound metastases following laparoscopic and open surgery for abdominal cancer in a rat model. Br J Surg 83:1087–1090
McDougall EM, Clayman RV, Eldshry OM (1996) Laparoscopic radical nephrectomy for renal tumour. The Washington experience. J Urol 155:1180

McMahon AJ et al (1994) Laparoscopic and minilaparotomy cholecystectomy: a randomised trial comparing post-operative pain and pulmonary function. Surgery 115:533–539

Ono Y, Katoh N, Kinakaw T (1997) Laparoscopic radical nephrectomy. The Nagoya experience. J Urol 158:719–724

Pagliaro AL et al (1983) Percutaneous blind biopsy versus laparoscopy with guided biopsy in diagnosis in cirrhosis. Dig Dis Sci 28:39–43

Parra O, Andrus CH, Boullier JA (1992) Staging laparoscopic pelvic lymph node dissection. Experience and indications. Arch Surg 127:1294–1297

Pietrabissa A, Shimi S, Cuschieri A (1993) Localisation of insulinoma by laparoscopic infragastric inspection of the pancreas and contact ultrasonography. Surg Oncol 2:83–96

Pezet D et al (1992) Parietal seedling of carcinoma of the gallbladder after laparoscopic cholecystectomy. Br J Surg 79:30

Rogers BM, Talbert JL (1976) Thoracoscopy for diagnosis of intra thoracic lesions in children. J Ped Surg 11(5):703–708

Rogers DA et al (1992) Thoracoscopy in children: an initial experience with an evolving technique. J Laparoendosc Surg 2:7–13

Ryckman FC, Rodgers BM (1982) Thoracoscopy for intra thoracic neoplasia in children. J Ped Surg 17:521–524

Sartorelli KH, Patrick D, Meagher DP Jr (1996) Port site recurrence after thoracoscopic resection of pulmonary metastasis owing to osteogenic sarcoma. J Ped Surg 31(10):1443–1444

Scherer U, Rothe R, Eisenburg J (1978) Diagnostic accuracy of CT in circumscript liver disease. Am J Roentgenol 130:711–714

Staren ED, Prinz RA (1996) Adrenalectomy in the era of laparoscopy. Surgery 120(4):706–709

Stillman R et al (1981) Ovarian failure in long term survivors of childhood malignancy. Am J Obstet Gynaecol 139:62–66

Takeda M, Go H, Watanabe R (1997) Retroperitoneal laparoscopic adrenalectomy for functioning adrenal tumours. Comparison with conventional transperitoneal laparoscopic adrenalectomy. J Urol 157:19–23

Tan HL et al (1993) Laparoscopic ovariopexy for pediatric pelvic malignancies. Pediatr Surg Int 8:379–381

Trokel MJ et al (1994) Preservation of immune response after laparoscopy. Surg Endosc 8:1385–1388

Vander Velpen GC, Shimi SM, Cuschieri A (1994) Diagnostic yield and management benefit of laparoscopy: a prospective audit. Gut 35:1617–1621

Waldhausen JHT, Tapper D (1997) Is pediatric laparoscopic splenectomy safe and cost-effective? Arch Surg 132:822–824

Watson RWG et al (1995) Exposure of the peritoneal cavity to air regulates early inflammatory response to surgery in a murine model. Br J Surg 82:1060–1065

Watt I et al (1989) Laparoscopy, ultrasound and computed tomography in cancer of the oesophagus and gastric cardia: a prospective comparison for detecting intra-abdominal metastases. Br J Surg 76:1036–1039

Waydhas C et al (1992) Inflammatory mediators, infection, sepsis, and multiple organ failure after severe trauma. Arch Surg 127:460–467

Welbourn CRB, Young Y (1992) Endotoxin, septic shock and acute lung injury: neutrophils, macrophages and inflammatory mediators. Br J Surg 79:998–1003

Part VII
Conclusion

CHAPTER 51

The Future of Endoscopic Surgery in Children

K.E. Georgeson

Minimal access pediatric surgery (MAPS) has gotten off to a slow start when compared to its adult counterpart. Many pediatric surgeons have dismissed the potential advantages of MAPS as unimportant except for minor cosmetic benefits.

Historically, medical caretakers of children have underappreciated their suffering. In 1975, in an extensive retrospective literature search, Eland found only 33 articles dealing with the importance of recognizing and alleviating pain in children published up to that time [1]. However, Gardiola and Banyos found almost 3000 articles published on the importance of pain in children in the 1980s [2]. Clearly an increasing awareness of the effects of stress and pain in children has developed.

Despite the old surgical aphorism that wounds heal from side-to-side and not along their length, the size of the access wound has been shown to be a determinant of perioperative morbidity. The postoperative stress response is influenced by the size of the surgical wound. The primary goal of minimal access pediatric surgery is to decrease the size of the surgical wound. In turn, the perioperative stress and pain, wound complications, systemic complications, scarring and perhaps even the time it takes to perform an operation may be decreased. The compelling reason for the application of minimal access surgery in children is to minimize the stress, pain and morbidity of the access incision. The cosmetic benefits are of secondary importance.

Several barriers resist the general application and acceptance of pediatric endoscopic surgery. Laparoscopy and thoracoscopy require complex technology which initially increases the cost per case. As with any new technology, the hardware is often upgraded making obsolete even the most recent acquisitions. Most instruments for laparoscopy and thoracoscopy were primarily developed for adults and are poorly suited to children. Just as important is the fact that operating skills are quite different using a two-dimensional perspective and long awkward instruments. The learning curve is gradual and requires intense devotion. Some inexperienced pediatric endoscopic surgeons reach beyond themselves and perform low quality surgical procedures or bungle into disastrous complications. With imperfect application of the craft, the early results of pediatric endoscopic surgery have been mixed.

It is appropriate to ask the question: how important a role will minimal access surgery play in the future of pediatric surgery?

It seems obvious that the application of minimally invasive techniques for children will progressively expand. The eventual goal of minimal access surgery is to convert many major surgical procedures into outpatient procedures. With the steady improvement of microendoscopic instruments and the increasing sophistication of the operative techniques, the potential for significant reduction in the surgical trauma for most major surgical procedures seems likely.

At the present time, many of the procedures described in other chapters of this book appear to be less traumatic using minimally invasive techniques instead of the traditional open approaches. As the instruments and surgical techniques become more sophisticated, most bowel resections with anastomosis, complex surgery for newborns and premature infants and even tumor surgery will be performed using minimally invasive approaches. Major surgical procedures outside the body cavities will also be performed in a minimally invasive fashion.

Potential improvements in minimal access pediatric surgery include the use of mechanical lifting devices in place of a pneumoperitoneum. These devices are currently being developed and evaluated in some pediatric surgical centers, particularly in Europe.

The development of long acting local anesthetics (24–48 h) when coupled with the use of microendoscopic instruments will help to further reduce the postoperative stress and pain of endoscopic surgery. With long-acting local anesthetics, the need for morphine derivatives for perioperative pain control should be diminished. As a consequence, gastrointestinal function and general morbidity should be favorably influenced.

The biology of wound healing has been under intense scrutiny over the past few years. Particularly attractive is the idea of scarless healing both in the body wall and within the body cavities. Smaller wounds can be more easily manipulated biologically than larger wounds. For this reason, endoscopic surgery seems well suited for cross-pollination with advances in wound healing.

Fetal surgery is another arena in which endoscopic techniques seem promising. Small puncture sites have been shown to elicit less uterine contractions than incisions in the uterine wall. Amniotic fluid allows for satisfactory visualization during the endoscopic fetal procedures. It seems likely that endoscopic techniques will play an increasingly important role in fetal surgery.

Minimal access pediatric surgery has elevated the therapeutic priority for some surgical procedures. The phenomena of changing indications for less invasive but equally effective therapy is quite common throughout medicine. CT has replaced exploration for traumatic solid organ injury in most pediatric surgery centers. Chemotherapy has replaced exenteration as the primary therapeutic modality for pelvic rhabdomyosarcoma with an improved posttreatment life style for the patient. Similarly, the diminished pain and morbidity associated with laparoscopic fundoplication when compared with open fundoplication has encouraged earlier referral for children with therapy-resistant asthma (J.J. Meehan, K.E. Georgeson, S.S. Rothenberg, personal communication, 1997). Other surgical indications are certain to follow in a similar pattern.

Some potential advances in pediatric endosurgery are still only a dream. These dreams include: (a) the development of transformer instruments which will be linear during insertion into body cavities but designed to be capable of internal transformation into useful robotic tools to aid in complex intracavitary surgical procedures; (b) devices or glues for rapid and precise tissue coaptation; (c) the creation of specimen removal systems which will allow resection of large intracorporeal organs or tissues which can be safely isolated and packaged for removal from the body through small ports; (d) the induction of inguinal hernia sac closure and closure of other internal spaces by injection of biologically active agents under endoscopic guidance; (e) the implantation of designer organs using endoscopic construction of biological scaffolding followed by the seeding of that scaffolding with stem cells which will grow and mature into immunocompatible organs; and (f) comparable advances of minimal access procedures in pediatric neurosurgery, cardiac surgery, orthopedic surgery, otolaryngology and plastic surgery.

Minimally invasive surgery does not require the use of scopes and cameras but includes all techniques that decrease the size and morbidity of the access wound for the performance of surgical procedures. It seems plausible that minimal access techniques will eventually dominate most operative procedures in children and adults.

The rapid growth of minimal access pediatric surgery has started. Pediatric surgeons are already experiencing the pain caused by this attractive but difficult surgical approach. General surgeons will become progressively less involved in the surgical care of children due to the highly technical nature of the application of minimal access surgery to children. It is the pediatric patient who has the most to gain from this cataclysmic change in their surgical care.

References

1. Eland JM, Anderson JE (1977) The experience of pain in children. In: Jacos A (ed) Pain: a sourcebook for nurses and other health professionals. Little and Brown, Boston (Context Link)
2. Gardiola E, Banyos JE (1993) Is there an increasing interest in pediatric pain? Analysis of the biomedical articles published in 1980's. J Pain Symptom Manage 8:449–450

Subject Index

A

abdominal pain   235
abdominal wall lift   21
achalasia, laparoscopy   157
-, preoperative preparation   158
-, preoperative workup   158
-, results   160
-, technique   159
acidosis   59 f, 62, 358
acute abdominal pain   138–141
acute appendicitis   139, 242
acute pelvic pain, laparoscopy   415
adhesiolysis   218, 219, 237
adhesions   4, 216, 218, 219
adnexal pathology, laparoscopy   415
-, complications   420
-, endometriosis   419
-, indications   415
-, oophorectomy/adnexectomy   419
-, oophoropexy   419
-, ovarian cystectomy   418
-, particularities in babies   420
-, results   420
-, technique   417
-, torsion   418, 422, 423
-, tubo-ovarian abscess   419
adnexectomy   419
adrenalectomy   381
alveolar deadspace   60
anatomy   14
anesthesia   5, 53
anesthetic technique during laparoscopy   64
anesthetic technique during thoracoscopy   75
antroplasty, laparoscopy   195
-, indications   195
-, personal experience   197
-, preparation   195
-, technique   196
apical subpleural blebs   102
appendicectomy, laparoscopy   49, 56, 234
-, abdominal wall complications   249
-, abscess   235, 250
-, advantages   247
-, aesthetic benefit   249
-, bowel obstruction   249, 250
-, contraindications   235
-, disadvantages   235
-, drain   243
-, hospital stay   249
-, indications   235
-, installation   237
-, postoperative care   244
-, preoperative preparation   237
-, residual abscesses   249, 251
-, shoulder pain   248
-, techniques   239
appendicitis   234, 235, 248, 416
-, abscess   235, 243
-, generalised peritonitis   235
-, infiltrate   243
-, obstruction   235
-, perforated   248
-, not perforated   248

Subject Index

appendix
-, carcinoid 244
-, normal 236
arachnoid cysts 444
archnoid cyst, fenestration 454
ascites 151
aspiration of gastric content 63, 65
atelectasis
-, Nissen 61
-, postoperative, thoracoscopy 66
azygos vein 122
-, thoracoscopic, catheterization 121

B

basic technique 14
biliary atresia 145
bladder emptying, (see also Credé, urinary catheter) 65
blood flow
-, adrenal 58
-, cerebral 58
-, diaphragm 58
-, inferior vena cava 54
-, kidney 58
-, liver 58
-, mesenteric 58
-, portal 58
-, regional 58
blunt abdominal trauma 150
body integrity 4
body wall
-, complications 3
-, loss of heat 3
-, loss of water 3
bowel activity 65
bronchiectasis 99
bronchodysplasia 62 f
bronchogenic cysts 66, 98, 104, 107
bronchoscopy 67

C

cameras
-, one chip 10
-, selection 10
-, two chip 10

-, 3-D imaging 10, 43
cannula (see trocar)
-, fixation 20
-, insertion
-, -, primary: closed method 17
-, -, primary: open method 19
-, secondary 21
-, for thoracoscopy 41, 77
-, position 38
-, site, closure 23
-, -, local anesthesia 23
capnography 63
cardiac disease 62
cardiac ouput 54–58
cardiorespiratory changes 53–57
cardiovascular changes during laparoscopy 57
cardiovascular changes during thoracoscopy 66 f
cardiovascular changes, cholecystectomy 54–56
cathecholamines 4
catheterisation 15
cell mediated function 5
cetrimide toxicity 364
cholangiography 145–147
cholecystectomy, laparoscopy 4, 55, 297
-, indications 297
-, operative technique 299
-, personal experience 305
-, preoperative preparation 299
-, special concerns in children 298
choledochal cyst 145
choledocholithiasis, laparoscopy 305
cholelithiasis 297
cholestasis 145
chronic abdominal pain 141–144
chronic abdominal syndrome 237
chronic appendicitis 142
chronic pelvic pain, laparoscopy 141, 417
chylothorax 89
chylous ascites 151

Subject Index

clips 12, 32
CO_2 17
-, arterial 57
-, diffusion 53, 59, 388
-, end-tidal 57, 59, 63 f, 67
-, excretion 54
-, elimination 59 f
-, insufflation 53 f, 58 f, 65, 388
-, resorption 53 f, 59 f, 388
-, retroperitoneal 60
-, thoracoscopy 78
-, tissue 59
colectomy (total), laparoscopy 254
-, anal mucosal dissection 258
-, descending colon/splenic flexure 255
-, ileoanal anastomosis with reservoir 257
-, ileoanal anastomosis without reservoir 259
-, postoperative care 259
-, rectal dissection 255
-, transverse colon/hepatic flexure 257
colectomy, total 254
colitis, ulcerative 254
compartment syndrome 5
compliance 60
complications, laparoscopy,
-, access 359
-, acidosis 358
-, cetrimide toxicity 364
-, dropped clips/staples 361
-, bleeding 22 f
-, dropped stones 361
-, gas embolism 357
-, hypothermia 358
-, hollow viscus perforation 23
-, inadvertant injury 22, 359 f
-, instrumentation 360
-, intraabdominal pressure 357
-, intracranial pressure 357
-, nausea/vomiting 361
-, pneumomediastinum 358
-, pneumoperitoneum 357

-, pneumopericardium 358
-, pneumothorax 358
-, port site bleeding 360
-, port site herniation 360
-, port site metastasis 360
-, specific operation 362
-, splanchnic perfusion 357
-, splenosis 363
-, subcutaneous emphysema 358
-, thromboembolism 357
-, tissue rupture/spillage 361
-, use of gas 357
-, venous stasis 357
-, Veress needle 357, 359
constrains in endoscopic surgery:
-, mechanical restrictions 36
-, visual limitations 36 f
contraindications 62
contralateral groin exploration
cortisol 4
cosmesis 5
cosmetic impact 4
c-reactive protein 4 f
Credé manoeuvre 237
cryptorchidism 49
cystic adenomatoid malformation 99, 107

D

débridement 93, 393
decortication 36
degrees of freedom of movement 36
diagnostic laparoscopy 137, 247
-, acute abdominal pain 138–141
-, -, indications 139
-, -, personal experience 141
-, -, placebo effect 143
-, -, technique 139, 143
-, cholestasis 145
-, chronic abdominal pain 141–144
-, -, indications 141
-, -, personal experience 143
-, gastrointestinal bleeding 144
-, liver biopsy 147

-, nonmalignant biliary tree
    pathology   145
-, nonmalignant liver pathology   145
-, oncology   149
-, regional enteritis   144
-, traumatology   149
-, -, indications   150
-, -, intracranial pressure   151
diagnostic peritoneal lavage   149
diagnostic thoracoscopy   83–91
diaphragm   321
diaphragmatic conditions,
    laparoscopy   323
diaphragmatic function,
    postoperative   61
diffuse pulmonary infilatrates   83, 87
diskectomy, lumbar,
    laparoscopic   435
dissection   24
dropped clips   361
dropped staplers   361
dropped stones   361
Duhamel, laparoscopy   259, 272
-, colostomy   278
-, extended aganglionosis   278
-, indications   272
-, preoperative workup   272
-, technique   273
-, personal experience   279
-, postoperative care   279
-, rectosigmoid aganglionosis   275

E

ectopic pregnancy   424
-, laparoscopy   417
electrocoagulation
-, bipolar   24
-, monopolar   24
empyema   92–97
-, indications, thoracoscopy   93
-, personal experience,
    thoracoscopy   94
-, postoperative care,
    thoracoscopy   96
-, preoperative preparation   95

-, preoperative workup   94
-, technique   95
endometriosis   424
-, laparoscopy   417
endorectal pull–through,
    laparoscopy   261
-, indications   261
-, personal experience   270
-, postoperative care   270
-, preparation   261
-, technique   262
endoscope-assisted
    microneurosurgery   455
endoscopic surgery in children,
    future   477
endoscopic linear stapler   88
enterogenous cyst   86
epidural blockade   64
ergonomics   35
esophageal atresia, thoracoscopic
    assisted repair   130–133
-, indication   130
-, personal experience   132
-, preoperative preparation   130
-, preoperative workup   130
-, technique   131
esophageal duplications   98, 104, 107
expandable cannula   9, 85, 88 f, 95

F

Fallopian tube, torsion   423
fiberoptic   67
fetal surgery   478
Fowler-Stephens   395
fundoplication
-, Nissen   163
-, Thal   184
-, Toupet   174

G

gallstones   297
gas embolism   17, 63 f
gastric heterotopia   226
gastroesophageal reflux   65, 163, 174,
    185, 203

Subject Index

gastrointestinal bleeding
   (unclear) 144
gastroparesis 203
gastrostomy, laparoscopy 191
–, indications 191
–, personal experience 194
–, preparation 191
–, technique 192
gonadal dysgenesis 394
–, pure 428
gonadectomy 400
graspers 11
gunshot wounds 150

H

haemostasis 27
Hasson's cannula 19
helium 5, 59
hemodynamic changes 5
hermaphroditism
–, pseudo, female 427
–, –, male 427 f
–, true 427
hernia
–, congenital diaphragmatic 323
–, –, laparoscopy 323
–, –, –, indications 323
–, –, –, personal experience 325
–, –, –, preoperative workup 324
–, –, –, technique 324
–, hiatal 109
–, inguinal
–, –, laparoscopy 331
–, –, –, contralateral groin
      exploration 331
–, –, –, indications 331
–, –, –, preparation 331
–, –, –, technique 332
–, Morgagni 327
–, –, laparoscopy, personal
      experience 327
–, –, –, preoperative workup 327
–, –, –, preoperative workup,
      technique 327
hiatal hernia 109

–, thoracoscopic repair, indications
–, –, preoperative workup 109
–, –, instrumentation 111
–, –, positioning 110
–, –, positioning of trocars 110
–, –, postoperative care 111
–, –, preoperative preparation 110
–, –, results 112
hiatus hernia 109
Hirschsprung's disease 261, 272, 281
–, total colonic 254
hospital stay 49
hydatid cysts, hepatic,
   laparoscopy 291
–, postoperative care 294
–, preoperative workup 291
–, results 295
–, specific instruments
–, technique 292
hydatid cysts, pulmonary 99, 106 f
hydrocephalus 63, 337, 444
–, endoscopic treatment
hydrojet 450
hypercapnia 53, 56, 58 f, 66
hyperhydrosis 49
hypertrophic pyloric stenosis 198
hypotension 67
hypothermia 3, 61 f
hypovolemia 34
hypoxia 65

I

imaging problems 34
implantation, malignant cells 5
injury, inadvertant 360
inspissated bile syndrome 145
instrumentation basic technique 8–13
instruments 8, 10, 35
–, for thoracoscopy 78
–, surgeon-instrument interface 44
insufflation 5
insufflation pressure 5
insufflators 10
interleukin 4
intersex

–, laparoscopy   417, 427
–, –, indications   427
–, –, results   428
–, –, technique   428
interstitial lung disease   73, 88
intestinal obstruction,
    laparoscopy   215
intestinal obstruction, laparoscopy
–, contraindications   215
–, indications   215
–, personal experience   217
–, preoperative workup &
    preparation   216
–, technique   216
intraabdominal pressure   53, 338, 340
intracranial hypertension   62
intracranial pressure   63, 338
intussusception, laparoscopy   229
–, equipment and instruments   229
–, postoperative care   232
–, preoperative preparation   229
–, results   232
–, technique   230
irrigation   27

J
jejunostomy, laparoscopy   204
–, preoperative workup   204
–, procedure   204

K
knotting: externally: Roeder;
    externally: Reef; internally   28

L
laparoscopy
–, anesthesia   63
–, intraoperative monitoring   63
laser   26
left ventricle afterload   55
left ventricle performance   57
left ventricle preload   56
lithotomy   381
liver biopsy   147
lobar emphysema   99, 107

lung biopsy   78, 83
lung distension   62
lung masses   99, 107
lymphangiectasia   151
lymphnodes in the chest   85
lymphomas   149

M
magnification   37
malignancies   5, 86, 465
malrotation, laparoscopy   207
–, findings   209
–, therapy   210
–, indications   207
–, postoperative care   11
–, preoperative workup   208
–, results   211
–, technique   208
Meckel's diverticulum,
    laparoscopy   221, 233
–, indications   221
–, installation   223
–, operative technique   224
–, postoperative care   225
–, preoprative preparation   222
–, resection   224
–, results   225
–, seach for   224
mediastinal cysts   98, 102 f, 107
mediastinal masses   83, 103
mediastinum   98
metastatic lesions   79
minilaparotomy   4 f
monitor   16
–, location   42
muscle relaxation   64
Müllarian inhibiting factor
    deficiency   428
myasthenia   100, 107

N
nasogastric tube   16, 65
nausea and vomiting,
    postoperative   361
needle drivers   12

Subject Index

needles 12, 29
nephrectomy, laparoscopy
–, equipment and instruments 372
–, indications and preoperative preparation 371
–, personal experience 376
–, postoperative care 375
–, potential complications 376
–, technique 372
nephrectomy, partial, retroperitoneal 379 f
nephrectomy, retroperitoneal 379 f
–, approach 382
–, indications 380
–, preparation 381
–, results 385
–, technique 381
nephroureterectomy, laparoscopy, transperitoneal 371
neuroendocrine system 5
neuroendoscopy 443
–, arachnoid cyst fenestration 454
–, bipolar coagulation electrode 449
–, camera/videosystem 445
–, complications 460
–, cyst fenestration 459
–, endoscope assisted procedures 460
–, endoscope-assisted microneurosurgery 455
–, fixation of the endoscope 446
–, grasping/biopsy forceps 447
–, hydrocephalus 453
–, hydrojet 450
–, indications 444
–, instruments 446
–, irrigation device 446
–, laser 448
–, light source 445
–, neuroendoscopes 444
–, personal experience 458
–, preoperative preparation 444
–, preoperative workup 444
–, puncturing needle 450

–, radiofrequency dissector 449
–, scissors 448
–, specific endoscopic techniques 452
–, technique 450
–, third ventriculostomy 459
–, tumor biopsy 460
–, ventricular cannula 447
–, ventricular tumors 455
neurogenic tumors 100, 102
neuromuscular blockade monitoring 64
Nissen fundoplication, laparoscopy
–, complications 170
–, equipment/ instruments 164
–, indications 163
–, postoperative care 169
–, preoperative preparation 163
–, results 169
–, laparoscopy, technique 165
nitrous oxide 64
nonpalpable testis, laparoscopy 393
–, diagnosis 397
–, gonadectomy 400
–, male pelvic anatomy 397
–, one stage orchidopexy 401
–, personal experience 404
–, preoperative preparation 395
–, preoperative workup 394
–, technique 396
–, two staged Fowler-Stephens 401
norepinephrin 57

O

omphaloenteric remnant 221
oncology 149, 465
oncology, endoscopic surgery
–, indications 466
–, instrumentation 468
–, outcome 470
–, preoperative preparation 467
–, techniques 468
one lung ventilation 66, 68, 87
oophorectomy 419
oophoropexy 419

orchidopexy 401
ovarian cyst 415 f, 421
ovarian cystectomy 418
ovarian transposition,
  laparoscopy 417
ovariopexia 149

P
pain 3, 5, 65, 81, 471
palmar hydrosis 125–129
pancreatic heterotopia 226
paraoophoric remnants 423
patent ductus arteriosus 114
–, percutaneous catheter
  closure 118
–, thoracoscopy,
  contraindications 119
–, –, indications 114
–, –, postoperative care 117
–, –, preoperative preparation 115
–, –, preoperative workup 115
–, –, procedure 115
–, –, results 117
patient preparation 15
peeping testis 394, 400
pelvic mass 416
pelvic tumours 423
penetrating trauma 150
pericadial drainage 114
pericadial window 102
peritoneal dialysis catheters 344
–, complications of laparoscopic
  insertion 351
–, indications 344
–, laparoscopic assisted
  insertion 348
–, –, contraindications 347
–, –, indications 346
–, –, operative techniques 347
–, –, preoperative workup 347
–, –, postopertive care 351
–, laparoscopic replacement of
  problematic catheters 352
–, laparoscopy 344
–, techniques of insertion 345

pleural debridement 93 f
pleural disorders 89
pleuropericardial cysts 98, 102, 104, 107
pneumomediastinum 358
pneumopericardium 358
pneumoperitoneum 14, 17–19
–, deflation 55, 64
–, insufflation 55, 57
pneumothorax 107, 126
–, artificial 66
–, CO_2, artificial 121
polyposis, familial 254
pooling of blood 64
port site bleeding 360
port site herniation 360
port site metastasis 360
position, patient 54
–, adverse effects 57
–, –, reverse Trendelenburg 57
–, –, Trendelenburg 61–64
–, –, –, cardiac barrier pressure 61
–, –, –, intracranial pressure 61
–, lateral decubitus 66
positioning for thoracoscopy 75
postoperative changes, diaphragmatic
  function 61
postoperative care, thoracoscopy 81
postoperative changes,
  respiratory function 60
postoperative considerations
–, laparoscopy 65
–, thoracoscopy 68
postoperative hypoxia 65
premature 62, 63
preoperative assessment,
  thoracoscopy 67
preoperative selection and assessment, laparoscopy 62
preparation patient 62
pressure
–, arterial 55–58, 64
–, central venous
–, filling 55
–, left atrial 55

–, right atrial   55
pulmonary biopsy   87
pulmonary lobectomy   106
pulmonary sequestrations   99, 102, 105, 107
pulmonary vascular resistance, thoracoscopy   66
pulmonary vasoconstriction, thoracoscopy   66
pulse oxymetry, postoperative   65
pyelo-ureteral junction stenosis   381
pyloromyotomy, laparoscopy   198
–, contraindications   198
–, instruments   199
–, personal experience   201
–, postoperative care   201
–, preoperative preparation   198
–, preoperative workup   198
–, technique   199

R
regional enteritis   144
respiratory changes during laparoscopy   58
respiratory changes during thoracoscopy   66
respiratory function, postoperative   60
retching   203
retrocaval ureter   381
retroperitoneal gas insufflation   58
retroperitoneal space   379
retroperitoneal surgery
–, adrenal exploration   387
–, nephrectomy see nephrectomy, retroperitoneal   382
–, varicocele   387
reverse Trendelenburg   57
right to left shunt, thoracoscopy   66
right ventricular failure   66

S
safety considerations   45
salpingitis   416, 423
scar

–, hypertrophic 4
–, paresthesia   3
scissors   12
scopes
–, angle   9, 40
–, diameter   9
–, length   9
–, magnification   38
–, selection   9, 40
shoulder pain   248
shoulder tip pain   358
sickle cell disease   61–63
single lung ventilation   75, 85, 89, 110
spinal diskectomy and fusion
–, anterior, thoracoscopic   433
–, operative technique   435
–, personal experience   439
–, preoperative preparation   434
splenectomy   311
–, laparoscopy, extracting the spleen   317
–, –, indications   312
–, –, lateral approach   316
–, –, postoperative care   319
–, –, preoperative preparation   313
–, –, preoperative workup   313
–, –, results   319
–, –, supine approach   315
–, –, technique   315
splenosis   363
spontaneous pneumothorax   89, 99, 105
stab wounds   150
staples   32
stapling devices   12
subacute pelvic pain   416
subcutaneous emphysema   358
suction   27
suturing   29
Swenson   281
sympathectomy, thoracoscopy   49, 125–129
–, results   128
–, technique   126

sympathetic stimulation 56
systemic vascular resistance 54–57

T
tactile feedback 36
Thal fundoplication 184
–, laparoscopy,
    contraindications 184
–, –, diagnostic workup 185
–, –, indications 184
–, –, personal experience 188
–, –, technique 185
theatre layout 15
thoracic duct interruption 114
thoracoscopy basic technique 73–83
thoracoscopy diagnostic 84
thoracoscopy
–, anesthesia 67, 75
–, basis technique 74–83
–, cannula placement 77
–, diagnostic 84–91
–, hemostasis 86
–, indications 73, 83
–, instruments 78
–, postoperative care 81
–, –, considerations 68
–, preoperative preparation 75
–, preoperative workup 74
–, technique 78
–, therapeutic, preoperative
    preparation 100
–, –, results 107
–, –, technique 103
–, video-assisted 81
thromboembolism 357
thymectomy 106 f
thymic disease 102
thymoma 100, 107
tissue rupture and spillage 37
tissue, retrieval 36 f
torsion, adnexal 415, 418, 423
Toupet fundoplication 174
–, laparoscopy, indication 174
–, –, postoperative care 178
–, –, preoperative preparation 175

–, –, preoperative workup 175
–, –, results 179
–, –, technique 177
training in paediatric endoscopic
    surgery 49–52
training
–, animals 50
–, bench trainer 50
–, course 50
–, qualified surgeons 51
–, residents 51
transanal eversion and perineal
    resection, laparoscopy 281
–, indications 281
–, operating room lay-out 282
–, postoperative care 286
–, preoperative preparations 282
–, preoperative workup 282
–, results 286
–, specific instrumentation 283
–, technique 284
–, trocar positioning 283
trauma, abdominal 49
traumatology 149–151
Trendelenburg 60
–, reverse 57
trocar, (see also cannula) 8
–, disposable 8
–, fixation, trocars, expandable 8 f
–, local anaesthesia
–, reusable 8
–, safety shield 8
–, screws 9
–, sleeves 9
–, spike 8
–, sutures 9
–, trumpet 8
–, valves 8
tubo–ovarian abscess 419
two lung ventilation 66

U
ultrasound 26, 216, 219
ureteral stenosis 381
ureteral valves 381

Subject Index

urinary bladder   15
urinary bladder catheterization   15
–, manual expression   16
uterovaginal malformations
–, laparoscopy   417
uterovaginal pathologies,
  laparoscopy   417

V

vanishing testis   394, 398
varicocele   381
–, laparoscopic see also varicocele,
  retroperitoneal surgery   408
–, –, indications   409
–, –, postoperative care   412
–, –, preoperative preparation   410
–, –, results   413
–, –, technique   411
vascular access
–, thoracoscopy   121–124
–, thoracoscopy, results   122
–, thoracoscopy, technique   121
vascular ring division   114
vasoactive hormones   56 f
vasopressin   57
venous return   54–56, 64
venous stasis   357
ventilation, minute   59, 64
ventricle compliance   56
ventricular tumors   455
ventriculocysternostomy   453
ventriculoperitoneal shunts   62

–, laparoscopy   337
–, –, insertion of the peritoneal
  part   337
–, –, –, contraindication   338
–, –, –, indication   338
–, –, –, preopartive preparation   338
–, –, –, preoperative workup   338
–, –, –, technique   338
–, –, shunt related intraabdominal
  complications   340
–, –, –, blockage   341
–, –, –, bowel obstruction   341
–, –, –, contraindications   340
–, –, –, indications   340
–, –, –, perforation   341
–, –, –, peritonitis   341
–, –, –, technique   341
ventriculostomy   453
Veress needle   9, 15, 17, 85, 88, 388
–, emphysema   19
–, insertion
–, penetrating injury   19
video-assisted thoracic surgery   114
video-assisted thoracoscopic
  surgery   81
vision, loss of binocular vision   37
vision, reduced field   38
volvulus   207

W

wedge resection, lung   104

Springer and the environment

At Springer we firmly believe that an international science publisher has a special obligation to the environment, and our corporate policies consistently reflect this conviction.

We also expect our business partners – paper mills, printers, packaging manufacturers, etc. – to commit themselves to using materials and production processes that do not harm the environment. The paper in this book is made from low- or no-chlorine pulp and is acid free, in conformance with international standards for paper permanency.

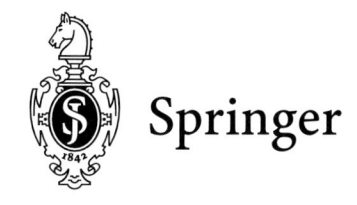

Springer

Computer to plate: Mercedes Druck, Berlin
Binding: Buchbinderei Lüderitz & Bauer, Berlin